Materials for Dye Degradation

Increased use of dyes compromises the visual quality of water sources and enhances the biochemical and chemical oxygen demand that promote toxicity, mutagenicity, and carcinogenicity of the environments. This book presents a broad-spectrum content of the functionalized materials and well-established methods, and a commercial perspective of various investigations conducted so far on dye degradation as an environmental cleaning application. It confines the emerging areas of advanced materials and efficient methods for the environmental remediation field as accommodating concepts.

- Describes fundamental as well as advancements in the field related to dye degradation and dye removal
- Discusses growth in the strategies to mitigate dye-related environmental issues through photocatalysis, electrocatalysis, and nanotechnology
- Covers photocatalysis micellar catalysis, electrocatalysis ion exchange materials, and nanomaterials
- Deals with various synthetic approaches and future perspectives for development of the advanced materials
- Focuses on pertinent green and sustainability aspects related to the environment.

This book is aimed at researchers and graduate students in environmental science, nanoscience, dyes, and chemistry.

Emerging Materials and Technologies

Series Editor: Boris I. Kharissov

The *Emerging Materials and Technologies* series is devoted to highlighting publications centered on emerging advanced materials and novel technologies. Attention is paid to those newly discovered or applied materials with potential to solve pressing societal problems and improve quality of life, corresponding to environmental protection, medicine, communications, energy, transportation, advanced manufacturing, and related areas.

The series takes into account that, under present strong demands for energy, material, and cost savings, as well as heavy contamination problems and worldwide pandemic conditions, the area of emerging materials and related scalable technologies is a highly interdisciplinary field, with the need for researchers, professionals, and academics across the spectrum of engineering and technological disciplines. The main objective of this book series is to attract more attention to these materials and technologies and invite conversation among the international R&D community.

Applications of Hybrid Nanofluids in Science and Engineering
Edited by A. K. Pandey, H. Upreti, O. D. Makinde, and A. J. Chamkha

Solar Cells Development and Fabrication
Edited by Shivani Dhall, Kapil Sood and Vinay Gupta

Geopolymers and Composites: Processing Technologies and Applications
Edited by Huirong Le, Kaibao Wang and Longyuan Li

Nanomaterials for Electrochemical Sensing
Edited by Syed Shahabuddin, Rama Gaur and Nandini Mukherjee

Organic-Inorganic Hybrid Nanomaterials: Energy Harvesting, Storage, and Advanced Applications
Edited by Srikanta Moharana, Bibhuti B. Sahu and Suresh Sagadevan

Nanocarbon to Polymer-Nanocarbon Composites: From Synthesis to Breakthrough Performance
Edited by Srikanta Moharana, Bibhuti B. Sahu and Suresh Sagadevan

Materials for Dye Degradation
Edited by Tarun Parangi and Soyebkhan Pathan

For more information about this series, please visit: www.routledge.com/Emerging-Materials-and-Technologies/book-series/CRCEMT

Materials for Dye Degradation

Edited by
Tarun Parangi and Soyebkhan Pathan

CRC Press
Taylor & Francis Group
Boca Raton London New York

CRC Press is an imprint of the
Taylor & Francis Group, an **informa** business

Designed cover image: Shutterstock

First edition published 2025
by CRC Press
2385 NW Executive Center Drive, Suite 320, Boca Raton, FL 33431

and by CRC Press
4 Park Square, Milton Park, Abingdon, Oxon, OX14 4RN

CRC Press is an imprint of Taylor & Francis Group, LLC

ISBN: 9781032444819 (hbk)
ISBN: 9781032578088 (pbk)
ISBN: 9781003441083 (ebk)

DOI: 10.1201/9781003441083

Typeset in Times
by Newgen Publishing UK

Contents

Figures

Tables

Preface

Chapter 1 of the book is a crucial foundational chapter that offers a comprehensive introduction to the world of dyes, including their classification, various uses in different industries, and the different techniques employed for dye degradation. This chapter serves as an essential guide for readers seeking to gain a broad understanding of dyes and their applications.

Chapter 2 provides a comprehensive overview of the advancements made in materials and techniques for removing industrial dyes through photocatalysis. This chapter takes into account the role of both organic and inorganic nanomaterials and heterostructures in dye treatment. Additionally, the chapter evaluates the effectiveness of different materials, their functionalities, and the obstacles associated with current approaches for dye treatment.

Chapter 3 presents a comprehensive literature review of the micellar catalytic degradation process, which is undeniably one of the most effective and cost-efficient methods available, owing to the remarkable electrostatic and hydrophobic interactions between dye and surfactant molecules, as well as environmental and toxicity factors. Furthermore, this chapter emphasizes the imperative need for future research in environmental remediation.

Chapter 4 delves into the crucial role of electrocatalysis in tackling the challenges posed by the extensive use of dyes in various industries. It provides a comprehensive overview of the principles of electrocatalysis, encompassing electrochemical fundamentals, key concepts, classifications of electrocatalysts, and selection criteria with a diversified focus. The mechanisms involved in dye degradation are also elaborated, including direct electron transfer, electrogenerated active species, and indirect oxidation by reactive species. Furthermore, the chapter explores into the challenges and limitations associated with catalyst stability, fouling, energy efficiency, and scaling up. It also examines regulatory and environmental considerations, supported by real-world case studies.

Chapter 5 is a comprehensive guide that explores the different functions of various types of ion-exchange materials when it comes to treating wastewater that has been contaminated with dye. The chapter provides an in-depth explanation of how ion-exchange materials have transformed the methods used to treat wastewater and dye, emphasizing the critical role they play in this field. It also discusses the different types of ion-exchange materials and their unique properties that make them effective in removing impurities from wastewater. The chapter also covers the factors that affect their efficiency. It is a valuable resource for anyone involved in wastewater treatment.

Chapter 6 explores the functionality of nanoparticles in various contexts, emphasizing their significance in biological, photocatalytic, and adsorption processes. The chapter also highlights ways to boost the efficiency of nanomaterials and identifies research gaps, proposing potential directions for future studies. This persistent endeavor to discover new applications for nanomaterials is critical for achieving sustainable environmental remediation.

Chapter 7 reviews the topic of pollution created by synthetic dyes and the impact it has on our environment. The chapter sheds light on the various techniques used to remove these dyes, detailing the effectiveness of each method and their practical applications. Additionally, it provides a comprehensive analysis of several case studies highlighting the severity of dye pollution in different parts of the world. Overall, the chapter aims to raise awareness of the pressing issue of dye pollution and encourage the adoption of sustainable practices to minimize its harmful effects.

The main theme of Chapter 8 is to highlight the importance of finding sustainable solutions for removing dyes by exploring different materials and emerging technologies. As economic and social factors play a crucial role, this chapter provides essential guidelines for selecting the most cost-effective processes. Furthermore, it emphasizes the need for educational programs to prepare for the emergence of new technologies and promote safer industrial practices.

Dr. Tarun Parangi

About the Editors

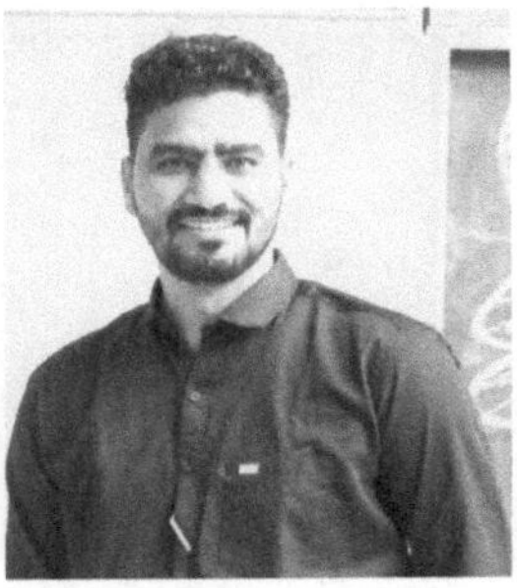

Tarun Parangi is currently working as Assistant Professor in the chemistry department, Shri Naranbhai Atmaram Patel Science College, Village Kakanpur, affiliated with the Shri Govind Guru University, Godhra. He completed his doctoral thesis work in the field of heterogeneous catalysis in applied chemistry and obtained his PhD degree from The Maharaja Sayajirao University of Baroda, Vadodara, in 2015. He worked as a UGC's Dr. D. S. Kothari postdoctoral research fellow in the chemistry department, Sardar Patel University, Vallabh Vidyanagar. His area of research focuses on developing functionalized inorganic catalytic materials for energy applications. Also, he is working on titania (TiO_2)-based photocatalysts for environmental cleaning applications. Parangi has published his research works in SCI and Scopus Journals such as *Comments on Inorganic Chemistry*, *Electrochimica Acta*, *Applied Catalysis A: Chem*, *ACS Industrial & Engineering Chemistry Research*, and *ACS Omega*, *Desalination & Water Treatment*. He has also delivered talks at international and national conferences/symposia and has acted as an active reviewer for several journals and conferences. He serves as a member of the Editorial Board of a prestigious publishing house. He has been honored by Rosalind Membership, *London Journal of Research in Science: Natural and Formal (LJRS)*, UK. Also, he has membership in various scientific associations and societies.

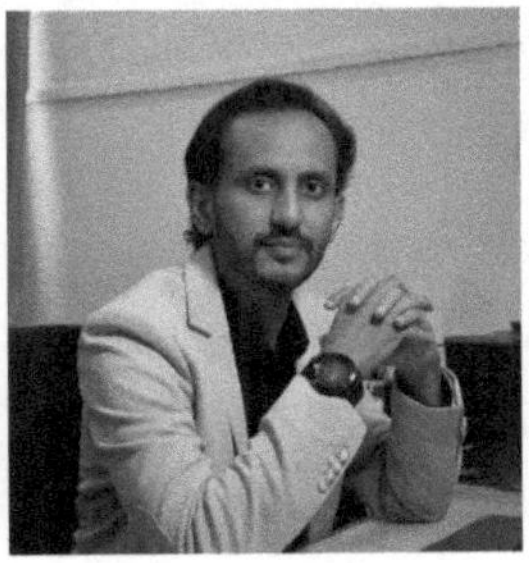

Soyebkhan Pathan has been working as a senior scientist cum assistant professor at the Research and Development Cell (RDC) and Parul Institute of Applied Sciences, Parul University, since September 2021. He earned his PhD in chemistry from The Maharaja Sayajirao University of Baroda in 2015. Prior to joining Parul University, he worked as a postdoctoral research fellow at Qatar Environmental & Energy Research Institute (QEERI) and as Research Associate-CSIR with the Polyoxometalates and Catalysis group at The Maharaja Sayajirao University of Baroda. Dr. Pathan's research focuses on developing heterogeneous as well as single-atom/controlled cluster catalysts, biomass and CO_2 valorization, green and sustainable chemistry, and polyoxometalates chemistry. He has received numerous fellowships and financial assistance from national funding agencies such as DST-SERB, UGC, and CSIR. Recently, he was awarded a Travel Grant from the Science and Engineering Research Board (DST-SERB), Govt. of India, to present his work at the 5th Annual UK Porous Materials Conference in the United Kingdom. Pathan has published his research work in reputable journals such as *Inorganic Chemistry*, *Catalysis Science and Technology*, *Chemical Engineering*

Journal, *Applied Catalysis A: Chem*, *Dalton Transactions*, *Microporous and Mesoporous Materials*, and *Industrial & Engineering Chemistry Research*. He has also delivered many talks at international and national conferences and acted as a reviewer for several journals. He serves as an associate editor for the journal *Frontiers in Catalysis* and has also acted as a co-convenor and organizing secretary for various national conferences.

Contributors

Anil Kumar Behera
Department of Chemistry, GITAM School of Science
GITAM (Deemed to be University)
Visakhapatnam, Andhra Pradesh, India

Malabika Borah
Bhola Nath College
Dhubri, Assam, India

Xuan Thang Cao
Faculty of Chemical Engineering
Industrial University of Ho Chi Minh City
Ho Chi Minh City, Vietnam

Dhruvi Chaudhari
Department of Chemical Science
Parul Institute of Applied Sciences
Parul University
Vadodara, Gujarat, India

Ravi Kumar Ganta
Department of Chemistry, GITAM School of Science
GITAM (Deemed to be University)
Visakhapatnam, Andhra Pradesh, India

Noble George
Parul Institute of Applied Sciences
Parul University
Vadodara, Gujarat, India

Srushti Jasani
Research & Development Cell
Parul University
Vadodara, Gujarat, India

Subodh Kumar
Department of Inorganic Chemistry, Faculty of Science
Palacký University Olomouc
Olomouc, Czech Republic

Shanta Raj Lakshmi
Department of Chemical Science
Parul Institute of Applied Sciences
Parul University
Vadodara, Gujarat, India

Harihara Padhy
Department of Chemistry, GITAM School of Science
GITAM (Deemed to be University)
Visakhapatnam, Andhra Pradesh, India

Shivani R. Pandya
Research & Development Cell & Parul Institute of Applied Sciences
Parul University
Vadodara, Gujarat, India

Tarun Parangi
Shri N. A. Patel Science College, Kakanpur
Shri Govind Guru University
Godhra, Gujarat, India

Kushan Parikh
Department of Chemical Science
Parul Institute of Applied Sciences
Parul University
Vadodara, Gujarat, India

Podilapu Atchutha Rao
Department of Chemistry, GITAM School of Science
GITAM (Deemed to be University)
Visakhapatnam, Andhra Pradesh, India

Preeti Nanda Sahu
Department of Chemistry, GITAM School of Science
GITAM (Deemed to be University)
Visakhapatnam, Andhra Pradesh, India

Anik Sen
Department of Chemistry, GITAM School of Science
GITAM (Deemed to be University)
Visakhapatnam, Andhra Pradesh, India

Brijesh Shah
Chemistry Division, School of Sciences
Navrachana University
Vadodara, Gujarat, India

Rahul Shukla
Department of Chemistry, GITAM School of Science
GITAM (Deemed to be University)
Visakhapatnam, Andhra Pradesh, India

Harjeet Singh
Research & Development Cell & Parul Institute of Applied Sciences
Parul University
Vadodara, Gujarat, India

Lalit Singh
Chemistry Division, School of Sciences
Navrachana University
Vadodara, Gujarat, India

Krishna Kumari Swain
Department of Physics
IIT Madras
Chennai, Tamil Nadu, India

Ravi Tejasvi
Department of Chemical Engineering
Pandit Deendayal Energy University
Gandhinagar, Gujarat, India

Setu Visavadia
Department of Industrial Chemistry
Parul University
Vadodara, Gujarat, India

Aim and Scope

The increasing global population leads to a high demand for textile materials. However, the process of dyeing these materials can have a significant impact on the environment. Textile dyes can compromise the visual quality of water sources and increase biochemical and chemical oxygen demand (BOD and COD). This, in turn, can lead to toxicity, mutagenicity, and carcinogenicity, which are harmful to human health. It is possible to remove the accumulation of used dye and other contaminants by using effective scientific operating procedures.

The book *Materials for Dye Degradation* provides a comprehensive overview of functionalized materials and established methods for dye degradation as an environmental cleaning application. The book's chapters cover various scientific horizons that are advantageous for commercial use, with the standards of day-to-day practices. This content is widely applicable to various scientific disciplines, such as material science, chemistry, environmental science, chemical engineering, nanotechnology, and green chemistry.

The book focuses on emerging areas of advanced materials and efficient methods for environmental remediation. It is an accommodating concept for researchers, chemical and pharmaceutical industries, and academic professionals. The book provides an updated ready reference for readers to understand the problems associated with dye removal processes and offers a probable explanation for the same.

1 Dyes as Pollutants

Setu Visavadia and Ravi Tejasvi

1.1 INTRODUCTION

"Colorant" is referred to a substance that imparts color to the object. Dyes and pigments are the ones that are used for the same. Dyes are generally chemical substances that impart color to textile, leather, paper, and many other materials. Dyes can bind with the substrate upon which it is being applied. Dyes are soluble in water or organic solvent. A dye is a colored substance, but all colored substances are not dyes [1]. The dye molecule is composed of chromophore and auxochrome. Chromophore is an unsaturated organic radical that can adsorb and reflect electromagnetic radiation in visible light regions and provides the color. Auxochrome is an electron-donating substituent that increases the dye molecule's overall polarity, intensifies the chromophore's color, and enhances dyed fiber's color fastness [2,3].

While pigments are insoluble in water and organic solvents, dye molecules are smaller than pigments. It can be imagined as dyes easily dissolve in clear water, making them colored, while pigments remain suspended in a binder.

Dyes and pigments differ in lightfastness – fading upon exposure to light. Dyes more easily fade/bleach upon exposure to ultraviolet (UV) or sunlight. That is because sunlight can break the bond of dye molecules and destroy their color; however, this process takes quite a long time. There is probably no dye that guarantees no change/alteration in its color. The shade and fastness of dye vary depending on the interaction of molecular orbitals of dye molecules with substrate/fiber [4]. At the same time, pigments can resist the fastening process. Dye and pigments differ in terms of their application. Dye is applied in terms of the solution, while pigments are applied in the form of paste in drying oil, where it is insoluble [4].

The blue wool test was used to test the fastness properties of dye and pigments. In brief, about the blue wool test, strips of colored fabric are placed in the laboratory under UV mimicked as sunlight. After a certain time, the fabric is observed and fading is rated on a scale from 1 to 8, where 8 resembles most fading. However, some colorless compounds are used as optical brighteners. These are called white dyes. They can absorb UV radiations and emit out visible light which fabric appears bright and improves the light fastness of the fabric [5].

DOI: 10.1201/9781003441083-1

1.2 CLASSIFICATION OF DYES

There have been several ways for classification of dyes.

1.2.1 Based on Source

Very common classifications of dyes are based on their origin. In this category, they can be classified as natural and synthetic. Natural dyes are the dye obtained/extracted from natural sources by long and elaborate processes. Natural dyes are discovered in woods, leaves, bark, and fungi [6,7]. Natural dyes were used till the 19th century; however, with synthetic dyes' advent, their use of them became less. As natural dyes were obtained from natural sources, they were ecofriendly and biodegradable, produced soft and soothing colors, and sometimes have antimicrobial and mosquito-repellent properties. In India, there are more than 450 plants that can give shades to a substrate [8,9]. However, because of the following problems, natural dyes are not quite used: extraction is time-consuming and not suitable for large-scale preparation, the yield is small compared to raw material being consumed, impurities in dyes produced cause color fading, difficult to produce the same shade, lack of availability of color, availability depending on the season. Examples: indigo, tyrain purple, alizarin, carminic acid.

Dyes that are made synthetically/chemically are referred to as synthetic dyes [1]. The demand for synthetic dye over natural dye has increased considerably because of its easy availability, easy application, color stability, and the same shade can be reproduced. In 1865, William H. Perkins was known as the founder of synthetic dyestuff and synthesized first synthetic dye called Mauve from aniline and sodium dichromate [10,11]. Later, many different chemists came up with synthetic dyes such as Bismarck brown (1865), aniline yellow (1869), and Congo red (1884) being an azo dye. During the same time, Graebe and Libermann, in 1868, synthesized alizarin-a mordant dye. Later in 1880, Baeyer synthesized indigo dye synthetically. Most dyes, synthesized in the 19th century, are derived from aromatic intermediate obtained from coal-tar distillation.

1.2.2 Based on Nature of Chromophore

Dyes have a different chemical structure based on their derivation from aromatic and heteroaromatic compounds. Dyes mainly differ from chromophore and auxochrome. Therefore, classification based on their structure is important. Also, it must be remembered that the same class of dyes may not have properties and modes of application.

1.2.2.1 Azo Dyes

These dye molecules consist of a (–N=N–) functional group as chromophore, also called azo linkage. There can be a symmetric/asymmetric non-azo alkyl/aryl group on either side. Azo dyes are prepared by coupling diazonium salt with amine or phenol. Out of the total dye being produced azo group consists of almost 60% of the total dye and the amount of dye being used in industries is almost 70% [4,12]. Researchers have demonstrated variety of intensity of shades with usage of same dye depending upon aromatic side groups [13]. Wide range of hues fall under category of azo dyes. Examples: methylene blue (MB), methyl orange (MO), mordant red, Congo red.

1.2.2.2 Nitro Dyes

The dye molecules, which consist of the functional group ($–NO_2$) as a chromophore and the hydroxyl group as auxochrome, are called nitro dye. Nitro dyes now have minor commercial importance but are of interest because of their smaller sizes which help to penetrate deep in dense fibers like polyesters. In earlier days, nitro dyes were used for dyeing natural and animal fibers like wool and silk. They are generally acidic in nature and yellowish in color. Because of low fastness properties, these dyes find limited application. Nitro dyes are of two types: acidic and dispersed dyes. Acidic dyes have a solubilizing agent as sulfonic acid, while disperse dyes do not have a solubilizing agent but have an o-nitro diphenylamine structure. Examples: acid yellow, disperse yellow, picric acid, Martius yellow.

1.2.2.3 Nitroso Dyes

The nitroso group contains the nitroso (–N=O) nitroso group as the chromophore. Dyes are complex metal derivatives of o-nitroso phenols. An iron complex of sulfonated group dye is of high commercial importance. These dyes are cheap and generally used for coloring paper. They are used with iron complex due to which gives green color. Examples: fast green, naphthol green, naphthol green-β.

1.2.2.4 Anthraquinone Dyes

These dyes are derivatives of anthraquinone, with the p-quinone dyes. These are the oldest type of dyes; evidence of anthraquinone dyes being used for wrapping mummies has been found (David warning). The position of the substituent in anthraquinone influences not only maximum absorption but also improves other properties' system being chromophore. Anthraquinone dyes are the second class of dyes after azo [14]. Anthraquinone is the colorless primary functional group, but electron donor groups such as amino and hydroxy are attached for creating commercially important dyes. These dyes have good fastness properties and are bright in color. These dyes can be used for non-textile materials like rubber, plastics, inks, paper, etc. However, these dyes are expensive [14]. Examples: alizarin, Vat blue 4.

1.2.2.5 Indigoid Dyes

These classes of dyes are the oldest known class of known dyes. Tyrian purple is the indigoid dye with the purple shade used by Romans. It was so expensive that only wealthy people could afford it. Therefore, the idiom "born to the purple" is used for wealthiness based on Tyrian dye. Out of many Indigoid dyes available, the indigo dye has industrial application to date. It can be used for dying denim jeans. Table 1.1 shows the classification of dyes based on their chemical structure.

1.2.3 Based on Method of Application

Dyes are applied on cellulosic materials such as viscose rayon, linen, cuprammonium rayon, and jute. In addition, dye and paper are also dyed. One of the important

TABLE 1.1
Classification of dye based on structure

Sr. no.	Class	Dye Chromophore	Example
1	Azo	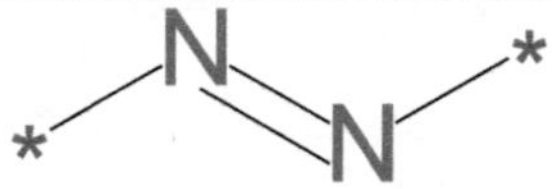	Congo red, methyl orange, methyl red
2	Nitroso	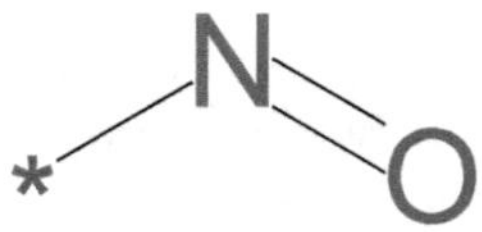	Fast green O, Gambine Y
3	Nitro	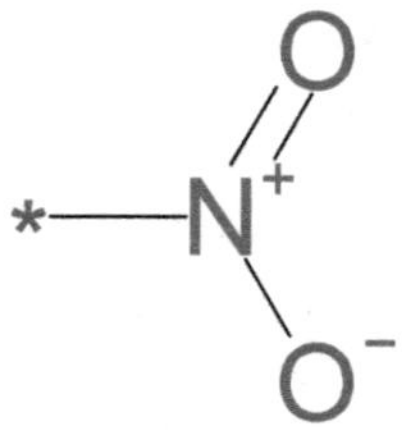	Naphthol yellow, picric acid, Martinus yellow
4	Indigo dye	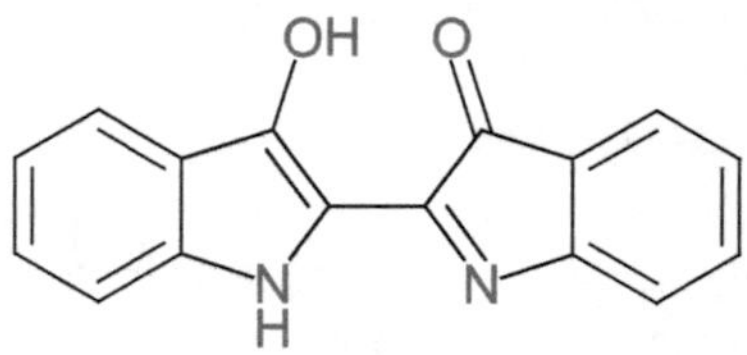	Vat blue 35
5	Anthraquinone dyes	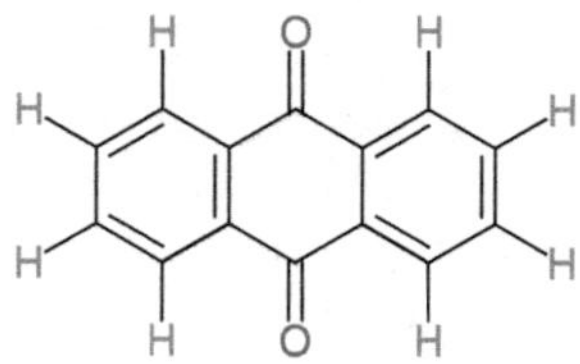	Uniblue, acid blue 129, alizarin
6	Triphenylmethane	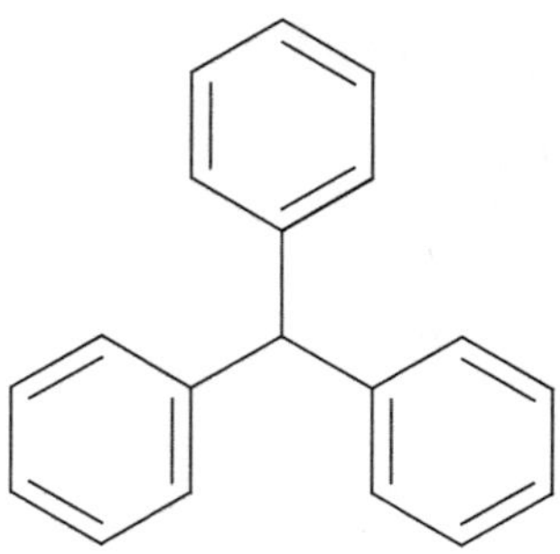	Crystal violet, malachite green

TABLE 1.1 (Continued)
Classification of dye based on structure

Sr. no.	Class	Dye Chromophore	Example
7	Phthalein dye	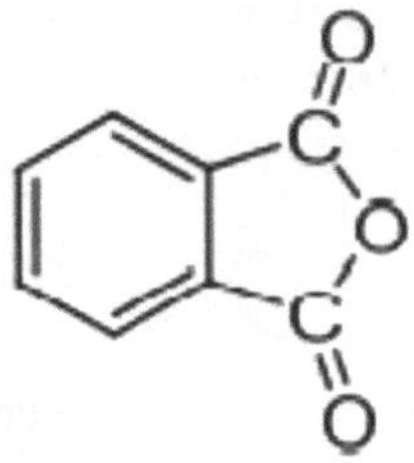	Phenolphthalein, indocyanine green

innovations that came to the textile industry was the introduction of fiber-reactive dye for cellulose. It was observed that a covalent bond was formed between cellulose and 2,4-dichloro-s-triazine dyes.

1.2.3.1 Reactive Dyes

Reactive dyes had been developed for wool and polyamide, but the most successful application was found for cotton. These types of dye react with fabrics and form covalent bonds; as a result, dye becomes a part of the fabric. These dyes are water soluble as they have a sulfonic group. Therefore, cotton fibers are attached to dyes from the solution and later heated in an alkaline atmosphere. The reactive dyes' chlorine atom reacts and can be used for dying cellulose, protein, and polyamide fibers. These produce bright colors and have excellent fastness properties. Dying of this fiber involves following steps: exhaustion of dye, fixation of dye over the surface, and washing off [14]. Reactive dyes are soluble with the cellulosic fiber's hydroxyl group, forming a covalent bond. Therefore, dye and fiber get attached by an ether linkage. Thus, dyes get fixed over the surface/fiber/substrate. Furthermore, fibers are washed with soap with the help of partially hydrolyzed reactive dye molecules [4]. The first commercially used dye for cotton was based on dichloro-s-triazine group [12].

1.2.3.2 Direct Dyes

These dyes are generally azo and are used directly on fabrics by placing them over the aqueous solution of dye-containing electrolyte. These anionic dyes have an affinity toward cellulosic fiber and get attached to fiber via h-bond. Generally used for cotton, it finds applications in leather and paper. Most small-scale dying industry uses direct dye because of its cheapness, easy application, and minimum requirement of chemicals. Examples: Martius yellow and Congo red.

1.2.3.3 Vat Dyes

Dyes applied on fabrics by the vatting process are called vat dyes. Vat dyes are water insoluble. They are made soluble by dissolving in an alkali medium and applied to the fabric. When such dyes are reduced by alkalis like sodium hydrosulfite and caustic soda, leuco is formed. The formed intermediate is soluble in alkali. Later the fibers are immersed in leuco, which has an affinity toward cellulosic fiber [4]. Further, it is kept in an air/oxidizing agent, regenerating its insoluble dye form. This process is called vatting. Vat dyes are used whenever there is a requirement for very high fastness and wet fastness properties [12]. Vat dyes have been found to have excellent chemical stability and color fastness properties. It accounts for 19% of the worldwide consumption of dyes. The disadvantage of vat dye is its cost and difficulty in application [14]. Example: indigo dye.

1.2.3.4 Mordant Dyes

Many natural dyes have a low affinity toward fiber; therefore, dyes require pretreatment with mordant – with the help of which dyes affinity toward textile fibers increases. Mordants are tannins or metallic salts that bond with specific dyes, increasing dyes' affinity and fastness toward fibers. The dyes applied through any metallic mordant are referred to as mordant dyes. Chromium commands mordant dyes in composition; therefore, these dyes are also called chrome dyes. Mordants comprise a functional group such as (–OH and –COOH), forming a coordinate complex with chromium inside the fiber. This complex helps improve the light-fastness properties of dye and wet treatment. Most mordant dyes are acid dyes based on their dyeing behavior. Mordant dyes generally have good light fastness, producing full color but giving dull shades for wool and nylon fibers. Dyes can be treated with mordant before or after the application of dye over fiber. Examples: alizarin, Eriochrome black T [4,14].

1.2.3.5 Sulfur Dyes

From the name itself, it can be concluded that sulfur dyes are called sulfur dyes. However, it is not the case. According to the definition, dyes that dissolve in and are reduced by sodium sulfide solution in the alkaline medium are called sulfur dyes. These dyes produce dull hues, black and blue dyes. In addition, yellow as well as full red dye is also possible to be produced. Little literature data are available for sulfur dyes compared to other known dyes. One of the reasons is that their fundamental structures are uncertain. The first commercial production of sulfur dye Cachou de Laval, in 1861, was obtained by heating bran and sawdust with sodium polysulfide at 300°C with the evolution of hydrogen sulfide. The chemistry of this product still needs to be clarified. The process of heating sulfur dye with sodium sulfide or sodium polysulfide is known as the nation. Yellow dyes were made by thionation of m-toluene diamine in the presence of benzidine, in this case, Immedial Yellow D. Upon increasing temperature from 190°C to 250°C, its color changes to orange. Therefore, it can be said that history is imprecise, and much attention has not been paid to an intermediate structure. Good red and violet dyes are unavailable in this class, but most black and blue shades are possible. Upon the thionation of indophenols, blue shades can be prepared. According to a study by Wang et al., half of the dyes being sued over cellulosic fibers are sulfur dyes put, of which almost 80% is contributed by black sulfur dyes [15].

1.2.3.6 Acid Dyes

These classes of dyes are water-soluble containing acidic groups like ($–SO_3H$) of a phenolic group. These classes of dyes have an affinity toward nylon, wool, and silk but do not towards cotton. These dyes are applied from an acidic bath having a pH range of 3–7 containing dilute sulfuric acid and acetic acids, where fibers hold dye molecules because of ionic bonds. Examples: picric acid, Metanil yellow, Orange 11.

1.2.3.7 Basic Dyes

These dyes have basic groups ($–NH_2$, $–NR_2$) and thus are cationic dyes. However, upon treatment with acid, they become anionic. They have poor affinity toward cellulosic fiber but can be applied to protein fiber such as silk and wool. Basic dyes have brilliant colors; however, they have poor fastness properties. Because of this, cellulosic fiber is treated initially with an intermediate called a mordant, such as tannin acid, and later is dyed with basic dyes. Mauve, the first synthetic dye, belonged to this category of dyes.

1.2.3.8 Disperse Dyes

Synthetic and semisynthetic fibers such as cellulose acetate and polyamides are hydrophobic. Hence such fibers cannot be dyed in an aqueous solution. For them, insoluble dyes are finely grounded and dispersed in water using some dispersing agents. These fine particles are applied to fibers with the help of organic carriers or high-pressure temperature conditions. Later, this fine particle gets diffused into fiber and is held by adsorption. Generally, nitro, azo, and anthraquinone dyes are used as dispersed dyes available as a mixture of insoluble dye and dispersing agent. These dyes are commercially available in mixtures for coloration [4]. Table 1.2 shows the classification of dyes based on application.

TABLE 1.2
Classification of dye based on application

Sr. no.	Dye Name	Properties	Examples	Application
1	Direct dye	Water-soluble compound, anionic in nature, affinity toward fibers in neutral and alkaline atmosphere, solubility increases with increase in temperature	Congo red, brilliant blue	Applied on rayon, silk, and wool
2	Vat dye	Insoluble in water but made soluble in water by treatment with base, find application on cellulosic fiber	Indigo dye, Vat blue 5	Cotton, rayon

(continued)

TABLE 1.2 (Continued)
Classification of dye based on application

Sr. no.	Dye Name	Properties	Examples	Application
3	Azo dye	Have azo linkage (–N=N–), insoluble in water, bright and high intensity color, fair to good fastness, cannot be directly applied to fiber	Methyl orange, methylene blue	Textile, leather, food, paper, paint
4	Reactive dye	High wet strength, anionic in nature, water soluble, alkaline condition is required for dyeing	C.I. Reactive red 120, C.I. Reactive black 5	Forms covalent bond with fibers. Used for dyeing nylon and wool
5	Sulfur dye	Sulfide linkage (–S–S–), highly colored, insoluble in water, needs to be converted to water-soluble state before application, bright black and brown shades	Indophenol and sulfur black	Cotton and rayon
6	Disperse dye	Insoluble in water, applied in form of dispersion with stabilizing agent, phenol, excellent fastness property	Disperse Orange 25, Disperse orange 1 Disperse orange 3	Synthetic fiber, polyester yarn
7	Acidic dye	Moderate to good fastness, bright color, soluble in water, amphoteric to fiber, anonic	Congo red, picric acid, acid orange 7	Nylon, wool, silk
8	Basic dye	Insoluble in water, poor fastness, cationic dye	C.I. Basic Yellow 1, C.I. basic Blue 9 and C.I. Basic Green 5	Acrylic materials, wool, silk fibers, inks

1.3 DYES USED IN VARIOUS INDUSTRIES

Dyes have been primarily used in the textile industry to color fibers. However, there have been other uses of dyes such as leather, paper, foodstuffs, drug, polymers, cosmetics, printing inks, varnishes, paints, oil, soaps, plastics, and many more. The structure of these dyes is like one used for textile fibers, but the choice must be made such that the resultant dyed substrate must be satisfactory.

1.3.1 Dye in Leather Industry

Leather is a protein-based substance and can be easily dyed with acid dyes, among other dyes available. Leather dyes have played a vital role in a glossy look to jackets, shiny black to shoes. and brilliant hues to bags. The dyeing of leather requires a solution to be penetrated deep to give uniform shade which causes the use of excess dye solution. Based on the application of dyes, acid and direct dyes have generally been used for dyeing leather with the help of mordant in alkaline conditions. In addition, basic dyes can also be used for dyeing leather, giving powerful, rich shades to a substrate. However, these dyes have an issue with the low fastness and become red upon dyeing with deep shades. However, when light shades are required upon leather, acid dyes can be used in the presence of formic acid. Based on the structure of dye, mostly azo dye is used. However, some acridine and aniline-based dyes also be used. Example: Chrysoidine Y. One of the prime things about leather dye is that it does not need to have excellent fastness properties but should not be sensitive to variation. Therefore, the color of the leather must be uniform over the substrate. Nowadays, the leather industry has developed the concept of aniline-dyed leather, which gives a natural look to the leather. Further, that also eliminates the need for the paint-finishing. Shoe-fine leather is finished with paint over the final surface, while clothing leather is dyed entirely and ensures that the color of the cut area is the same as that of the surface. Examples: Bismarck brown, orange dye. Metal complexes are also useful for leather dyeing, e.g., Igenal brown dye. It is a copper complex azo dye prepared by heating the dye in an aqueous copper sulfate and ammonia solution. Dye has shown good level and penetrating power over vegetable-tanned and chrome leather. Along with the copper complex, the chromium complex can also be used for dyeing leather.

1.3.2 Paper Dyes

One of the oldest applications of dye and pigments remains in the paper industry. The paper industry includes copier paper, facial tissue paper, envelope grades, cover papers, corrugated cases, specialty papers, decorated laminated papers, and packaging in addition to normal paper taken into consideration. The paper is a non-woven material made up of cellulose; dyes get adsorbed over these fibers because of the affinity of cellulose. Primarily, the dyeing of paper is done by dipping or impregnation. Most dyes used for paper dyeing are direct cationic dyes and sulfur dyes. Pulp is a negatively charged surface; therefore, cationic direct dye is more suitable for dyeing paper. In addition, its planar structures and extended surface conjunction aid in easy adsorption of dye over the paper pulp. Carbon paper is made by coating paper with a mixture of wax, oil, and oil-soluble dye. Most carbon paper contains carbon black and blue colors to compensate for the shade of carbon black. The selection of dye over paper pulp is specific. A selection must be based on the dye and paper pulp charge, its affinity toward cellulose, light fastness, bleed fastness, right shade, and clear background. The colored paper must have high fastness properties toward light, acid, alkali, and temperature as they find a wide range of applications. A plastic laminate sheet must have excellent color fastness properties as they are often exposed to sunlight. Paper that can be used for writing must have fastness toward acid as ink applied over can be acidic. The paper used for alkaline storage materials such as soap and detergents must have fastness properties towards alkali. Examples: basic blue dye, methyl violet 10 BNS, Safranine T.

1.3.3 Food Color

Food helps to give nutrition to humans as well as animals. But still, its acceptance depends on color. Natural colors such as chlorophyll, cochineal, saffron, and turmeric were used. They still are accepted, but synthetic food has also been widely accepted and used in industry because of their low cost and easy availability. Synthetic color may be added to food during any of the following processes production, processing treatment, and transport and storage. Synthetic color has been used instead of natural color because it would improve aesthetically with the uniform color distribution. At times, it becomes possible that natural color tends to get removed during the process. Although food color has no nutritional value, it is only used to make it attractive. Color is used in the food industry such as bakeries, confectionery, beverages, dairy and ice cream, meat and seafood, etc. [16].

It has been observed that food color over the specific limit has potential health hazards. The study has shown that consuming synthetic food colors higher than the limit can cause irritability, restlessness, difficulty sleeping, and depression in children. Red 40, Yellow 5, and Yellow 6 have shown carcinogenic effects at a higher level of consumption in humans; similarly, the Yellow 5 dye, also called tartrazine, causes allergies. One can remain safe by removing processed food from the diet [16]. Examples: tartrazine, amaranth, erythrosine, naphthol yellow, fast red. Alternatively, biocolorants are used as coloring agents. Biocolorants are dyes made from renewable sources, while most are naturally obtained from plants. Along with color, these biocolorants can also act as preservatives. Certain biocolorants are antagonist of bacteria, fungi, and virus; therefore, it protects food from microbial contamination [17,18].

1.3.4 Solvent Dyes

This type of dye is soluble in an organic solvent derived from azo, anthraquinone, and phthalocyanine. This type of dye is used in printing inks, pen inks, polymer, fat, oil, and wax. Examples: Sudan orange, brown dye.

1.3.5 Wood Dyes

These types are applied to wood. These dyes are applied on wood to match color according to requirements. These dyes are allowed to dissolve in solvents like water, alcohol, thinner, etc.; when the wood is painted with said dye, wood soaks with solvent or evaporates, which results in the drying of the color of the wood.

1.3.6 Medicinal Dyes

Ehrlich first discovered the possible application of dye in the medical field. It was then he found out that MB has the ability for staining nerve calls selectively [8,9]. Drawing inspiration from this, it was later established that dyes could also have medicinal use. It has been observed that the skin can absorb the therapeutic effects of medicinal plants. Madder roots are red-colored and have anthraquinone as their main constituent. Now anthraquinone is antimicrobial and antibacterial, which is useful for the human body. Other dyes like chamomile, yarrow, wormwood, wood, turmeric, goldenrod, rosemary, and marigolds exemplify plant-based dyes that have their medical importance along with their utility as natural colorant [8]. Mercurochrome and acriflavine have antiseptic properties. In addition, other dyes with limited applications such as bactericides are crustal violet, malachite green, and methyl violet. Furthermore, Prontosil and Neo Prontosil are azo dyes in nature that are used for the treatment of sleep sickness [9].

1.3.7 Photography Dyes

Generally, photographic films are sensitive to specific colors, such as violet and blue, depending on their wavelength. However, if a certain color is added to the emulsion, the film becomes sensitive toward the visible spectrum and near-infrared region. The dyes added that enhance sensitivity are called photographic sensitizers. To achieve the effect of sensitivity, the added dyes must be in their purest form and applied in dilute nature. Cyanine is one of the oldest photographic dyes known. Its sensitizing property is enhanced by coupling with a coupler such as ammonium or alkali aurous thiocyanate [4]. Generally, dyes having shades of cyan, greenish blue, magenta, and yellow are used. Examples: ethyl red, pinacycnol.

1.3.8 Dyes Used in Cosmetics

Color can attract attention; therefore, they are added to cosmetics to attract consumers. Dyes have been added to cosmetic items such as face powders, lipsticks, nail polish, hair color, etc. Before using dye in these products, it must be made sure that they are non-toxic, not harmful to the skin, and resist perspiration. Out of the class of dyes, azo dyes are most widely used in consumer products because of their easy availability and lower cost. However, dyes have been found to have mutagenic, genotoxic, and carcinogenic effects. Much of the human exposure is by dermal contact with synthetic dyes, which, on larger exposure, causes harm to the human body. Literature has shown that triaryl methanes can enter the bloodstream upon adsorption. Xanthene's dyes, such as Acid Red 92 and Erythrosine which give red color and are quite popular in cosmetics, have proved to cause skin roughness upon reacting with skin proteins. Usage of tartrazine-azo structure-based dye has been put to limited use as it is prone to cause dermatitis, itching of the lips, and tongue [19]. In addition, yellow-6 dye can cause concentration disorder and hyperactivity among children and allergic reactions that may lead to anaphylaxis. Further, Acid Red 13 is prone to cause damage to the DNA chain and amaranth dyes cause hormonal imbalance [19]. Looking at such harmful effects, regulations are applied over the use of dyes across the globe in cosmetics [20]. In addition to that, Rhodamine-B (RhB) dye is being used in lipsticks whose concentration needs to be kept in check according to standards.

1.4 DYE DEGRADATION: THE NEED

In most industries like paper, pharmaceutical, petroleum, rubber, ceramic, and textile, abundant water and effluent wastewater are sent directly to water reservoirs without much pretreatment. Water contains oil, toxic heavy metals, solids, salts, organic and

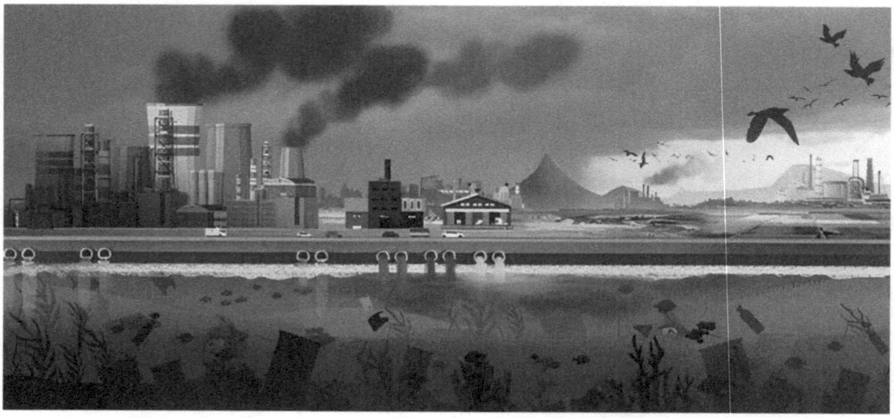

FIGURE 1.1 Schematic representation of water pollution originating from industrial effluents [25].

inorganic chemicals, pathogens, and dyes. Because of such waste disposal, the quality of surface water and the environment deteriorates. Dyes remain a serious concern of all these impurities/pollutants [7,21,22]. Practically looking into matter, dyes are the first contaminant which is recognized in wastewater due to their appearance [23]. Low dye concentration, i.e., <1 ppm concentration, can also be detected easily. Dyes are released from textiles, paper, paints and pigments, and food. These dyes are non-biodegradable, toxic, and may have carcinogenic effects. Dyes are color-imparting organic molecules with higher molecular weight, water-soluble, carcinogenic, and inhibit sunlight [7]. According to the literature, about 1,00,000 different types of dye are currently used in the textile industry, causing worldwide 7×10^5 tons of dye effluent annually. About 17–20% of water pollution is caused by the textile industry. About 10,000 tons of dye effluent per year is produced by textile industries worldwide [24,25]. A schematic of the same is shown through Figure 1.1. During the dying operation, chemicals, dye, and water are mixed. After completion of the operation, excess dyestuff is rejected into the environment. This leftover dye is about 85% of the total dyestuff prepared for operation [26,27]. The presence of dye in water peril aquatic life by color, which hinders the biological process and growth of aquatic life. Dyes also affect human health; upon contact, nausea or vomiting while intake causes irritation to the skin, extreme sweating, confusion, and mouth burns, and upon consumption by any source, damage kidney, liver, and brain and disrupt the nervous system [6,28,29].

1.5 DYE DEGRADATION: THE TECHNIQUES

Thus, to soothe the harmful effects of dyes on the environment and satisfy demands for quality drinking water, many physical, chemical, and biological approaches have been employed [27]. Out of the three techniques, mainly applied is the physical technique. The physical method includes adsorption, coagulation or flocculation, ion exchange, and membrane filtration. These techniques generally refer to transferring pollutants from one to another media. In addition, techniques such as adsorption and treatment of solid are necessary for regeneration which adds cost to the process [23,26,27]. Chemical treatment includes oxidation, ozonation, electrochemical, and UV irradiation. The chemical removal method is less attractive as it requires specific equipment and higher electrical energy; in addition to this chemical required, disposal of intermediates and effluent after treatment causes issues and needs to be treated before disposal, which adds to the cost of operation [30,31]. While least used is a biological method, an in situ method combines aerobic and anaerobic processes. The biological method uses adsorption by microbial biomass, algae degradation, enzyme degradation, and microbial culture. However, biological processes alone are not sufficient for the complete removal of dyes and are slow processes operating only under specific conditions [32].

Considerable research has been done on techniques to address technical and economic issues. The advanced oxidation process (AOP) has gained popularity because it can detoxify recalcitrant substances from wastewater. AOP is a competent technique to degrade organic compounds by generating reactive oxygen species (ROS) [33]. ROS are produced in situ and can oxidize any compound in the water matrix. Hydroxyl ($\cdot OH$) and superoxide ($\cdot O_2^-$) are well-known radicals with oxidation potentials of 2.7 and −2.3 eV, respectively. On the other hand, oxidation potential for organic compounds varies from −1 to 2 eV. Due to the variation in potential between ROS and organic species, an organic species containing ROS would enter a reactor and can gain or lose electrons spontaneously and convert to two or smaller compound [34]. A comparative study was undertaken between chemical treatment and AOP. Chemical oxygen demand (COD) for the chemical method was found to be 60%, while for AOP, it was 90%. Moreover, AOP removed 95% of color while chemical treatment with the ferrous substrate removed 49% [27,33]. Out of the different AOP techniques available, photocatalysis emerged as one of the effective subcategories of AOP for degradation of harmful pollutants [35,36].

Photocatalysis is an AOP that uses light energy to excite the catalyst to accelerate the oxidation reactions. The photocatalysis process is based on the generation of redox species for the degradation of pollutants [37,38]. Photocatalysis has flourished since the first time in 1972 Honda and Fujishima used TiO_2 as a photocatalyst for H_2 generation from water [39–41]. A schematic of the mechanism of photocatalysis is shown in Figure 1.2.

A semiconductor has an energy bandgap between the conduction valence band (VB) and high energy conduction band (CB), and the gap between them is called a bandgap or forbidden band. At absolute zero, VB is filled with minimum energy, while CB is empty and possesses maximum energy [42–44]. This size of the bandgap determines the optical properties of semiconductors. When the energy of the source is larger than the bandgap of the semiconductor, electrons of VB are excited to CB, generating holes in VB. An electric field separates these photogenerated electrons and holes. Photogenerated pores have a substantial oxidizing property and can be oxidized substances. These electron–hole pairs can recombine themselves, which reduces performance; therefore, the recombination of carriers must be avoided [45,46].

The typical photocatalysis procedure starts with transporting contaminants from the surroundings to the photocatalyst surface, where dye molecules get adsorbed on the surface. Further oxidation–reduction reactions occur when products are desorbed

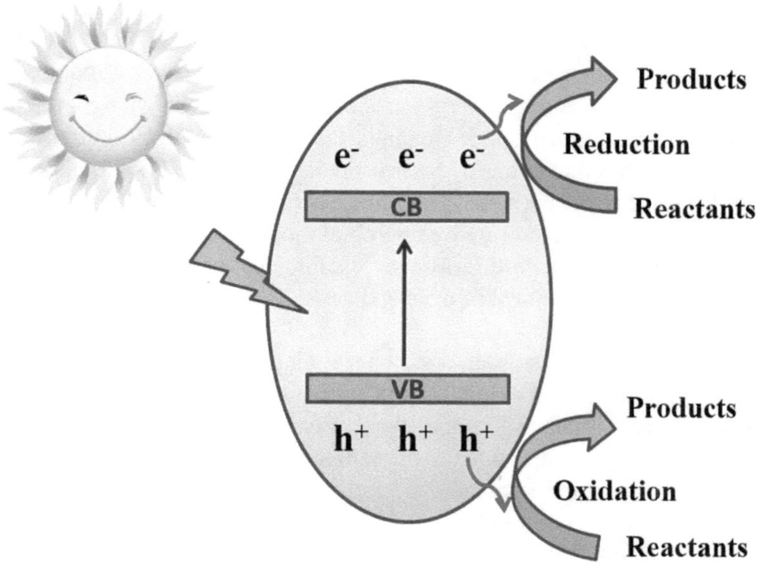

FIGURE 1.2 Schematic of photocatalytic mechanism [40].

from the surface to bulk fluid. The reaction for photocatalytic dye degradation is shown below [33]:

$$\text{Photocatalyst} + hv \rightarrow h^+_{VB} + e^-_{CB}$$

$$h^+_{VB} + e^-_{CB} \rightarrow hv$$

$$H_2O + h^+_{VB} \rightarrow \cdot OH\ (\text{hydroxyl radical}) + H^+$$

$$O_2 + e^-_{CB} \rightarrow O_2^-$$

$$O_2^- + H^+ \rightarrow HO_2^{\cdot}$$

$$HO_2^{\cdot} + O_2^{\cdot} \rightarrow OH_2^- + O_2$$

$$2OH_2^- \rightarrow H_2O_2 + O_2$$

$$H_2O_2 + hv \rightarrow 2OH^{\cdot}$$

$$OH^{\cdot} + \text{Pollutants} \rightarrow \text{Degraded products}$$

It forms electron–hole pair when exposed to energy by an equal or higher energy source than the bandgap. A hole in CB oxidizes pollutants or water molecules forming hydroxyl radicals, while in VB, electrons can reduce dissolved oxygen in water or oxygen adsorbed over the surface [47]. However, during operation, there are chances where electron and hole gets recombined. This seriously affects the process. Recombination of electrons and hole is considered a drawback of the photocatalysis process. In addition to the photoactivity of these semiconductors, nanoparticles (NPs) are constrained to the UV range of the solar spectrum, which consists of only 5–7% of the total spectrum. There are a few ideal properties that are sought in any good photocatalyst. These key properties include low bandgap, high photon absorption, low electron–hole recombination, high surface area, low cost, and high chemical stability. There is hardly any single material that has all these properties [48].

Studies revealed that dye degradation by photocatalyst is successful. However, certain drawbacks are large bandgap, low absorption of light, recombination of electrons and holes, reducing practical application. Thus, certain modifications are done to look for these matters, such as doping, formation of heterojunction, Z-scheme, and dye sensitization. Various techniques have been developed to tailor a suitable photocatalyst. Many pristine and modified semiconductors have been used as photocatalysts for pollution degradation. All these materials were processed using one or more of the following techniques to enhance their photocatalytic properties.

1.5.1 Doping

Doping is attributed to intentionally adding impurities into semiconductors to vary their properties. Composite formed may be a multicomponent system made of two or more different phases separated by a distinct interface [49]. By introducing heteroatoms, the bandgap value of the compound can be tuned to increase the photoresponse range. This would decrease the resistance between layers and accelerate charge separation, increasing photocatalytic activity [44,50,51]. The main motive of doping is to reduce bandgap and to bring absorption range in visible spectrum [23,52,53]. A schematic illustration of doping in catalysts is shown in Figure 1.3. Doping can be done by metal, non-metal, and precious metal. Notably metal

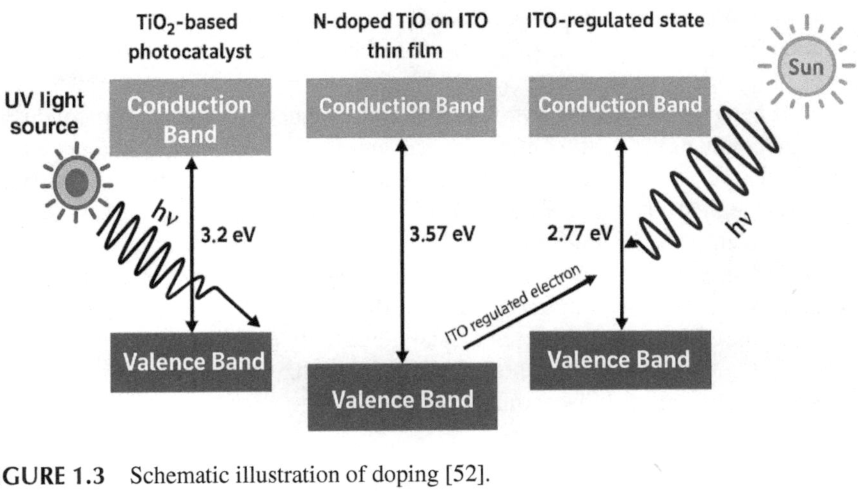

FIGURE 1.3 Schematic illustration of doping [52].

and non-metal doping shows considerable effects on photoexcitation process [54,55]. The doping of metals such as Pt, Ag, Pd, and Au over photocatalyst is an efficient method to reduce the recombination of excitons, thereby increasing the photocatalytic efficiency [46,56]. However, the entire mechanism still needs to be sorted out. But it is a known fact that metals are electron sinks that load and shuttle photogenerated electrons resulting in charge separation. A doped structure having less recombination can be known from photoluminescence spectra. For example, TiO_2 widely used photocatalyst has a bandgap of 3.2 eV, which responds to the UV range. Quite a lot of work has been done over TiO_2 to improve its efficiency through modifications. Precious metal platinum (Pt) was used for doping TiO_2, which enabled to use of TiO_2 photocatalyst under visible light due to the formation of new energy levels and improved and stable nanocrystalline structure.

1.5.2 Heterojunctions

Heterojunction is one of the excellent ways to enhance photocatalyst efficacy. Two or more semiconductors with suitable band edge potential can be integrated to form a heterojunction [57]. The variation in potential between these semiconductors causes band bending. Due to this band bending internal electric field is produced, which drives holes and electrons. As a result, the separation and migration of charge carriers is enhanced. Band edge positions are known from Mulliken electronegativity theory, which is the geometric mean of the electronegativity of the constituent atoms. Schematics of different types of heterojunctions are shown in Figure 1.4.

Type-I heterojunctions have band positions set in a straddling arrangement. The VB of semiconductor 1 has a higher potential than the VB of semiconductor 2 and the CB of semiconductor 1 has a lower potential than the CB of semiconductor 2. Thus, both VB and CB of the semiconductor are restricted in the energy gap of semiconductor 2. Upon irradiation, the photoexcited electrons from CB semiconductor 2 transfer to CB semiconductor 1 due to variation in their reduction potential. The holes from VB of semiconductor 2 also shift to VB of semiconductor 1 due to their oxidation potential differences. As electrons and holes pile up in one semiconductor, chances of recombination increase [58].

Type-II heterojunction have the band positions staggered between semiconductor 1 and semiconductor 2. In this, both the CB and the VB of semiconductor 2 are a greater potential than semiconductor 1. When such a semiconductor is irradiated, the photogenerated electrons transfer from the CB of semiconductor 2 to the CB of semiconductor 1. The holes transfer from the VB of semiconductor 1 to the VB of semiconductor 2. Therefore, semiconductor 1 becomes affluent in electrons, and semiconductor 2 becomes affluent in holes. Because of this, charge separation is achieved, which further upgrades photocatalytic activity [58].

Type-III heterojunction have tinted bandgaps and charge transfer is hindered. The bandgaps do not overlap and use tunneling effect [58].

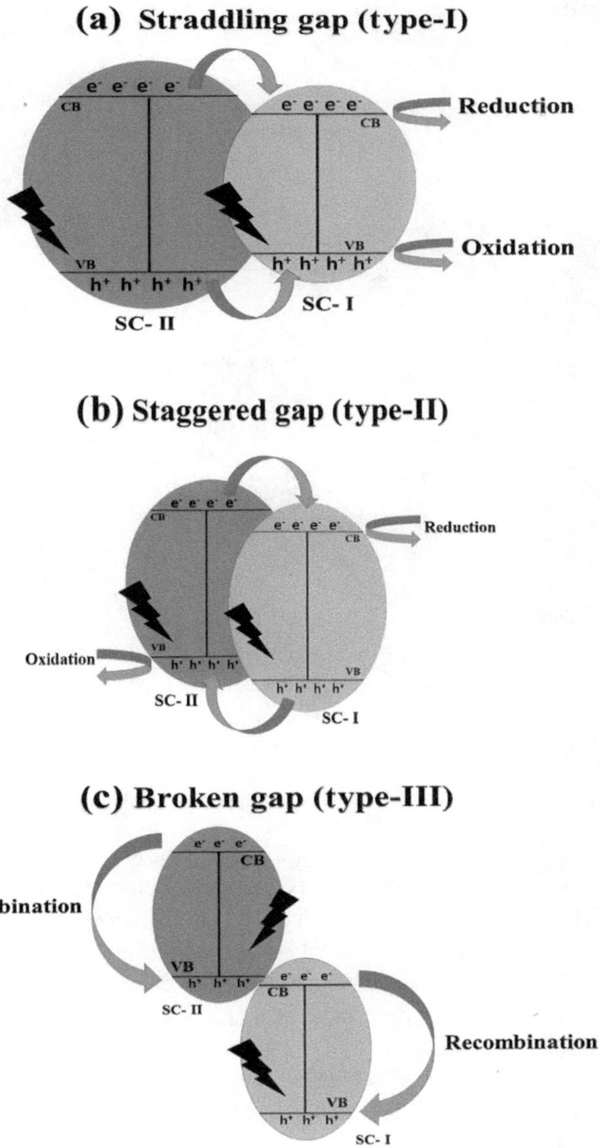

FIGURE 1.4 Schematic representation of (a) straddling gap (type-I), (b) staggered gap (type-II), and (c) broken gap (type-III) [58].

1.5.3 Z-Scheme

Z-scheme formation is a promising method for decreasing the recombination of excitons. On irradiation, both the semiconductors form electrons and holes. The semiconductor with a more negative CB potential generates the electrons. The

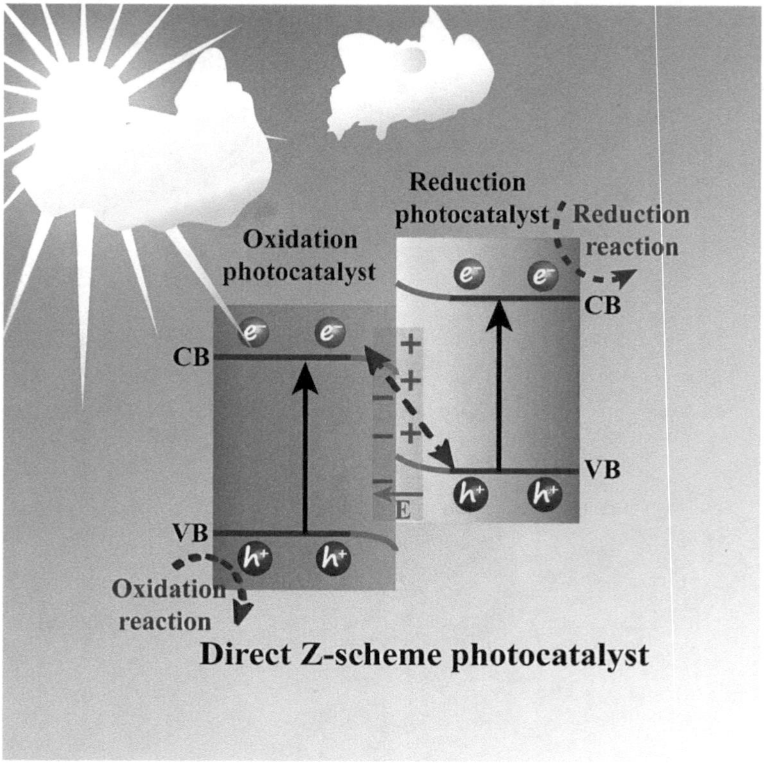

FIGURE 1.5 Schematic illustration of Z-scheme photocatalyst [57].

semiconductor with a more positive VB provides photogenerated holes, thereby separating the charges. Photogenerated electrons from CB of semiconductor A transfer to VB of semiconductor B due to electrostatic attractions. This causes charge carrier separation in both individual photocatalysts. The e^- in the CB of semiconductor B upon reducing O_2 forms oxygen radicals as has CB potential is more negative than the standard redox potential of $O_2/\cdot O_2^-$, whereas the VB potential of semiconductor A is more positive compared to the standard redox potential of $O_2/\cdot O_2^-$ and the H^+ reacts with OH^- or H_2O to form OH• [56]. The schematic illustration of Z-scheme is shown in Figure 1.5.

1.6 LITERATURE REPORT

Moiz et al. [59] undertook a study for the degradation of MB dye with Mn/ZnO as a photocatalyst and found 91% degradation of MB dye at 30 mg/L of 6% Mn/ZnO at pH 4 in the existence of H_2O_2. They also found that MB dye was sensitive toward the H_2O_2 atmosphere . Shekofteh-gohari and Habibi-yangjeh [60] synthesized Fe_2O_3/ ZnO/WO_3 composite to study RhB dye. However, they had accrued out a study to study the effect of photocatalyst and photocatalyst and another composite. Under

50 W LED lamp, 0.1 g of photocatalyst and 1.0×10^{-5} of dye, Fe_2O_3, Fe_2O_3/ZnO, Fe_2O_3/$CoWO_4$, and Fe_2O_3/ZnO/$CoWO_3$ showed 23.8%, 16.4%, 52.34%, and 98.3% dye degradation. Mechanism of degradation of RhB is undertaken by the deterioration of the aromatic ring .

Hitam and Jalil [7] synthesized photocatalyst by depositing Fe_2O_3 and tungsten oxide NPs on a graphene sheet using a hydrothermal process. The synthesized photocatalyst WO_3-Fe_2O_3-rGO showed 94% degradation of RhB and 98% MB dye in the presence of H_2O_2 in 40 minutes. Dumbbell (D) and cone-shaped (C) ZnO nanostructures were hybridized with g-C_3N_4 to form g-C_3N_4/ZnO by Mamba et al. [42] for degradation of MB dye. MB degradation was close to 99% within 140 minutes in the presence of known quantities of dye and photocatalyst. Composite g-C_3N_4/ZnO (D) shows four times higher degradation efficiency than g-C_3N_4, while g-C_3N_4/ZnO (C) shows three times higher efficiency than g-C_3N_4.

A comparative study by Alakhras et al. [61] noted that the zeolite-TiO_2 mixture had better performance for dye degradation compared to zeolite-ZnO under UV radiation. The facile solvothermal technique was used to synthesize CQD/TiO_2/α-Fe_2O_3 (CTF) for dye degradation of MB by Zhang et al. [62] CQD refers to carbon quantum dots. To degrade 20 mg/L MB dye, 0.05 g of the photocatalyst was used with a 300 W Xe arc lamp. Around 86.5% degradation has taken place in 180 minutes for C20TF, where 20 refers to 20 mL of CQD.

Babar et al. [63] conducted a comparative study for dye degradation of 20 ppm of MO using g-C_3N_4 & g-C_3N_4–Fe_2O_3. For 100 mg of photocatalyst and 20 ppm of dye, using g-C_3N_4-Fe_2O_3 showed 99% degradation, while for g-C_3N_4, it was 38%. Khan et al. [64] synthesized CuO/nano clay (NC) by mixing $CuCl_2{\cdot}2H_2O$ (0.5 M) and 4 g NC in a flask and was sonicated for 10 minutes. To maintain pH at 9, 2M NaOH was mixed. Later, it was refluxed for 4 hours under stirring. The mixture was cooled, filtered, and washed. Subsequently heating to 150°C gives CuO/NC. A comparative study was done between CuO/NC and CuO/NP for degradation of MO having 30 ppm concentration under a UV source. Results revealed that CuO/NC has an efficiency of 95.96% and 97.18% in 1 and 4 minutes, respectively, while in the case of CuO/NP, it was 62.36% and 68.32% for the same interval of time. In other study undertaken by Liu et al. [65], porous Fe_2O_3 nanorods (NR) were synthesized by facile chemical reaction method. Under 500 W Xe lamp, 15 mg of porous Fe_2O_3 NR was successful for degradation of RhB dye having initial concentration 10 mg/L. Results showed that 97% of RhB was degraded in 270 minutes. These porous Fe_2O_3 NRs could be recycled readily. No significant loss of activity for photocatalyst after five cycles of operation of degradation of RhB dye was observed.

Mohamed et al. [66] made ternary composites of Fe_2O_3/GO/WO_3 which were named FWG in the study. α-Fe_2O_3 was synthesized with help of aqueous flaxseed extract as templating agent. WO_3 nanomaterial was prepared by dropwise addition of 2 M (50 mL) of HCl solution into 50 mL of sodium tungstate $Na_2WO_3{\cdot}H_2O$. Fe_2O_3/WO_3 nanocomposites were prepared ex situ by varying molar ratio of α-Fe_2O_3 and WO_3. Similarly, Fe_2O_3/GO/WO_3 was prepared using different ratio of GO (5, 10, 30, 50, 100). Ternary composites was denoted as FWG 5, FWG 10, FWG 30, FWG 50, and FWG 100, where 5, 10, 30, 50, and 100 represent % of GO. These ternary composites of different compositions were used for dye degradation of MO with 1 g/L of photocatalyst and 20 ppm of dye. Figure 1.6 shows results of degradation. Results were in favor that the order of photoactivity is FWG 5 < FWG 10 < FWG 30 whereas in case of FWG 50, photoactivity decreased.

Gupta et al. [67] checked for activity of Ag^+ doped TiO_2 photocatalyst. Decoloration efficacy was shown to be >99% for basic violet and methyl red in 90 minutes of irradiation, whereas it had 86% of mineralization. Minchi et al. [68] synthesized 5 wt. % Ca doped TiO_2 nanofibers which increased dye degradation from 73% to 95% within 100 minutes. Zhang et al. [45] reported studies that prepared Fe^{+3} doped TiO_2. Semiconductor showed high photocatalytic efficiency under solar lamp. Time taken for Fe^{+3} doped TiO_2 to decompose MB by 98.8% is 120 minutes. It was also reported that some other studies prepared Mg, Zn, and Cr codoped TiO_2 nanocrystals using co-precipitation method to degrade Congo red dye. Experimental results highlighted that the MgZnCr–TiO_2 catalyst had noteworthy catalytic performance in the visible range. These samples have great recyclability and are stable even after five cycles. It has been also noted out that doped TiO_2 has improved stability [69].

Research groups [70,71] have studied the effect of Ag doped on ZnO for degradation of acid blue 13 dye. At 20 ppm initial concentration of dye, catalyst dosage of 0.15 g/L for 75 minutes of irradiation, it was observed that with increase in concentration of Ag from 0.04 mol% to 3.5 mol%, degradation improved from 60% to 95%. In addition, Ag-doped ZnO had better recyclability. Optimum dosage was found to be 3.5 mol%. However, upon increasing Ag mol% from 4.2% to 4.9% extended degradation to 60%.

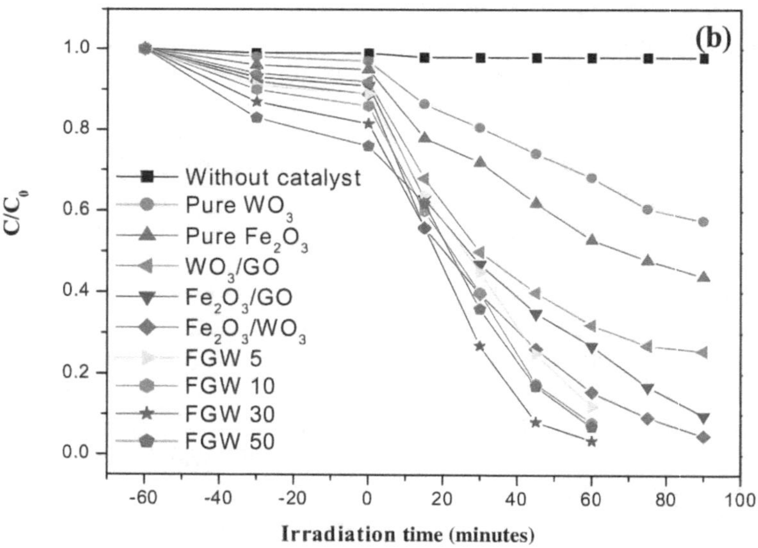

FIGURE 1.6 Photocatalytic degradation efficiency of MB in the presence of Fe_2O_3/WO_3 nanocomposites with different Fe_2O_3:WO_3 ratios [66].

Babar et al. [63] synthesized Fe_2O_3 from waste of toner printer and combined with g-C_3N_4 and form heterojunction. Photocatalytic performance of synthesized g-C_3N_4–Fe_2O_3 was tested against MO and textile effluent under action of sunlight. In experiment 100 mg of synthesized photocatalyst was suspended in 20 mg/L of MO solution and stirred in dark for 30 minutes to attain adsorption/desorption equilibrium. g-C_3N_4 and Fe_2O_3 showed 38% and 8% degradation of MO dye, whereas g-C_3N_4–Fe_2O_3 showed excellent 99% degradation efficiency. From these results, it can be concluded that addition of g-C_3N_4 to Fe_2O_3 enhanced performance by formation of heterojunctions. Selected results of this study are shown in Figure 1.7.

Researchers [72] have further synthesized ternary composites like NZVI@BiFe_2O_3/g-C_3N_4 by hydrothermal method for photocatalytic degradation of RhB dye. $BiFeO_3$ was doped by non-zero valent iron and then composite with g-C_3N_4 was formed which was assumed to enhance photocatalytic property. In photocatalytic experiment, if photocatalyst was added to 100 mL of 10 mg/L of RhB dye solution before irradiating against solar power meter, samples were stirred in dark for adsorption/desorption equilibrium for 30 minutes and activity of NZVI@BiFe_2O_3/g-C_3N_4 was tested against pH value from 2 to 11. It was observed that in acidic range degradation was not sufficient while with an increase in pH there is increase in degradation efficiency. RhB being cationic dye, under basic condition surface, is negatively charged

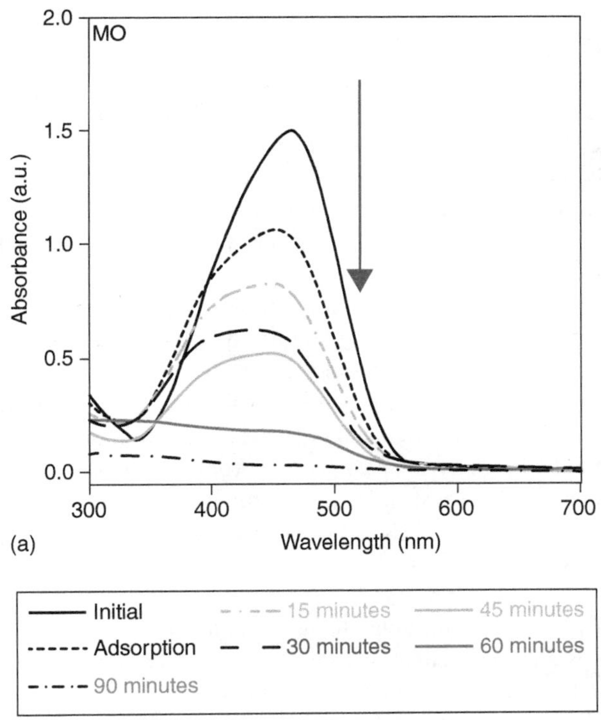

FIGURE 1.7 UV–visible spectral changes with time of MO upon photocatalytic degradation with g-C_3N_4–Fe_2O_3 [63].

which effectively improves dye adsorption and thus, photocatalytic degradation. To find optimum dosage of photocatalyst (2–18 mg) in 100 mL was added it was found that maximum degradation took place at 10 mg. in general with increase in dosage of photocatalyst, degradation increased up to optimum value and later decreased. This decline is attributed to overlapping of photocatalyst surface which reduces light penetration. At optimized condition, degradation efficiency increased with time. After 120 minutes, 97% dye degradation took place with NZVI@$BiFe_2O_3$/g-C_3N_4 catalyst.

α-Fe_2O_3 possesses excellent photocatalytic property and recently has been used for pollution remediation purposes. It had been noted that Fe_2O_3 can also enhance adsorption site. Heterojunction of α-Fe_2O_3/g-C_3N_4 can enhance performance and surface area. Looking at these aspects, Wang et al. synthesized α-Fe_2O_3/g-C_3N_4-R composite, where R = % of Fe_2O_3 for photocatalytic degradation of MO and MB. Synthesized Fe_2O_3/g-C_3N_4-0.5 (15 mg) were added to 60 mL of 50 mg/L of MO maintained at pH of 3 and 60 mL of 18 mg/L of MB at pH 7 where samples were stirred in dark for adsorption/desorption equilibrium and photocatalytic degradation starts when solution is irradiated to 300 W Xe lamp. After 150 minutes, photocatalyst was able to degrade 79.5% of MO and 80.9% of MB. α-Fe_2O_3/g-C_3N_4-0.5 showed excellent photocatalytic efficiency compared to pristine g-C_3N_4. For practical applicability of photocatalyst, same catalyst had been reused and showed decrease in removal of MO from 79.49% to 71.63% while in case of MB it was 80.93% to 72.75% after four cycles. Thus, it can be concluded that photocatalyst is stable and can be reused [73].

Ag_3VO_4/g-C_3N_4 heterojunction was synthesized for performance of malachite green, basic fuchsin, and crystal violet. Under visible light irradiation, malachite showed 97% degradation within 1 hour of irradiation, whereas basic fuchsin and crystal violet showed slower degradation. After 240 minutes of operation basic fuchsine showed 97% while crystal violet showed 75% degradation. The higher performance of Ag_3VO_4/g-C_3N_4 can attributed as potential of CB for g-C_3N_4 was high (–0.73 eV) which could generate superoxide anion while VB of Ag_3VO_4 had potential for hydroxyl radical. These ROS further reacts with organic pollutants and convert then to non-toxic components [33].

Huang et al. [74] synthesized ultrathin g-C_3N_4/AgI heterojunctions via in-situ growth method for photocatalytic degradation of RhB. In a typical photocatalytic experiment, 20 mg of synthesized photocatalyst was dispersed in 30 mL of 20 mg/L of RhB dye solution and stirred in dark for 40 minutes. Later it was irradiated using a 500 W Xe lamp. Prepared photocatalyst was efficient in removal of dye; however, UCNA-70 where 70% represents mass ratio of AgI to UCN showed excellent photocatalytic efficiency with almost degrading within 60 minutes compared to another composite. The performance of UCNA-70 was compared with pure AgI and g-C_3N_4 where results showed that UCNA-70 has 2.62 and 4.02 times better ability compared to pure AgI and g-C_3N_4. For reusability study, photocatalyst was used for four consecutive cycles where no noticeable change in efficiency was observed. However, a slight change was due to deactivation of active sites and minor mass loss during separation. Selected results of this study are shown in Figure 1.8.

Looking at favorable results of Fe_2O_3 upon coupling with semiconductor, Ghane et al. [75] synthesized g-C_3N_4–Fe_2O_3 nanocomposite from solution combustion

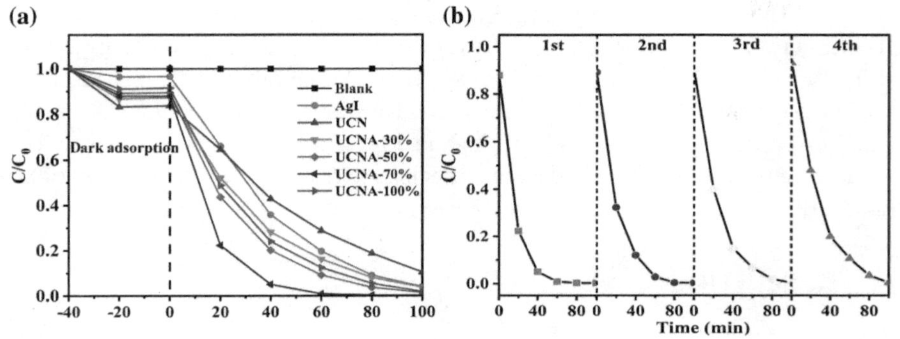

FIGURE 1.8 (a) Adsorption and photocatalytic activities of as-prepared AgI, UCN, and UCNA-X% samples for RhB degradation; (b) recycling tests of UCNA-70% composite [74].

synthesis method for photocatalytic dye degradation of MB. Here, g-C_3N_4 was produced from direct calcination of melamine at 550°C and later g-C_3N_4 powder was added to DI water and different amount of $Fe(NO_3)_3 \cdot 9H_2O$ and urea were added to suspension. The solution was heated at 80°C and gel was formed which was further heated to 250°C. The obtained powder was hand-crushed and washed with water and ethanol. The obtained powder product was denoted as CNFe-w, where w refers to wt. of $Fe(NO_3)_3 \cdot 9H_2O$ which was 0.31, 0.70, 1.21, and 2.52 g for photocatalytic experiment, 50 mg of powdered photocatalyst was added to solution of MB having initial concentration of 5.5 mg/L and was stirred in the dark for 30 minutes to attain adsorption/desorption equilibrium. Later, a light source of 30 W LED was used to initiate photocatalytic reactions. From these results, it was concluded that CNFe-1.21 has better photocatalytic ability compared to other composite formed. Pure g-C_3N_4, Fe_2O_3, and CNFe-1.21 showed 22.10%, 8.03%, and 66.79% degradation efficiency, respectively, for the same given time intervals. However, pure Fe_2O_3 has negligible photocatalytic activity upon coupling with g-C_3N_4, and showed threefold improvement compared to pure g-C_3N_4. This enhanced performance is attributed to light harvesting and lowering recombination of charge carriers. Mechanism presumed that the photogenerated e^- migrates from the CB of g-C_3N_4 migrate to the CB of Fe_2O_3 whereas photogenerated h^+ is migrates the opposite way, from the VB of Fe_2O_3 to the VB of g-C_3N_4. This charge separation leads to enhanced photoactivity.

Balu et al. [76] synthesized g-C_3N_4/ZnO@α-Fe_2O_3 ternary nanocomposite by sol–gel method, which can be used for efficient visible range photocatalyst for degradation of organic pollutants. In photocatalytic experiment, 0.05 g of synthesized photocatalyst was added to 100 mL solution of 10 mg/L of tartrazine and the solution was stirred in dark for 15 minutes to obtain adsorption/desorption equilibrium. Later it was irradiated using a 350 W mercury Xenon lamp. Results showed that g-C_3N_4/ZnO@α-Fe_2O_3 ternary composite degrades 99.34% of tartrazine dye within 35 minutes. Degradation with g-C_3N_4, ZnO, ZnO@α-Fe_2O_3, g-C_3N_4/ZnO@α-Fe_2O_3, and without catalyst nanocomposite was 76.55%, 48.59%, 64%, 99.34%, and 8%, respectively. Plausible mechanism for ternary Z-scheme is given as g-C_3N_4, which has more negative CB compared to ZnO and α-Fe_2O_3. Photogenerated electrons in CB of ZnO@α-Fe_2O_3 migrate to g-C_3N_4 via Z-scheme structure. This electron reacts with adsorbed oxygen to form superoxide anion. On the other hand, VB of ZnO is more positive compared to Fe_2O_3 and g-C_3N_4. Thus, photogenerated holes formed in g-C_3N_4/α-Fe_2O_3 migrate to the VB of ZnO, and these holes react with water to form hydroxyl radical (·OH). These oxidative species are responsible for oxidation of tartrazine dye.

1.7 CONCLUSION

This chapter briefly overviews the fundamental concepts related to dyes, their classification, and the introduction of photocatalysts. Through investigation of the mechanism behind photocatalysis, we gain insight into the potential of this process in environmental applications. The literature review on dye degradation using photocatalysts highlights the extensive research and development in this field, showcasing the promising results of various catalysts in removing dyes from wastewater.

It is evident that the use of photocatalysts holds great potential for addressing the global issue of dye pollution. The wide range of available catalysts and their varying degrees of efficiency underscore the need for continued research and optimization. Additionally, the importance of understanding the specific interactions between dyes and photocatalysts must be considered, as this knowledge will guide the design of more effective and sustainable treatment processes.

We must focus on bridging the gap between theoretical understanding and practical implementation as we move forward. Real-world applications of photocatalytic dye degradation should be explored, considering factors such as reactor design, catalyst immobilization, and scalability. Moreover, exploring synergistic approaches, combining photocatalysis with other treatment methods holds promise for even more efficient and cost-effective dye removal.

In conclusion, this chapter sets the stage for a deeper exploration into the practical applications and advancements in photocatalytic dye degradation, offering a solid foundation for further research and innovation in this critical area of environmental science and engineering.

Authors declare there is no conflict of interest.

REFERENCES

[1] Alegbe, E. O.; Uthman, T. O. "A Review of History, Properties, Classification, Applications and Challenges of Natural and Synthetic Dyes". *Heliyon*, 2024, *10* (13), e33646. https://doi.org/10.1016/j.heliyon.2024.e33646.

[2] Melghit, K.; Al-Rubaei, M. S.; Al-Amri, I. "Photodegradation Enhancement of Congo Red Aqueous Solution Using a Mixture of $SnO_2 \cdot xH_2O$ Gel/ZnO Powder". *J. Photochem. Photobiol. A Chem.*, 2006, *181* (2–3), 137–141. https://doi.org/10.1016/J.JPHOTOCHEM.2005.11.015.

[3] Khaled, A.; El Nemr, A.; El-Sikaily, A.; Abdelwahab, O. "Treatment of Artificial Textile Dye Effluent Containing Direct Yellow 12 by Orange Peel Carbon". *Desalination*, 2009, *238* (1–3), 210–232. https://doi.org/10.1016/j.desal.2008.02.014.

[4] Chatwal, G. R. *Synthetic Dyes*, 1st ed.; Himalaya Publishing House, 2009.

[5] Ghosh, A.; Mal, P. "Testing of Fibres, Yarns and Fabrics and Their Recent Developments". In *Fibres to Smart Textiles*; CRC Press: Boca Raton, 2019; pp. 221–256. https://doi.org/10.1201/9780429446511-12.

[6] Mohd Adnan, M. A.; Muhd Julkapli, N.; Amir, M. N. I. I.; Maamor, A. "Effect on Different TiO_2 Photocatalyst Supports on Photodecolorization of Synthetic Dyes: A Review". *Int. J. Environ. Sci. Technol.*, 2019, *16* (1), 547–566. https://doi.org/10.1007/s13762-018-1857-x.

[7] Hitam, C. N. C. N. C.; Jalil, A. A. A. "A Review on Exploration of Fe_2O_3 Photocatalyst towards Degradation of Dyes and Organic Contaminants". *J. Environ. Manage.*, 2020, *258* (October 2019), 110050. https://doi.org/10.1016/j.jenvman.2019.110050.

[8] Islam, S. R.; Alam, M. K.; Alassod, A.; Ahmed, T.; Yousif, A. H. D.; Rashid, M. M.; Kamal, S. A. Bin; Mia, R. "Natural Dyes and Pigments as a Source of Medicine". *Renew. Dye. Pigment.*, 2024, 177–232. https://doi.org/10.1016/B978-0-443-15213-9.00009-0.

[9] Santiago, D.; Cunha, J.; Cabral, I. "Chromatic and Medicinal Properties of Six Natural Textile Dyes: A Review of Eucalyptus, Weld, Madder, Annatto, Indigo and Woad". *Heliyon*, 2023, *9* (11), e22013. https://doi.org/10.1016/j.heliyon.2023.e22013.

[10] Benkhaya, S.; M' rabet, S.; El Harfi, A. "A Review on Classifications, Recent Synthesis and Applications of Textile Dyes". *Inorg. Chem. Commun.*, 2020, *115*, 107891. https://doi.org/10.1016/j.inoche.2020.107891.

[11] Sharma, J.; Sharma, S.; Soni, V. "Classification and Impact of Synthetic Textile Dyes on Aquatic Flora: A Review". *Reg. Stud. Mar. Sci.*, 2021, *45*, 101802. https://doi.org/10.1016/J.RSMA.2021.101802.

[12] Benkhaya, S.; Harfi, S. El; Harfi, A. El. "Classifications, Properties and Applications of Textile Dyes: A Review". *Appl. J. Environ. Eng. Sci.*, 2022, *3* (3), 2022.

[13] Al-Rubaie, L. A. A. R.; Mhessn, R. J. "Synthesis and Characterization of Azo Dye Para Red and New Derivatives". *E-Journal Chem.*, 2012, *9* (1), 465–470. https://doi.org/10.1155/2012/206076.

[14] Ooyama, Y.; Yagi, S. *Progress in the Science of Functional Dyes*, 1st ed.; Ooyama, Y., Yagi, S., Eds.; Springer Singapore: Singapore, 2021. https://doi.org/10.1007/978-981-33-4392-4.

[15] Maulik, S. R.; Bhattacharya, A.; Roy, P. P.; Maiti, K. "Reactive Dye and Its Advancements". In *Textile Dyes and Pigments*; Pandit, P., Singha, K., Maity, S., Ahmed, S., Eds.; Wiley, 2022; pp. 17–44. https://doi.org/10.1002/9781119905332.ch2.

[16] Dey, S.; Nagababu, B. H. "Applications of Food Color and Bio-Preservatives in the Food and Its Effect on the Human Health". *Food Chem. Adv.*, 2022, *1* (January), 100019. https://doi.org/10.1016/j.focha.2022.100019.

[17] Molina, A. K.; Corrêa, R. C. G.; Prieto, M. A.; Pereira, C.; Barros, L. "Bioactive Natural Pigments' Extraction, Isolation, and Stability in Food Applications". *Molecules*, 2023, *28* (3), 1200. https://doi.org/10.3390/molecules28031200.

[18] Thakur, M.; Modi, V. K. "Biocolorants in Food: Sources, Extraction, Applications and Future Prospects". *Crit. Rev. Food Sci. Nutr.*, 2024, *64* (14), 4674–4713. https://doi.org/10.1080/10408398.2022.2144997.

[19] Wargala, E.; Sławska, M.; Zalewska, A.; Toporowska, M. "Health Effects of Dyes, Minerals, and Vitamins Used in Cosmetics". *Women*, 2021, *1* (4), 223–237. https://doi.org/10.3390/women1040020.

[20] Guerra, E.; Llompart, M.; Garcia-Jares, C. "Analysis of Dyes in Cosmetics: Challenges and Recent Developments". *Cosmetics*, 2018, *5* (3), 47. https://doi.org/10.3390/cosmetics5030047.

[21] Saggioro, E. M.; Oliveira, A. S.; Moreira, J. C. "Heterogeneous Photocatalysis Remediation of Wastewater Polluted by Indigoid Dyes". *Textile Wastewater Treatment*, 2016, *93*, 93–114. https://doi.org/10.5772/63790.

[22] Rono, N.; Kibet, J. K.; Martincigh, B. S.; Nyamori, V. O. "A Comparative Study between Thermal Etching and Liquid Exfoliation of Bulk Graphitic Carbon Nitride to Nanosheets for the Photocatalytic Degradation of a Model Environmental Pollutant, *Rhodamine B". J. Mater. Sci. Mater. Electron.*, 2021, *32* (1), 687–706. https://doi.org/10.1007/s10854-020-04849-8.

[23] Ajmal, A.; Majeed, I.; Malik, R. N.; Idriss, H.; Nadeem, M. A. "Principles and Mechanisms of Photocatalytic Dye Degradation on TiO_2 Based Photocatalysts: A Comparative Overview". *RSC Adv.*, 2014, *4* (70), 37003–37026. https://doi.org/10.1039/C4RA06658H.

[24] Rodríguez-Couto, S.; Osma, J. F.; Toca-Herrera, J. L. "Removal of Synthetic Dyes by an Eco-friendly Strategy". *Eng. Life Sci.*, 2009, *9* (2), 116–123. https://doi.org/10.1002/elsc.200800088.

[25] Velusamy, S.; Roy, A.; Sundaram, S.; Kumar Mallick, T. "A Review on Heavy Metal Ions and Containing Dyes Removal Through Graphene Oxide-Based Adsorption Strategies for Textile Wastewater Treatment". *Chem. Rec.*, 2021, *21* (7), 1570–1610. https://doi.org/10.1002/tcr.202000153.

[26] Katheresan, V.; Kansedo, J.; Lau, S. Y. "Efficiency of Various Recent Wastewater Dye Removal Methods: A Review". *J. Environ. Chem. Eng.*, 2018, *6* (4), 4676–4697. https://doi.org/10.1016/j.jece.2018.06.060.

[27] Solayman, H. M.; Hossen, M. A.; Abd Aziz, A.; Yahya, N. Y.; Leong, K. H.; Sim, L. C.; Monir, M. U.; Zoh, K.-D. "Performance Evaluation of Dye Wastewater Treatment Technologies: *A Review". J. Environ. Chem. Eng.*, 2023, *11* (3), 109610. https://doi.org/10.1016/J.JECE.2023.109610.

[28] Rafatullah, M.; Sulaiman, O.; Hashim, R.; Ahmad, A. "Adsorption of Methylene Blue on Low-Cost Adsorbents: A Review". *J. Hazard. Mater.*, 2010, *177* (1–3), 70–80. https://doi.org/10.1016/j.jhazmat.2009.12.047.

[29] Rafiq, A.; Ikram, M.; Ali, S.; Niaz, F.; Khan, M.; Khan, Q.; Maqbool, M. "Photocatalytic Degradation of Dyes Using Semiconductor Photocatalysts to Clean Industrial Water Pollution". *J. Ind. Eng. Chem.*, 2021, *97*, 111–128. https://doi.org/10.1016/j.jiec.2021.02.017.

[30] Kumar, S.; Karthikeyan, S.; Lee, A. F. "G-C3N4-Based Nanomaterials for Visible Light-Driven Photocatalysis". *Catalysts*, 2018, *8* (2), 74. https://doi.org/10.3390/catal8020074.

[31] Mandal, R. K.; Saha, P.; Majumder, T. P. "Structural, Optical Characterization of the Synthesized Fe Doped CdO Nano Particles, Its Application as a Promising Photocatalyst for Degradation of the Hazardous Methyl Violet Dye". *Optik (Stuttg).*, 2021, *246* (August), 167795. https://doi.org/10.1016/j.ijleo.2021.167795.

[32] Sardar, M.; Manna, M.; Maharana, M.; Sen, S. "Green Adsorbents to Remove Metals, Dyes and Boron from Polluted Water". In *Green Adsorbents to Remove Metals, Dyes and Boron from Polluted Water*; Inamuddin, Ahamed, M. I.; Lichtfouse, E.; Asiri, A. M.; Eds.; Environmental Chemistry for a Sustainable World; Springer International Publishing: Cham, 2021; Vol. 49, pp. 377–403. https://doi.org/10.1007/978-3-030-47400-3.

[33] Anwer, H.; Mahmood, A.; Lee, J.; Kim, K.-H. H.; Park, J.-W. W.; Yip, A. C. K. K. "Photocatalysts for Degradation of Dyes in Industrial Effluents: Opportunities and Challenges". *Nano Res.*, 2019, *12* (5), 955–972. https://doi.org/10.1007/s12274-019-2287-0.

[34] Weinberg, N. L.; Weinberg, H. R. "Electrochemical Oxidation of Organic Compounds". *Chem. Rev.*, 1968, *68* (4), 449–523. https://doi.org/10.1021/cr60254a003.

[35] Ahmad, K.; Ghatak, H. R.; Ahuja, S. M. M. "A Review on Photocatalytic Remediation of Environmental Pollutants and H2 Production through Water Splitting: A Sustainable Approach". *Environ. Technol. Innov.*, 2020, *19*, 100893. https://doi.org/10.1016/j.eti.2020.100893.

[36] Ahmad, N.; Anae, J.; Khan, M. Z.; Sabir, S.; Yang, X. J.; Thakur, V. K.; Campo, P.; Coulon, F. "Visible Light-Conducting Polymer Nanocomposites as Efficient Photocatalysts for the Treatment of Organic Pollutants in Wastewater". *J. Environ. Manage.*, 2021, *295* (June), 113362. https://doi.org/10.1016/j.jenvman.2021.113362.

[37] Tejasvi, R.; Sharma, M.; Upadhyay, K. "Passive Photo-Catalytic Destruction of Air-Borne VOCs in High Traffic Areas Using TiO_2-Coated Flexible PVC Sheet". *Chem. Eng. J.*, 2015, *262*, 875–881. https://doi.org/10.1016/j.cej.2014.10.040.

[38] Fawzi Suleiman Khasawneh, O.; Palaniandy, P. "Removal of Organic Pollutants from Water by Fe_2O_3/TiO_2 Based Photocatalytic Degradation: A Review". *Environ. Technol. Innov.*, 2021, *21* (xxxx), 101230. https://doi.org/10.1016/j.eti.2020.101230.

[39] Zada, A.; Humayun, M.; Raziq, F.; Zhang, X.; Qu, Y.; Bai, L.; Qin, C.; Jing, L.; Fu, H. "Exceptional Visible-Light-Driven Cocatalyst-Free Photocatalytic Activity of g-C3N4 by Well Designed Nanocomposites with Plasmonic Au and SnO_2". *Adv. Energy Mater.*, 2016, *6* (21), 1601190. https://doi.org/10.1002/aenm.201601190.

[40] Zhang, J.; Hu, W.; Cao, S.; Piao, L. "Recent Progress for Hydrogen Production by Photocatalytic Natural or Simulated Seawater Splitting". *Nano Res.*, 2020, *13* (9), 2313–2322. https://doi.org/10.1007/s12274-020-2880-z.

[41] Singh, A.; Tejasvi, R.; Karmakar, S.; Basu, S. "α-Fe_2O_3 Nanorods Decorated with NiMnO3 Co-Catalyst as Photoanode for Enhanced Oxygen Evolution Reaction in Photoelectrochemical Water Splitting". *Mater. Today Commun.*, 2021, *27*, 102231. https://doi.org/10.1016/j.mtcomm.2021.102231.

[42] Mamba, G.; Mishra, A. K. K. "Graphitic Carbon Nitride (g-C_3N_4) Nanocomposites: A New and Exciting Generation of Visible Light Driven Photocatalysts for Environmental Pollution Remediation". *Appl. Catal. B Environ.*, 2016, *198* (July), 347–377. https://doi.org/10.1016/j.apcatb.2016.05.052.

[43] Tejasvi, R.; Basu, S. "Formation of Thin Film like Assembly of Exfoliated C_3N_4 Nanoflakes by Solvent Non-Evaporative Method Using Centrifuge". *Appl. Surf. Sci.*, 2017, *424*, 9–14. https://doi.org/10.1016/j.apsusc.2017.03.067.

[44] Tejasvi, R. "Shape Tailoring of TiO_2 Nanostructures during Thermochemical Synthesis by Etchant-Oxidant Combinatorics". *Mater. Today Proc.*, 2022, *57* (1), 130–134. https://doi.org/10.1016/j.matpr.2022.02.073.

[45] Zhang, F.; Wang, X.; Liu, H.; Liu, C.; Wan, Y.; Long, Y.; Cai, Z. "Recent Advances and Applications of Semiconductor Photocatalytic Technology". *Appl. Sci.*, 2019, *9* (12), 2489. https://doi.org/10.3390/app9122489.

[46] Tejasvi, R.; Basu, S. "Thermochemical Method of Synthesizing Stemmed Nanoflower TiO_2/eC_3N_4 Heterojunction Structures with Enhanced Solar Water Splitting". *J. Phys. Energy*, 2020, *2* (3), 035002. https://doi.org/10.1088/2515-7655/ab8912.

[47] Saravanan, A.; Kumar, P. S.; Vo, D.-V. N. V. N.; Yaashikaa, P. R.; Karishma, S.; Jeevanantham, S.; Gayathri, B.; Bharathi, V. D. "Photocatalysis for Removal of

Environmental Pollutants and Fuel Production: *A Review". Environ. Chem. Lett.*, 2021, *19* (1), 441–463. https://doi.org/10.1007/s10311-020-01077-8.
[48] Sarkar, B.; Daware, A. V.; Gupta, P.; Krishnani, K. K.; Baruah, S.; Bhattacharjee, S. "Nanoscale Wide-Band Semiconductors for Photocatalytic Remediation of Aquatic Pollution". *Environ. Sci. Pollut. Res.*, 2017, *24* (33), 25775–25797. https://doi.org/10.1007/s11356-017-0252-3.
[49] Sagadevan, S.; Lett, J. A.; Weldegebrieal, G. K.; ud Dowla Biswas, M. R.; Oh, W. C.; Alshahateet, S. F.; Fatimah, I.; Mohammad, F.; Al-Lohedan, H. A.; Paiman, S.; et al. "Enhanced Gas Sensing and Photocatalytic Activity of Reduced Graphene Oxide Loaded TiO2 Nanoparticles". *Chem. Phys. Lett.*, 2021, *780* (April), 138897. https://doi.org/10.1016/j.cplett.2021.138897.
[50] Song, J.; Seo, M. J.; Lee, T. H.; Jo, Y.-R. R.; Lee, J.; Kim, T. L.; Kim, S. M. S. Y. S.-M. S.-Y.; Kim, S. M. S. Y. S.-M. S.-Y.; Jeong, S. Y.; An, H.; et al. "Tailoring Crystallographic Orientations to Substantially Enhance Charge Separation Efficiency in Anisotropic BiVO4 Photoanodes". *ACS Catal.*, 2018, *8* (7), 5952–5962. https://doi.org/10.1021/acscatal.8b00877.
[51] Hasija, V.; Raizada, P.; Sudhaik, A.; Sharma, K.; Kumar, A.; Singh, P.; Jonnalagadda, S. B.; Thakur, V. K. "Recent Advances in Noble Metal Free Doped Graphitic Carbon Nitride Based Nanohybrids for Photocatalysis of Organic Contaminants in Water: *A Review". Appl. Mater. Today*, 2019, *15*, 494–524. https://doi.org/10.1016/j.apmt.2019.04.003.
[52] Albert, P.; Narayanan, J.; Arockiadoss, T. "Indium-Tin Oxide Regulated Band Gap of Nitrogen-Doped Titanium Oxide Thin Films for Visible Light Photocatalyst". *Appl. Phys. A*, 2021, *127* (12), 900. https://doi.org/10.1007/s00339-021-05053-z.
[53] Arunachalam, P.; Nagai, K.; Amer, M. S.; Ghanem, M. A.; Ramalingam, R. J.; Al-Mayouf, A. M. "Recent Developments in the Use of Heterogeneous Semiconductor Photocatalyst Based Materials for a Visible-Light-Induced Water-Splitting System—*A Brief Review". Catalysts*, 2021, *11* (2), 160. https://doi.org/10.3390/CATAL11020160.
[54] He, X.; Liu, Y.; Butch, C. J.; Lee, B. R.; Guo, F.; Wu, J.; Wang, Z.; Lu, Q.; Jeong, J. H.; Wang, Y.; et al. "One-Pot Exfoliation of Graphitic C3N4 Quantum Dots for Blue QLEDs by Methylamine Intercalation". *Small*, 2019, *15* (44), 1902735. https://doi.org/10.1002/smll.201902735.
[55] Zhang, Y.; Yuan, J.; Ding, Y.; Liu, B.; Zhao, L.; Zhang, S. "Research Progress on g–C3N4–Based Photocatalysts for Organic Pollutants Degradation in Wastewater: From Exciton and Carrier Perspectives". *Ceram. Int.*, 2021, *47* (22), 31005–31030. https://doi.org/10.1016/j.ceramint.2021.08.063.
[56] Bisaria, K.; Sinha, S.; Singh, R.; Iqbal, H. M. N. "Recent Advances in Structural Modifications of Photo-Catalysts for Organic Pollutants Degradation–A Comprehensive Review". *Chemosphere*, 2021, *284* (December 2020), 131263. https://doi.org/10.1016/j.chemosphere.2021.131263.
[57] Xu, Q.; Zhang, L.; Yu, J.; Wageh, S.; Al-Ghamdi, A. A.; Jaroniec, M. "Direct Z-Scheme Photocatalysts: Principles, Synthesis, and Applications". *Mater. Today*, 2018, *21* (10), 1042–1063. https://doi.org/10.1016/j.mattod.2018.04.008.
[58] Jindal, H.; Kumar, D.; Sillanpaa, M.; Nemiwal, M. "Current Progress in Polymeric Graphitic Carbon Nitride-Based Photocatalysts for Dye Degradation". *Inorg. Chem. Commun.*, 2021, *131* (May), 108786. https://doi.org/10.1016/j.inoche.2021.108786.
[59] Moiz, M. A.; Mumtaz, A.; Salman, M.; Mazhar, H.; Basit, M. A.; Husain, S. W.; Ramzan, M. "Enhancement of Dye Degradation by Zinc Oxide via Transition-Metal

Doping: *A Review*". *J. Electron. Mater.*, 2021, *50* (9), 5106–5121. https://doi.org/10.1007/s11664-021-09093-2.

[60] Shekofteh-Gohari, M.; Habibi-Yangjeh, A. "Fe3O4/ZnO/CoWO4 Nanocomposites: Novel Magnetically Separable Visible-Light-Driven Photocatalysts with Enhanced Activity in Degradation of Different Dye Pollutants". *Ceram. Int.*, 2017, *43* (3), 3063–3071. https://doi.org/10.1016/j.ceramint.2016.11.115.

[61] Alakhras, F.; Alhajri, E.; Haounati, R.; Ouachtak, H.; Addi, A. A.; Saleh, T. A. "A Comparative Study of Photocatalytic Degradation of Rhodamine B Using Natural-Based Zeolite Composites". *Surfaces and Interfaces*, 2020, *20* (May), 100611. https://doi.org/10.1016/j.surfin.2020.100611.

[62] Zhang, J.; Kuang, M.; Wang, J.; Liu, R.; Xie, S.; Ji, Z. "Fabrication of Carbon Quantum Dots/TiO_2/Fe_2O_3 Composites and Enhancement of Photocatalytic Activity under Visible Light". *Chem. Phys. Lett.*, 2019, *730* (May), 391–398. https://doi.org/10.1016/j.cplett.2019.06.011.

[63] Babar, S.; Gavade, N.; Shinde, H.; Gore, A.; Mahajan, P.; Lee, K. H.; Bhuse, V.; Garadkar, K. "An Innovative Transformation of Waste Toner Powder into Magnetic g-C_3N_4-Fe_2O_3 Photocatalyst: Sustainable e-Waste Management". *J. Environ. Chem. Eng.*, 2019, *7* (2), 103041. https://doi.org/10.1016/j.jece.2019.103041.

[64] Khan, I. I.; Khan, I. I.; Usman, M.; Imran, M.; Saeed, K. "Nanoclay-Mediated Photocatalytic Activity Enhancement of Copper Oxide Nanoparticles for Enhanced Methyl Orange Photodegradation". *J. Mater. Sci. Mater. Electron.*, 2020, *31* (11), 8971–8985. https://doi.org/10.1007/s10854-020-03431-6.

[65] Liu, X.; Chen, K.; Shim, J.-J. J.; Huang, J. "Facile Synthesis of Porous Fe_2O_3 Nanorods and Their Photocatalytic Properties". *J. Saudi Chem. Soc.*, 2015, *19* (5), 479–484. https://doi.org/10.1016/j.jscs.2015.06.009.

[66] Mohamed, H. H. "Rationally Designed Fe_2O_3/GO/WO_3 Z-Scheme Photocatalyst for Enhanced Solar Light Photocatalytic Water Remediation". *J. Photochem. Photobiol. A Chem.*, 2019, *378* (March), 74–84. https://doi.org/10.1016/j.jphotochem.2019.04.023.

[67] Gupta, A. K. K.; Pal, A.; Sahoo, C. "Photocatalytic Degradation of a Mixture of Crystal Violet (Basic Violet 3) and Methyl Red Dye in Aqueous Suspensions Using Ag+ Doped TiO_2". *Dye. Pigment.*, 2006, *69* (3), 224–232. https://doi.org/10.1016/j.dyepig.2005.04.001.

[68] Minchi, L.; Cao, F.; Xinni, Z.; Youqiang, C.; Xuhua, L. "Photocatalytic Activity of Ca-TiO2 Nanofibers with Different Concentrations of Calcium". *Chem. Phys. Lett.*, 2019, *736* (September), 136807. https://doi.org/10.1016/j.cplett.2019.136807.

[69] Gopinath, K. P.; Madhav, N. V.; Krishnan, A.; Malolan, R.; Rangarajan, G. "Present Applications of Titanium Dioxide for the Photocatalytic Removal of Pollutants from Water: A Review". *J. Environ. Manage.*, 2020, *270* (June), 110906. https://doi.org/10.1016/j.jenvman.2020.110906.

[70] Guo, Z.; Li, P.; Che, H.; Wang, G.; Wu, C.; Zhang, X.; Mu, J. "One-Dimensional Spindle-like $BiVO_4$/TiO_2 Nanofibers Heterojunction Nanocomposites with Enhanced Visible Light Photocatalytic Activity". *Ceram. Int.*, 2016, *42* (3), 4517–4525. https://doi.org/10.1016/j.ceramint.2015.11.142.

[71] Weldegebrieal, G. K. "Synthesis Method, Antibacterial and Photocatalytic Activity of ZnO Nanoparticles for Azo Dyes in Wastewater Treatment: A Review". *Inorg. Chem. Commun.*, 2020, *120* (June), 108140. https://doi.org/10.1016/j.inoche.2020.108140.

[72] Rahman, M. U.; Qazi, U. Y.; Hussain, T.; Nadeem, N.; Zahid, M.; Bhatti, H. N.; Shahid, I. "Solar Driven Photocatalytic Degradation Potential of Novel Graphitic Carbon Nitride Based Nano Zero-Valent Iron Doped Bismuth Ferrite Ternary

Composite". *Opt. Mater. (Amst).*, 2021, *120* (March), 111408. https://doi.org/10.1016/j.optmat.2021.111408.

[73] Wang, L.; Hou, Y.; Xiao, S.; Bi, F.; Zhao, L.; Li, Y.; Zhang, X.; Gai, G.; Dong, X. "One-Step, High-Yield Synthesis of g-C_3N_4 Nanosheets for Enhanced Visible Light Photocatalytic Activity". *RSC Adv.*, 2019, *9* (67), 39304–39314. https://doi.org/10.1039/C9RA08922E.

[74] Huang, H.; Li, Y.-X. X.; Wang, H.-L. L.; Jiang, W.-F. F. "In Situ Fabrication of Ultrathin-g-C_3N_4/AgI Heterojunctions with Improved Catalytic Performance for Photodegrading Rhodamine B Solution". *Appl. Surf. Sci.*, 2021, *538* (September 2020), 148132. https://doi.org/10.1016/j.apsusc.2020.148132.

[75] Ghane, N.; Sadrnezhaad, S. K. K.; Hosseini H., S. M. "Combustion Synthesis of g-C_3N_4/Fe_2O_3 Nanocomposite for Superior Photoelectrochemical Catalytic Performance". *Appl. Surf. Sci.*, 2020, *534* (May), 147563. https://doi.org/10.1016/j.apsusc.2020.147563.

[76] Balu, S.; Velmurugan, S.; Palanisamy, S.; Chen, S.-W. W.; Velusamy, V.; Yang, T. C. K.; El-Shafey, E.-S. S. I. "Synthesis of α-Fe_2O_3 Decorated g-C_3N_4/ZnO Ternary Z-Scheme Photocatalyst for Degradation of Tartrazine Dye in Aqueous Media". *J. Taiwan Inst. Chem. Eng.*, 2019, *99*, 258–267. https://doi.org/10.1016/j.jtice.2019.03.011.

2 Photocatalysis for Dye Degradation

Subodh Kumar and Xuan Thang Cao

2.1 INTRODUCTION

A substantial number of industrial dyes (>3000) are being used to solve the dying purposes in different industries besides the additional supplementary chemicals. The irreplaceable role of dyes in textiles, leather, packaging, and other industries can be accounted for on the basis of their enormous requirement in tons per year [1,2]. However, the main problem is the discharging of dye residues in the effluent during the coloring processes. This dye-contaminated effluent is a potential threat to the environment including aquatic and human life [3, 4]. Synthetic dyes are categorized based on their chromophores and/or auxochrome groups responsible for the origin of color. Moreover, the availability of other functional groups can also affect the properties of dye molecules, i.e., acidic groups are found to increase the solubility in water. Apart from the dye, other chemicals may also be present in the effluent that may cause serious problems to the environment including aquatic life. Therefore, treatment of the industrial effluent is necessary before discharging it into the natural water sources or the fields to avoid possible harmful effects on nature. The contribution of the textile industry in releasing dyes in the water bodies is more than half of total dye effluent contamination. However, textile and other industries have their own importance in the daily life of humans and thus cannot be replaced. Therefore, it would be important to either use natural dyes or separate/convert the residual synthetic dyes into non-harmful or useful chemicals. Although natural dyes are the best candidates for coloring purposes because of their biocompatibility and nontoxic nature [5,6], natural dyes cannot fill the huge demand of various industries [7]. Therefore, the efficient treatment of the effluent is a mostly accepted way to counter this problem at the current time. In fact, several methods including physical or chemical methods have shown their competency to eliminate the dyes from the industrial wastewater stream [8,9]. However, the complexity of effluents due to the existence of different chemicals besides dye residues is the main cause for the incapability of a single method in the treatment of all types of effluents. In fact, in some cases, it is better to combine two or more treatment processes to make a hybrid process to achieve the best results in terms of water quality and the feasible cost of the process at the industrial level [10–13]. Therefore, it is required to develop a material or method keeping in mind that during the dye removal process, no other harmful chemicals are formed as a side

DOI: 10.1201/9781003441083-2

or end product. The main methods for dye removal can be characterized based on their removal mechanism. Mainly biological [14, 15] chemical [8,16], and physical treatments [17,18], are important methods that are generally used for dye removal [19]. These methods can be further subdivided into various subcategories [20]. However, all these methods have their pros and cons and can be applied based on the chemicals and physical nature of the effluents. Moreover, the cost, feasibility, and efficiency of the process are also principal factors in determining the best methods for the treatment of the particular effluent. Many review articles have already been published covering the different aspects of dye treatment processes applying various strategies (chemical, physical, biological, and hybrid) and materials for efficient dye removal from contaminated industrial spent water [21–23]. In this chapter, we focus on compiling the results and presenting concise research in similar fields. Moreover, the present chapter discusses in detail the importance of the photocatalytic degradation process and materials used for dye removal.

2.2 METHODS

Dyes are colored organic compounds that have different chromophores and auxochromes responsible for absorbing visible light yielding different colors. Various industries such as textile, leather, cosmetics, plastic, packaging, and many more procure these dyes for coloring purposes. However, a great amount spent on residual dyes is discarded without prior treatment. Except for natural dyes, most of the dyes are harmful to the groundwater, ecosystem, and humans. Therefore, there is continuous thrust to develop technologies to treat industrial effluents to reduce the harmful effects of synthetic dyes. Nevertheless, a number of techniques have been developed and applied to treat the dyes containing industrial effluent. However, the chemical nature of industrial effluents in terms of the type of dye and its concentration are important parameters for choosing the effective strategy to overcome the associated challenges (Table 2.1). In this section, we have discussed varied materials and methods used for the treatment of industrial wastewater to remove the dye.

2.2.1 Biological Treatment

In this process, microorganisms (bacteria, algae, yeast, and fungi) are employed, thus excluding the requirement of hazardous chemicals and can be performed under aerobic and anaerobic conditions. Microorganisms transform synthetic dyes into competitively less harmful chemical compounds or sludge. Therefore, it is comparatively an economical and environmentally friendly process. Bacteria are generated as a result of the fermentation process. Many bacteria have been reported to decolorize/degrade industrial dyes efficiently owing to a high specific growth rate. However, dye treatment conditions are the main parameters to determine their effectiveness in the dye removal process. Krishnan et al. degraded the mixture of three dyes from the water using bacterial culture while modulating the pH, dye concentration, and column dosage to get the optimum results using response surface methodology. They successfully achieved more than 31.2%, 71.5%, and 87.6% removal efficiency for

TABLE 2.1
Classification of dyes based on their solubility, applications, and eco-toxicological effects

Type of Dye	Examples	Structure Example	Water Solubility	Dye Application	Toxic Effects	References
Acid dye	Tartrazine, Acid red 87, Acid orange 7, Acid Blue 7	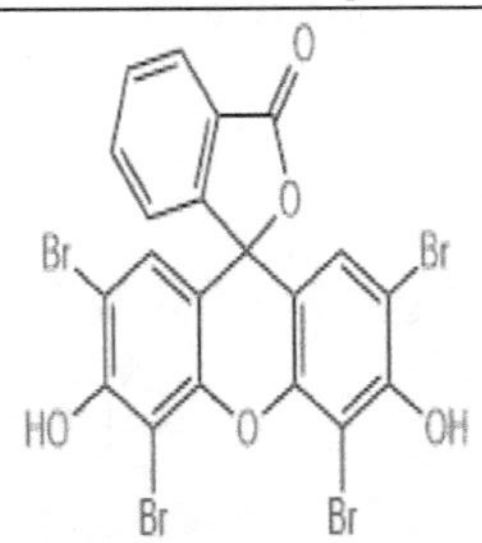 Acid Red 87	Soluble	Pharmaceutical, leather and textile industries; nylon wool, silk, and modified acrylics	Diarrhea, vomiting, nausea, carcinogenic and mutagenic effects	[4, 20–23]
Vat dye	Anthraquinone derivatives, vat blue 1, vat acid blue 74	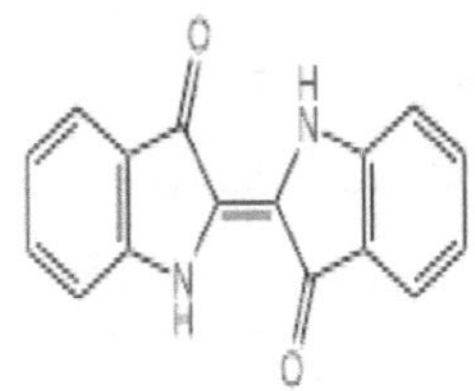 Vat blue 1	Insoluble	Coloring cellulosic fibers: cotton, fibers natural fibers	Allergic conjunctivitis, rhinitis, and other allergic reaction	[4, 20, 21, 24–26]

(continued)

TABLE 2.1 (Continued)
Classification of dyes based on their solubility, applications, and eco-toxicological effects

Type of Dye	Examples	Structure Example	Water Solubility	Dye Application	Toxic Effects	References
Basic dye	Basic Blue 9, Basic red 1, Basic red 118	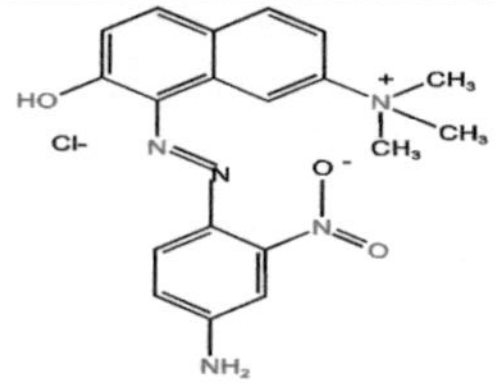 Basic red 118		Paper, polyacrylonitrile-modified nylons, and modified polyesters	Devastating effects on flora and fauna. Detrimental effects on water bodies.	[4, 20, 24]
Direct dye	Congo red (CR), Direct red 28, Brilliant yellow, Direct black 38	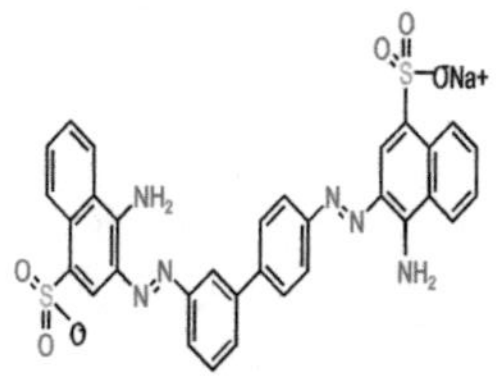 Direct red 28	Soluble	Biological materials, coloring paper products	Carcinogenic; mutagenic, and dermatitis. Dangerous to aquatic life.	[4, 20, 27, 28]
Dispersed dye	Disperse red 9, Disperse Violet 1, Disperse red 60	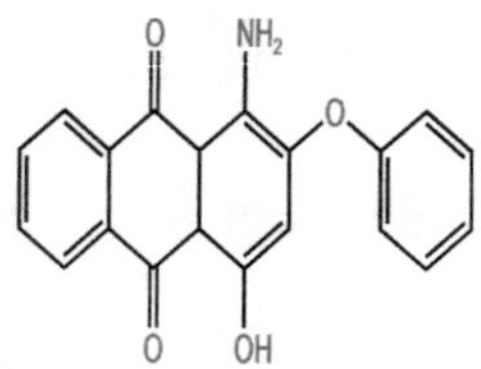 Dispersed red 60		Polyester, nylon, cellulose acetate, and acrylic fibers	Mutagenic; carcinogenic; causes soil and water pollution	[4, 20, 29]

Reactive dye	C.I. reactive red 120, C.I. reactive Black 5, C.I. reactive blue 19	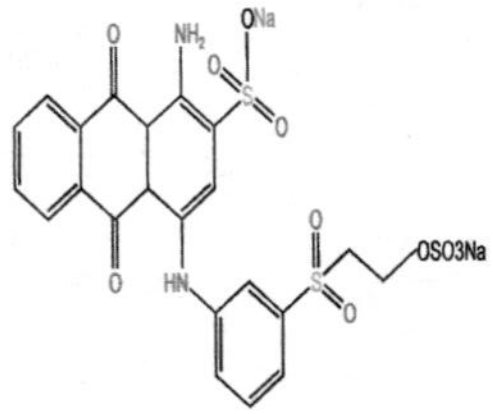 C.I Reactive Blue 19	Dyeing cellulosic, silk, and wool fibers	Allergic reaction in eyes, skin, mucous membrane, and the upper respiratory tract	[4, 20]
Mordant dye	Mordant red 11, Mordant Black 17	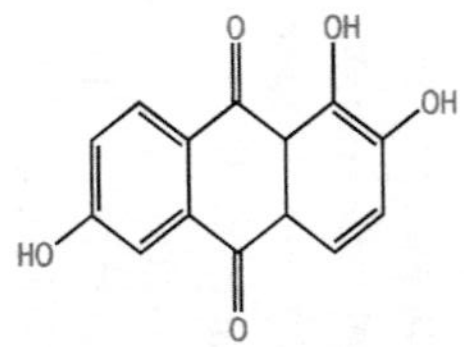 Mordent red 4	Textile fibers such as wool, silk, and leather	Allergic reactions, especially skin	[4, 20, 30, 31]
Azo dye	Direct Black 22, Disperse Yellow7, Acid Orange 20, Methyl red, Methyl orange (MO), Trypan blue	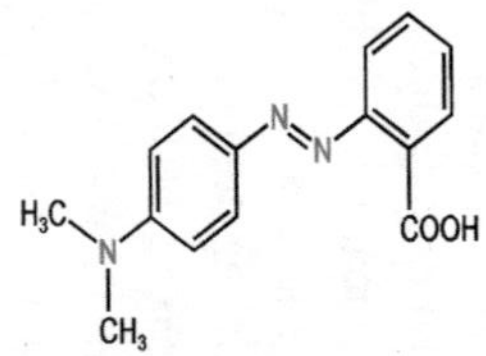 Methyl red	Textile industry for dyeing, process and food coloring	Carcinogenic to humans and animals. Hazardous when inhaled or swallowed: affects the eye, skin, digestive tract. Disturbs aquatic life.	[4, 20, 21, 32, 33]

RBRX-3B, DB-6, and DB-19, respectively [24]. Roy et al. [25] identified a new bacterium (*Enterobacter* sp. CV–S1) and used it to degrade the crystal violet (CV) dye from the mineral salt medium. Decolorizing efficiency was examined at the different reaction temperatures, pH, dye concentration, and inoculum size using a photoelectric colorimeter. Complete decolorizing was achieved at 35°C and pH 6.5 for the 150 mg/L of CV dye in 72 hours. In another report by Rames and coworkers, three different bacterial strains were employed to degrade the azo dyes [26]. The bacterial consortium was found to decolorize dye-containing solution (200–800 mg/L of dye) with effectivity up to 93% within 18 hours under optimized pH, salt levels, and temperature. Cell-free extracts of the strains showed azo reductase activity and accordingly breakdown the azo bond which was confirmed by the presence of reductive products (4-aminonaphthalene-1-sulphonic acid and 5-amino-6-hydroxynaphthalene-2-sulphonic acid) in the treated reaction mixture during high-performance liquid chromatography (HPLC) and UV–Vis analysis. Moreover, the phytotoxicity test showed a steep decrease in the toxicity level of the treated medium. Although bacteria can degrade or decolorize the dye, they sometimes produce carcinogenic and mutagenic amines. Therefore, the choice of bacteria is important to avoid the formation of such harmful by-product chemicals. Moreover, yeast species have been reported mostly as adsorbents due to their high growth rate and stable nature under treatment conditions [27]. Soh et al. have used the spent yeast from the brewery as a biosorbent to eliminate Congo red dye from the effluent. The biosorbent (4 g/L) exhibited optimum adsorption capacity for Congo red dye (50 mg/L) [28]. Adsorption kinetics followed a pseudo-second-order model. Interestingly, 100% Congo red dye was recovered in the desorption process by applying sonication. M. S. Mahmoud tested Baker's yeast strain (*Saccharomyces cerevisiae*) to decolorize real industry effluent in a repeated batch process [29]. To facilitate the separation of yeast after the adsorption of dye from the wastewater, Azeez and Al-Zuhairi [30] have presented a highly effective technique to remove the methyl orange dye from wastewater by using immobilized yeast cells on the magnetic nanoparticles as biosorbent. The immobilization strategy enhanced not only the surface area which in turn increased the sorption capacity but also its facile separation. Under the optimized condition, the maximum removal efficiency was recorded to be 96.52 %. Enzymes cost is comparatively higher and therefore less attractive for dye treatment. However, a recent study shows that enzymes can either degrade the dye into other valuable products or remove it via the precipitation process [31,32]. Ariaeenejad et al. covalently immobilized a model enzyme on the surface of amine-functionalized magnetic graphene oxide (GO) [33]. The synthesized material was then investigated for dye removal from the water and compared its activity with the free enzyme. It was evident that the immobilization of the enzyme enhanced its adsorption and degradation competence. Moreover, free enzymes were found to be deactivated on storage but not immobilized. Bio-based peroxidases are always desirable for the treatment of wastewater thanks to their sustainable nature. Chiong et al. [34] employed plant-based peroxidase enzymes to treat methyl orange-contaminated water samples. In this study, luffa skin peels and soybean hulls were used to obtain the respective peroxidase (*Luffa acutangula* peroxidase and soybean peroxidase). Soybean peroxidase performed better in terms of decolorization efficiency under the optimized conditions. These results are important to develop a comparatively cheap dye removal process utilizing the enzymes.

2.2.2 Chemical Treatment

Chemical processes are comparatively more energy-intensive than biological and physical treatments. It requires electrical energy, harmful chemicals, and equipment, and produces hazardous end products as a result of dye degradation which are difficult to dispose of further. Advanced oxidation processes (AOPs) are one of the chemical processes that are performed to treat dye-contaminated water by utilizing in situ generated oxidizing species [35,36]. These methods include ozonation [37], Fenton, photo-Fenton [38], photocatalysis [39], electrochemical oxidation [40], ultrasound [41], plasma [42], and coagulation–flocculation methods [43]. Moreover, coagulation–flocculation methods require coagulants to reduce or neutralize the charge of dispersed particles and flocculants to aggregate the particles to form larger particles which are easy to remove by sedimentation. Although some natural materials such as *Moringa oleifera*, *Tamarindus indica,* and *Musa* genus have also shown coagulation properties, flocculants are generally polymers. Electrochemical treatment involves two metal electrodes and a current source. Oxidation and reduction reactions occur at the surface of electrodes while in situ generation of coagulants. This process can be divided into electro-Fenton and anodic oxidation methods. The electro-Fenton method is the fusion of two processes (oxidation and coagulation) with the added advantages of fewer by-products, chemical requirements, and better process control. Alternatively, the anodic oxidation process either involves the dye's adsorption at the anode surface, which is then degraded through electron transfer reactions, or strong oxidizing species are generated electrochemically and used further for the oxidation reaction. This process is efficient but not economically viable because of high cost and less stability.

2.2.3 Physical Treatment Process

Physical methods rely on the mass transfer mechanism and offer some advantages such as basic design and better efficiency (85–99%). In the adsorption techniques, physisorption and chemisorption of adsorbate occur at the surface of the adsorbent, involving different types of interactions, such as H-bonding, electrostatic attraction, van der Waals forces, and hydrophobic interactions [44–47]. Although the materials with high surface area and suitable pore size distribution are a better choice due to the facile mass transfer, high efficiency, and reusability are also important for an adsorbent to remove the dye from the water efficiently [48, 49]. Importantly, the adsorption efficiency of materials can be tuned by modulating their chemical and physical nature. Activated carbon [50], alumina [51], and silica gel [52] have been applied to treat the wastewater due to their abundance and comparatively low cost. However, the complete regeneration of these materials is difficult. Therefore, the development of sorbents is the area of interest providing effective sorbents that may serve the purpose of industries. Apart from synthetic materials, natural materials (clays, biopolymers, and food waste), along with hybrid magnetic materials, have been excellent choices because of their biodegradable nature and ease of recovery from the effluent after the treatment [53,54]. Moreover, their surface functionalities or chemical nature can be modified accordingly with the aim of enhancing the total adsorption capacity. Membrane filtration technology is also a physical method to remove the dyes by passing the contaminated water through the membrane [55,56]. The working principle of a membrane is simple and based on the size of its pores. Only smaller molecules with a lower size than the pores are allowed to pass through the membrane, thus giving an exempted solution. However, the bigger solutes deposited on the surface of the membrane create a layer of filter cake that can restrict the facile filtration process. Therefore, periodic removal of this unwanted layer from the membrane surface is necessary. This technique is further categorized as a micro-filtration membrane technique based on the size of the pores (micrometer, ultrafiltration, and nanometer) of the membrane. However, as the size of the pores decreases, the working pressure increases. Moreover, one of the most important membrane-based technologies used in industries to treat wastewater is reverse osmosis which requires a semi-permeable membrane. Importantly these techniques require no thermal energy or chemicals to treat the wastewater and are thus considered to be comparatively safe and cost-effective. The important aspect of membrane technology is the modification of membranes using various materials (activated carbons, silica, based materials, natural polymeric materials, etc.) to develop a hybrid system. Another physical treatment process is the ion exchange which works on the principle of interaction of the dye molecules owing various functional groups with the ion exchange resin [57]. This method is comparatively efficient and cheap.

2.2.4 Hybrid Treatment Process

To develop an efficient dye treatment process, researchers may require the help of more than one technique due to the complexity of industrial effluents. In fact, researchers have combined more than one technique to develop a more efficient hybrid treatment process. Hybrid treatment processes are designed to get the most from the combination of different treatment techniques, thus avoiding the drawbacks of individual treatment processes. In these processes, effluent is processed sequentially to achieve higher efficiency while modulating the individual treatment process within one reactor. This feature makes this technique cost and time effective requiring comparatively less space and energy. Hybrid technologies mainly include chemical–chemical, chemical–physical, and chemical–biological processes [10,11].

2.2.5 Photocatalytic Process

The treatment of dye-contaminated water is a major challenge for the scientific community around the globe as dyes are continuously participating in a huge amount of polluted freshwater during various industry processes. Therefore, several methods have been developed and implemented including photocatalytic degradation methods. Photocatalysts are semiconductor materials that use only light

(UV or visible) to degrade the dyes and thus have the potential to be implemented at the industrial level. Theoretically, photocatalytic dye degradation may occur via three pathways: (1) dye sensitization via charge transfer reactions, (2) dye degradation via oxidation/reduction, and (3) photolysis of dye. The type of dye degradation mechanism depends on the features of catalysts and reaction parameters. Moreover, the efficiency of photocatalyst for the dye degradation is determined by numerous factors including catalyst amount, concertation of dyes, pH, and light source. The dye sensitization mechanism involves the absorption of light in the form of photons with threshold energy and generates charge carriers (electrons and holes) at valence (VB) and conduction (CB) bands. The respective holes and electrons convert the dye molecules to anionic and cationic radicals which get decomposed spontaneously to harmless products. The indirect mechanism also involves the formation of electrons and holes on exposing photocatalysts to light. However, in this case, these charge carriers generate oxygenated radicals via a series of reactions. These radicals function as potential nonselective oxidizing agents and thus contribute to the degradation of dye molecules. On the other hand, the direct photolysis mechanism has comparatively slow kinetics and does not depend on the type of catalyst.

2.3 PHOTOCATALYSTS FOR DYE DEGRADATION

It is evident that the role of catalysts is paramount in the efficient photolysis of dyes. Therefore, several methods have been developed to produce diverse photocatalysts involving metal oxides, organic polymers, functionalized carbon-based nanostructures, and other nanomaterials. Moreover, the integration of two or more materials to construct photoactive hetero-structures is one of the effective strategies to improve the electronic properties for obtaining optimum dye degradation ability. In this part, we will discuss the advancement in the synthesis of several types of photocatalysts and their application for light-driven dye degradation. Decolorization of benzidine-based azo dyes has been studied using a solar-driven photo-Fenton process for real textile wastewater showing 56% and 63% of color and chemical oxygen demand (COD) removal, respectively [58]. For scaling up the wastewater treatment, 100 L of real wastewater was completely decolored in 1 hour using 7 m^2 of solar irradiation.

2.3.1 Coupled Photocatalysts

Coupled photocatalysts are the combination of two or more individual materials with diverse electronic, chemical, and physical properties. Therefore, coupled photocatalysts are believed to have collaborative properties, which certainly assist in enhancing the photocatalytic activity. Different approaches have been implemented to construct such efficient coupled photocatalysts by using various nanomaterials. Caixia et al. have integrated the metal-organic framework (MOF) (NH_2-UiO-66) into $ZnIn_2S_4$ to fabricate a high surface area bi-functional photocatalysts (NU66/ZIS) for the dye (malachite green (MG)) degradation and hydrogen evolution reaction [59]. In this process, the mixing of NH_2-UiO-66 and $ZnIn_2S_4$ under ultra-sonication energy followed by solvent thermal treatment resulted in the formation of coupled photocatalysts, NU66/ZIS. Based on characterization results, heterostructure NU66/ZIS demonstrated a high surface area with exposed activity sites for the redox reactions. Moreover, heterojunction formation facilitated the charge separation and their transfer and broadened the light absorption range. The synthesized photocatalyst demonstrated 98% degradation efficiency of MG dye and improved hydrogen evolution rate up to 2199 μmol/h g. The vitro cytotoxicity assay results revealed that the synthesized catalyst is safe for the environment and humans. Moreover, theoretical calculation finds out that Zr and In sites at NU66 and $ZnIn_2S_4$ interface respectively, were the main active sites. Further, Ding et al. [60] have coupled UiO-66(Zr) and Bi_2MoO_6 in different molar ratios via electrostatic interaction to obtain Bi_2MoO_6/UiO-66(Zr) composites for RhB degradation under the visible-light irradiation. Bi_2MoO_6/UiO-66(Zr) composite with 2:1 molar ratio of Bi:Zr (BMUO-2) demonstrated excellent photocatalytic activity, stability and recyclability. The enhanced photoactivity could be attributed to the enhanced solar response and diminished recombination rate of charge carriers due to the constructive collaboration between individual materials: UiO-66(Zr) and Bi_2MoO_6. The high electrical conductivity of UiO-66(Zr) might also be contributing to suppressing the recombination rate. These reports are a clear example of the importance of the integration of two materials to construct photocatalysts with higher activity and chemical stability for water treatment processes. Fundamentally, photocatalytic degradation of dye requires either visible or UV light to produce the reactive oxygen species (ROS) (superoxide or hydroxyl radical). Lakshmi Prasanna and Rajagopalan [61] have developed an interesting nanocomposite utilizing ZnO_2 and polypyrrole that can produce ROS even in the dark. Therefore, the synthesized material (ZnO_2/ppy) was able to degrade the dyes (Rhodamine B (RhB) and methylene blue (MB)) in the presence of light as well as in dark via an advanced oxidation process excluding the requirement of any external reagents. It was found that the coupling of polypyrrole with ZnO_2 resulted in tuned physio-chemical constructive collaboration which enhanced the efficiency of dye removal. The availability of free electrons on polypyrrole and specific features of ZnO_2 participated together in the generation of ROS. Notably, ZnO_2 and polypyrrole itself failed to degrade the mentioned dye molecules even in the presence of visible light. In another report, three photoactive nanocomposites, TiO_2-Pt, TiO_2-Pt/GO, and TiO_2-Pt/reduced GO, were synthesized by a combined chemical-thermal method [62]. Their photo-activity was tested for the degradation of azo dyes in UV as well as natural sunlight. The integration of GO with TiO_2-Pt resulted in a shifting of absorption range towards the visible region which in turn enhanced photocatalytic activity following a pseudo-first-order kinetic. Metal oxide and its heterostructure are well-known photoactive materials. Lan et al. [63] have prepared a hybrid composite via thermal decomposition of Zn–In layered double hydroxide (ZnIn-LDH) in the presence of melamine. Morphological and optical results of the synthesized composites indicated that the in situ formation of g-C_3N_4 sheets was uniformly decorated with ZnIn-MMO nanoparticles and showed better visible light absorption. It was found that unique ternary semiconductor coupling facilitated charge transportation and their separation thus resulting in constant production of ROS to degrade the RhB under visible light irradiation. For the synthesis of composites, ZnIn-LDH was ground with melamine with different mass ratios. Next, the resulting powder material was calcined at 550°C for 4 h under N_2 gas environment. The current study presents a straightforward way to construct a g-C_3N_4-based visible-light-active semiconductor composite for the degradation of pollutants via advanced oxidation processes. TiO_2 is one of the most explored metal oxides in the photocatalysts. A lot of research has been conducted to modify its structure and chemical nature to tune its electronic properties. Moreover, their integration with other materials to prepare the heterostructures with enhanced photocatalytic activity is an area of interest. In this regard, Zalfani et al. [64] have synthesized the composites involving $BiVO_4$/3DOM and TiO_2 to degrade the RhB dye in an aqueous solution under visible light irradiation. A hydrothermal strategy was applied to the construction of $BiVO_4$/3DOM TiO_2 nanocomposites by dissolving stoichiometric amounts of $Bi(NO_3)_3{\cdot}5H_2O$ and NH_4VO_3 in a stoichiometric volume of ethylene glycol and water mixture. The resulting solution was stirred until a clear solution was obtained. Next, the required amount of 3DOM TiO_2 was added, sonicated, and stirred to obtain a yellow-colored mixture, which was transferred into a Teflon-sealed autoclave and heated at 160°C for 24 hours. The solid was separated, washed, and vacuum-dried, and finally calcined at 300°C for 1 hour. $BiVO_4$ was used as a visible light sensitizer and its amount in $BiVO_4$/3DOM TiO_2 nanocomposites was found to affect the photoactivity and reach a maximum of 0.2. Moreover, improvement in photocatalytic activity was also due to the facile electron transfer at the interface of the coupled materials, the presence of channels, and the high surface area to allow easy mass transfer resulting in high accessibility to the active sites. Chemical composition, morphological, textural, and optical properties revealed that $BiVO_4$ content can control the densities of charge carriers and thus the rate of photocatalytic degradation. Second, the proportion of 3DOM TiO_2 in the nanocomposite is responsible for the high surface area.

Moreover, $BiVO_4$-based heterostructures have also displayed excellent photoactivity towards dye degradation. Based on the literature, the probable reason for the enhanced photocatalytic activity is the formation of a high-efficiency heterojunction that improves the charge transfer and their separation (Figure 2.1). This strategy might help to design a more efficient heterostructure-based photocatalyst to degrade the dyes and organic pollutants. Ming et al. have construed a novel $BiVO_4/Ag_3VO_4$ heterojunction via hydrothermal and precipitation processes to degrade the RhB under visible light [65]. Heterostructure with a molar ratio of 10:1 of $BiVO_4{:}Ag_3VO_4$ showed higher activity indicating that the composition of individual materials plays a significant role in photocatalytic performance. For the synthesis, $AgNO_3$ was mixed into the water dispersion of $BiVO_4$ and stirred for 0.5 hours. Next, an aqueous solution of Na_3VO_4 was added dropwise into the above solution under continuous stirring in the dark for 7 hours. Finally, the solid material was separated by centrifuging, washing, and drying at 60°C for 12 hours. The higher activity might be due to the effective separation of charge carriers at the heterojunction. The authors also proposed the photocatalytic mechanism by trapping the active species (h^+ and •OH) through ESR, as shown in Figure 2.2.

It is evident the photocatalytic activity of the semiconductor material can be improved by the integration of another semiconductor. Mohini et al. [66] have grown

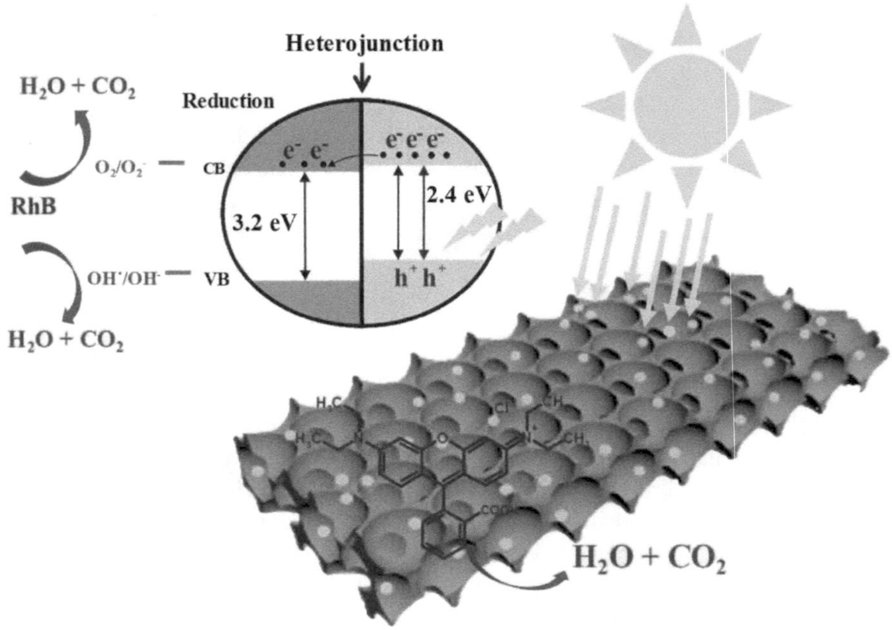

FIGURE 2.1 Band diagram and charge transfer process for $BiVO_4$@3DOM TiO_2 nanocomposite.

mesoporous TiO_2 nanoparticles on the surface of carbon nitride to obtain coupled semiconductor-based photocatalysts. The synthesized composite (g-C_3N_4/TiO_2) was investigated for methyl orange dye degradation. An improvement in the photocatalytic activity of the composite is observed due to the large surface area and efficient charge separation, which was evident by the photoluminescence (PL) results.

The binary photocatalyst of MoS_2/WO_3 was synthesized for degradation of RhB and thiamethoxam (TM) yielding an efficiency of 90.2% and 92.6% after 120 minutes, respectively, under real solar light. Moreover, the percent chemical oxygen demand (% COD) and the percent total organic carbon (% TOC) removal of the real industrial wastewater were to be 80% and 78.9%, respectively [67]. The bismuth ferrite-coated nickel/nickel oxide foam (BFCNF) was also prepared for photocatalytic degradation of MG and MB in a real industrial wastewater treatment study. The catalyst showed a degradation efficiency of 99% for both MG and MB [68].

2.3.2 Metal-Organic Frameworks

Porosity is the required feature for the photocatalysts to allow the facile movement of substrates and their adsorption at the active centers. MOFs are one of the few fascinating materials that have high surfaces with the possibility of pore designing. Therefore, the application of MOFs as photocatalysts for dye degradation is significantly being researched. In this section, we will discuss the synthesis methods of

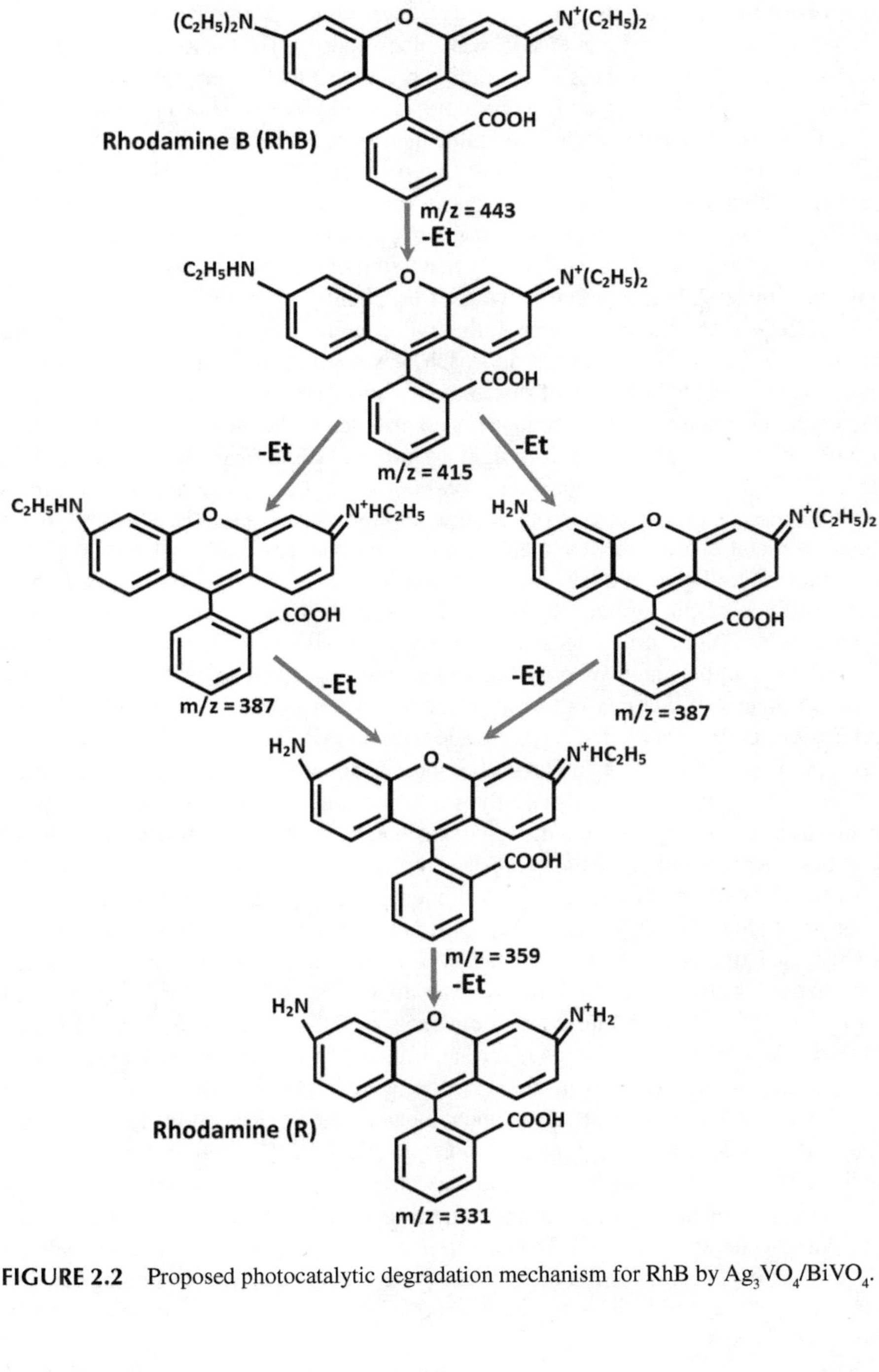

FIGURE 2.2 Proposed photocatalytic degradation mechanism for RhB by $Ag_3VO_4/BiVO_4$.

MOFs-based photocatalysts aiming for dye degradation. Alamgir et al. synthesized a new functional mixed ligand MOF with block shaped, BUT-206, via on pot controllable solvothermal process to degrade the CV and RhB dyes [69]. Zinc nitrate, 2,5-furan dicarboxylic acid, and 1,2-bis(4-pyridyl) ethylene were taken and dissolved using DMF solvent with the help of ultrasonic energy. The resulting solution was sealed in a Pyrex vial and then put into the oven at 100°C for 48 hours. The final material is obtained as solid crystals which were separated by filtration and washed with organic solvents (DMF and acetone). Prepared BUT-206 were evaluated under different reaction conditions (pH, catalyst amount, concentration) for degrading dye molecules under UV irradiation. It worked excellently with good recyclability and without involving photosensitizer following pseudo-first-order kinetic equation. In another report, a hydrothermal approach was applied to synthesize two visible-light responsive 3D Cu-MOFs of different structures procuring 4,4′-bipyridine [70]. Cage-type morphology of the frameworks contributed to the photocatalytic reduction of MB dye molecule using visible light by providing the channels to the reaction substrates. Moreover, it is found that the photocatalytic degradation follows first-order kinetics and rate enhanced by adding an electron acceptor (H_2O_2) through the ligand-to-metal charge transfer mechanism. Functionality plays a vital role in efficient photodegradation of dyes. Therefore, the designing of novel MOFs with diverse functionalities is gaining interest. Porphyrin-based MOFs could be a suitable choice as they have a high surface area as well as the possibility of tuning the functionality. Chen et al. [71] have reported a novel porous porphyrin-based MOF consisting anionic framework that can not only selectively adsorb cationic dyes (MB^+, RhB^+, and astrazone pink (FG^+)) but also degrade them by generating singlet oxygen ($^1O_2$) and superoxide radicals ($^{\cdot}O_2^-$). The porous nature and high surface area of MOF allow the selective adsorption of cationic dyes. On the other hand, functional porphyrin groups participate in generating the oxygenated active species under light irradiation. A stable (thermal and chemical) copper (I)-based MOF (CuTz-1) was successfully constructed by using $Cu(NO_3)_2$ and 3,5-diphenyltriazolate via hydrothermal reaction in the presence of H_2SO_4 solution [72]. During the process, Cu(II) ions were reduced to Cu(I) and triazole was deprotonated even under the acidic medium. The extensive characterization of CuTz-1 featured an unprecedented secondary building unit in the form of a Cu5Tz6 cluster, with channels of 8.3 Å in diameter. The prepared MOF displayed a semiconductor nature and thus excellently worked for the photocatalytic degradation of dyes in the presence of hydrogen peroxide generating supplementary OH active species. This phenomenon was explained by suggesting that Cu(I) interacted with photo-generated holes to yield Cu (II), which functions as a catalytic site to generate extra $^{\cdot}OH$ radicals via a Fenton-like reaction (Figure 2.3). Moreover, hydrogen peroxide also participates in producing $^{\cdot}OH$ radicals by scavenging photo-generated electrons. Hence, this excess amount of $^{\cdot}OH$ radicals which are the most active species for the degradation of dye molecules (methyl orange (MO), MB, methyl blue, and RhB) was found responsible for enhancing photolytic activity under natural light and Xe lamp.

Sarkar et al. [73] have replicated the first single-crystal zinc version of $[M_3(BTC)_2(H_2O)_3]{\cdot}xH_2O$ (HKUST-1) MOF. The synthesized MOF was grown by

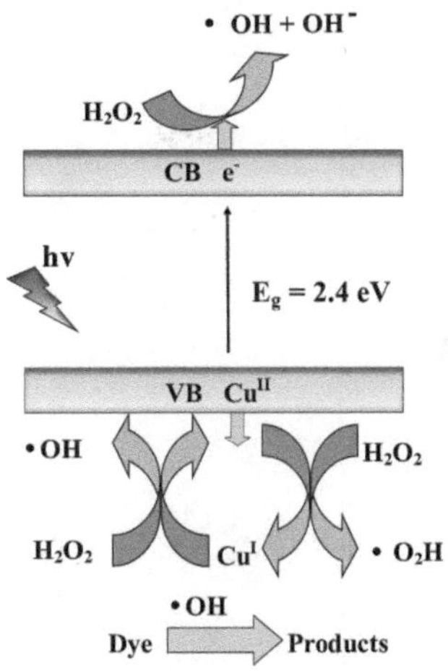

FIGURE 2.3 Suggested mechanism for the photocatalytic degradation of dyes over CuTz-1.

heating $ZnCl_2$ and 1,3,5-benzenetricarboxylic acid in DMF maintaining pH 8.2 using triethylamine. Single-crystal XRD data disclosed that a 3D polymeric unit is constructed by paddlewheel secondary building units (SBUs) consisting of large pores (~8.35 × 8.35 Å^2). The synthesized single-crystal MOF exhibited not only excellent iodine uptake but also photocatalytic degradation of dyes (RhB, MB) in aqueous solution under the irradiation of visible light in the presence of hydrogen peroxide. Utilization of hydrogen peroxide as an electron scavenger in photocatalytic degradation of dyes is required to facilitate the degradation process by generation of oxygenated active species. However, its use is not sustainable in terms of economic and environmental concerns. Therefore, new catalysts and methods are being developed to exclude the H_2O_2 requirement during the photocatalytic degradation processes to achieve high photocatalytic efficiency. In this journey, a novel 2D zinc (II) MOF was obtained via a solvothermal process by dissolving $N(NO_3)_2{\cdot}6H_2O$ and 4-(pyridine-4-yl) phthalic acid in DMA/H_2O (3/2, v/v) [74]. The constructed MOF displayed a 3D supramolecular framework connected via H-bonding and worked as a stable and reusable photocatalyst for the degradation of organic dyes (RhB and MO) in aqueous solution. MOF characterization data revealed its semiconductor nature having a band gap of 3.282 eV (Figure 2.4). The photocatalytic degradation of dyes was accomplished under the light of a 300 W Xe lamp at a fixed temperature (25°C) using a cryogenic thermostatic tank without adjusting the pH value. Notably, neither any photosensitizer and co-catalyst nor electron acceptor H_2O_2 was used during the process. The higher activity could be due to the generation of a higher number of $\cdot O_2^-$ species which are the effective oxidant for the dye degradation. Mechanistically, photo-generated electrons and holes interacted with O_2 and H_2O molecules to give $\cdot O_2^-$ and $\cdot OH$, H^+ species, respectively. The $\cdot O_2^-$ and $\cdot OH$ species react with dye molecules to give CO_2, water, and other products as a result of degradation (Equations 2.1–2.4).

$$MOF + hv \rightarrow h^+ + e^- \quad (2.1)$$

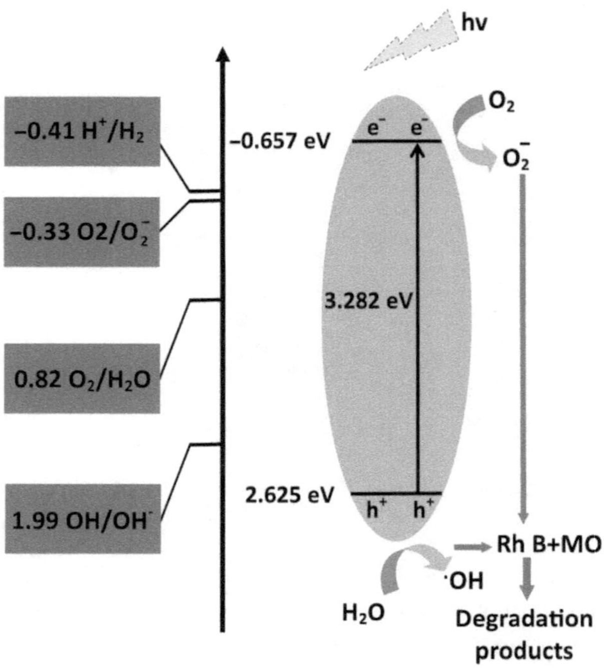

FIGURE 2.4 Schematic representation of the energy position and dye degradation over MOF.

$$h^{+} + H_2O \rightarrow HO\cdot + H^{+} \tag{2.2}$$

$$O_2 + e^{-} \rightarrow O_2^{\cdot-} \tag{2.3}$$

$$RhB / MO + O_2^{\cdot-} + HO\cdot \rightarrow CO_2 + H_2O + Others \tag{2.4}$$

The integration of third material with the MOF has gotten lots of attention in a short time to alter their chemical and electronic nature. Yu et al. have constructed a core–shell type hybrid, via grinding which efficiently degraded the organic dyes (MB, MO, and RhB) photocatalytically [75]. Its photocatalytic performance in terms of degradation efficiency exceeded 90% in 140 minutes was attributed to the high number of active species, hydroxyl radicals, which were responsible for the dye degradation under UV light irradiation (mercury lamp).

2.3.3 Doped Metal Oxide-Based Photocatalysts

Doping is an important approach to tailor the electronic as well as chemical properties of any material including semiconductors. Various metal oxide semiconductor materials used as photocatalysts have been doped to improve their photocatalytic activity by boosting charge carrier separation and light absorption capacity and range of the solar spectrum. Doping can be done by using a nonmetal or metal species. In this section, we will discuss the doped photocatalysts focusing on the role of dopants on their photocatalytic activity towards dye degradation. Among the various semiconductor materials, ZnO has been reported as a photocatalyst for dye degradation. However, the modification of ZnO in terms of morphology, chemical properties, and electronic properties has been well-reported to enhance photocatalytic efficiency. Priyanka and Srivastava [76] have doped the zinc oxide with iron via the solution combustion method for the photocatalytic treatment of acid red 1 dye-bearing wastewater. $Zn(NO_3)_2{\cdot}6H_2O$, $Fe(NO_3)_3$, and dextrose were dissolved (stoichiometric amount) in water and stirred to get a homogeneous mixture. The resulting solution was heated at 400°C for a brief time to achieve a solid product after cooling in a desiccator. Structural, morphological, and optical characterization were performed to investigate the changes in properties (chemical, physical, and electronic) of zinc oxide after iron doping. The photocatalytic activity of iron-doped ZnO was then evaluated under the 125 W UV bulb (365 nm) irradiation for the degradation of the dye solution. For this, the catalyst is first dispersed in the dye solution and placed on the hot plate to provide a constant temperature during the experiment. Hydrogen peroxide was added after 30 minutes, the experiment was stopped, and the concentration of dye solution was measured. The whole assembly was guarded by a wooden box and aluminum foil. Moreover, the effect of various parameters including the doping amount pH of the dye solution was evaluated to get the optimum dye removal (71%), degradation (94%), and total organic carbon removal (41%). It was found that the different amounts of iron doping alter the band gap energy (E_g) in the range of 3.14–3.24 eV. It is well known that the doping of every metal induces some characteristic properties in the resulting materials in terms of electronic and chemical nature. Subsequently, the concept of co-doping is being applied to tune the catalytic activity of the catalyst not only in photocatalysis but also in the other fields of catalysis. In this regard, several studies have been reported with the aim of finding an effective combination of co-dopants to enhance photocatalytic activity. Alam et al. co-doped ZnO nanoparticles with yttrium (Y) and vanadium (V) by applying a sol–gel strategy and used as photocatalysts to degrade dyes (RhB and MB) under the irradiation of visible light [77]. The characterization of synthesized material clarified the co-doping of Y and V. The maximum photocatalytic performance was witnessed in the case of 3%Y/1%V-ZnO and attributed to the effective light absorption and separation of charge carriers. The enhanced activity was explained by the fact that vanadium doping creates a mid-energy level and thus facilitates visible light harvesting capacity and diminishes the recombination of holes and electrons. In addition, yttrium can control nanoparticle growth by the surface enrichment property. A. T. Kuvarega et al. have performed the metal (Pd) and nonmetal (N) co-doping of TiO_2 by the calcination of a hydrolyzed mixture of titanium *iso*-propoxide with $NH_3{\cdot}H_2O$ for the enhanced dye degradation from contaminated water under visible light [78]. Crystalline doped TiO_2 particles (10–20 nm) with mainly anatase phase were formed exhibiting a redshift absorption and thus lowering the band gap. Consequently, the co-doped material displayed better photocatalytic degradation efficiency for the Eosin Yellow dye than only N- or Pd-doped TiO_2 material and commercial TiO_2 (Degussa P25). It was observed that the dopant amount is crucial and needs to be optimized for higher efficiency. The higher concentration of dopants may follow the charge recombination centers. The high activity was attributed to the cooperative effects of N- and Pd- co-doping to enhance the visible light energy and promote the separation of photo-generated charge carriers while Pd sites functioned as electron traps. Moreover, nonmetal co-doping has also been found effective. Han et al. [79] reported the S-doped WO_3 nanowires (S-WO_3) as an effective photocatalyst for dye degradation under visible light irradiation. Hydrothermal method and low-temperature solid-state annealing treatment approach were used to synthesize S-WO_3 with different loading, uniform size, and high purity. The photocatalytic activity was investigated under visible light using a 420 nm cut-off filter for MO degradation in an aqueous solution, and the concentration of the reaction solution was monitored at different time intervals by measuring UV–Vis spectra at 464 nm. S doping was found to enhance the light-harvesting capacity which in turn enhances the photodegradation efficiency of the doped WO_3 nanowires for the methyl orange dye. In another report by Sudrajat et al. [80], N-doping (interstitial and substitutional) was performed in ZrO_2 via the thermal decomposition method which significantly altered the optical nature of the materials. In this process, the thermal decomposition of the zirconium hydroxide-urea complex resulted in N-doped ZrO_2 material with a high crystalline monoclinic structure and optically responsive for the broader light spectrum. N-ZrO_2 performed better than the bare ZrO_2 in terms of photocatalytic activity for the degradation of two dyes (MB and amaranth) in UV as well as visible light irradiation. The author concluded that a narrow band gap, smaller crystalline size, high specific area, and higher availability of surface hydroxyl groups could be the possible reasons for this enhanced activity. The co-doping approach is also applied to tailor the electronic nature of the semiconductor materials. J. H. Shah et al. [81] have doped tungsten oxide (WO_3) and manganese oxide (Mn_2O_3) nanoparticles with N and N-B through precipitation and hydrothermal process. Co-doping of WO_3 and Mn_2O_3 resulted in 3.5 and 3.0 times higher photocatalytic activity against the photodegradation of MB dyes respectively, than their bare counterparts. The incorporation of N and B atoms into the monoclinic crystal lattice of WO_3 and the cubic lattice of Mn_2O_3 decreased the crystallite size. N-doping created the levels near the VB and N-B doping narrowed the band gap by hybridizing with the orbital of O_2p thus resulting in better light absorption and photocatalytic degradation of MB under visible light. Moreover, the developed material showed excellent reusability without showing any significant decrease in efficiency. Scavenger molecules were found to inhibit MB degradation, indicating photo-generated charge carriers were necessary to degrade the dye molecules. Besides the general dopants, carbon-based materials are also used to dope the metal oxide. GO is a graphitic material with high conductivity. It has been used to tailor the band gap of the MgO for photocatalytic degradation of dyes [82]. MgO was doped with GO via the chemical precipitation method to yield a cubic structure with enhanced light absorption. Band gap was calculated to be 4.8 eV which was lower than the undoped MgO (5.0 eV). Based on the HRTEM results, doping induced two types of morphology (cubic and hexagon) showing rode-like growth with a decrease in diameter. Moreover, PL intensity was diminished accompanied by a blue shift indicating a hampered recombination rate of excitons. The photocatalytic activity was assessed towards dye degradation in acidic conditions and achieved 45% degradation.

2.3.4 Plasmonic Photocatalysts

Plasmonic metal nanoparticles-based photocatalysts are significantly investigated for the development of solar–fuel technologies due to the surface plasmon resonance (SPR) effect. SPR facilitates absorption of radiation from visible to infrared region, effective charge separation, solar energy storage, and transfer of plasmonic energy, thus making an efficient system in terms of high conversion efficiency. In fact, a plasmonic-based photocatalyst has been found to be effective for various photo-induced reactions including dye degradation due to the cascade charge transfer effect. There are many ways to synthesize plasmonic nanoparticles. Biosynthesized plasmonic nanoparticles are synthesized using bio extract and utilized as a constructive photocatalyst for the effective degradation of industrial dye in the aqueous media. Singh et al. [83] have synthesized spherical plasmonic silver nanoparticles with size between 15 and 25 nm and SPR band at 430 nm by employing extracts (stem) of *Nepeta leucophylla*. Moreover, a face-centered cubic structure with a crystal size of 10 nm was obtained. The natural presence of phenol in the extracts reduced the silver ions to nanoparticles while protein helped as an overlaying agent in preventing their agglomeration. The photocatalytic degradation of dyes results proved that biosynthesized silver nanoparticles exhibited good photocatalytic activity in visible light and liquid phase. In another report by Mehata [84], various bio extracts such as *Zingiber officinale*, *Ocimum sanctum*, plant nectar fructose *Azadirachta indica*, pomegranate peel extracts and were used to synthesize the plasmonic silver nanoparticles with enhanced SPR. Ag NPs synthesized with *Zingiber officinale* extract found to be efficient in terms of higher formation rate of Ag nanoparticles, strong SPR and well controlled by physicochemical properties. Subsequently, they exhibited excellent dye (MB) degradation activity in the presence of $NaBH_4$. In another report, *Sargassum ilicifolium* is used to synthesize silver and gold plasmonic nanoparticles in sunlight. The synthesized nanoparticles were used to degrade the cationic dyes (MB and MG) [85]. Other methods such as precipitation followed by reduction are also frequently used with the aim to develop plasmonic catalysts with diverse electronic and chemical properties. Xu et al. [86] synthesized a novel silver-based plasmonic photocatalysts through precipitation and in situ photoreduction process. The deposition of AgCl NPs on the $NaTaO_3$ was performed by the mixing of $NaTaO_3$ nanocubes and $AgNO_3$ in distilled water followed by adding an excess amount of HCl solution. The resulting material was then subjected to light irradiation (300 W xenon lamp) to reduce the Ag^+ ions into Ag(0). The synthesized photocatalyst was visible light active and showed better activity towards dye degradation (MB and RhB) than their counterparts ($NaTaO_3$ nanocubes and Ag/AgCl NPs). Electronic and electrochemical characterization suggested that charge separation ability and enhanced light absorption were the reasons behind the higher activity of the photocatalysts. Various composites have been investigated for dye degradation and their efficiency depends on the plasmonic effect and charge separation efficiency. In fact, better interfacial interaction among the individual substrates of composites can facilitate electron transfer and thus enhance the lifetime of the charge carriers. Pattappan et al. [87] have reported the preparation of Au-based ternary composites (Au/$ZnFe_2O_4$@rGO) to degrade bromophenol blue and RhB dyes under sunlight. The author concluded that the interfacial contact between Au, $ZnFe_2SO_4$, and rGO, diminished the recombination process by speeding up the electron transfer process from the CB of $ZnFe_2O_4$ to rGO which in turn enhances the quantum efficiency. Moreover, ROS experimental data showed that $O_2^{\cdot-}$ species were mainly responsible for the effective degradation of dye. In another report, a core–shell nanostructure was constructed via a two-step process involving hydrothermal and seed-mediated growth of Ag nanoclusters with [111] facets onto the surface of ZnO nanorods with [001] facets [88]. The morphology and structure of the synthesized hybrids were investigated through state-of-the-art characterization techniques (XPS, TEM, and SEM) to ensure the formation of the core–shell model. Moreover, the electronic properties were also evaluated by measuring the UV-Vis and PL spectra. The appearance of the SPR band with characteristic excitonic peaks of ZnO in the UV–Vis spectrum and quenching of UV emission in the PL spectrum not only signify the successful construction of hybrid nanostructure but also verify their role in the suppression of charge recombination. Accordingly, Congo red, R6G, and amino black 10B dyes as well as real-time samples from industrial textile effluent were photo catalytically reduced using the ZnO@Ag core–shell nanorods as photocatalyst in presence of solar and UV light.

Evidently, ZnO@Ag core–shell nanorods exhibited better photocatalytic activity than the bare ZnO nanorods due to an increase in oxygen-related defects and interfacial charge transfer. Moreover, plasmonic Ag nanoclusters helped in inducing the formation of holes and electrons in VB and CB respectively, by acting as sinks for charge carriers (Figure 2.5). The integration of plasmonic nanomaterial with other materials of different properties (electronic, physical, and chemical) is desirable to reduce the cost and enhance the efficiency of the photodegradation process. Xu et al. [89] have introduced the piezotronic effect to develop a more efficient plasmonic photocatalysis and synthesized Aux/$BaTiO_3$ plasmonic photocatalysts by precipitating Au nanoparticles (<8 nm) on the surface of piezoelectric $BaTiO_3$ nanocubes. This approach significantly broadens the visible light absorption range (300–600 nm) of the resulting heterostructure and thus its photocatalytic activity was investigated to degrade the methyl orange dye. Based on the experimental data, Au content, SPR, and piezoelectric potential of the $BaTiO_3$ were the main factors for the enhanced photocatalytic activity. The piezoelectric field significantly contributed to separating photon-generated charge carriers and facilitated the formation of $^{\cdot}OH$ radicals, thus exhibiting better oxidizing ability of organic dyes. Furthermore, the content of plasmonic metal significantly affects the photocatalytic activity of the resulting materials. D'Amato et al. [90] have investigated the role of Au content on the band gap of the polypropylene-coated plasmonic Au/TiO_2 materials. In this study, Au nanoparticles were formed by taking advantage of the reducing power of the dispersing agent, acetylacetonate present in the TiO_2 paste thus excluding the involvement of any further reducing agents. Based on the characterization, 0.006 wt.% of Au content provided a smaller band gap of 2.97 eV than the band gap of 3.1 eV of the parent material. Accordingly, photodegradation efficiency was found to be enhanced 2.45 times higher than unmodified material. Importantly, each Au concentration was specific for the types of Au nanoparticles and, therefore, exhibited photocatalytic activity

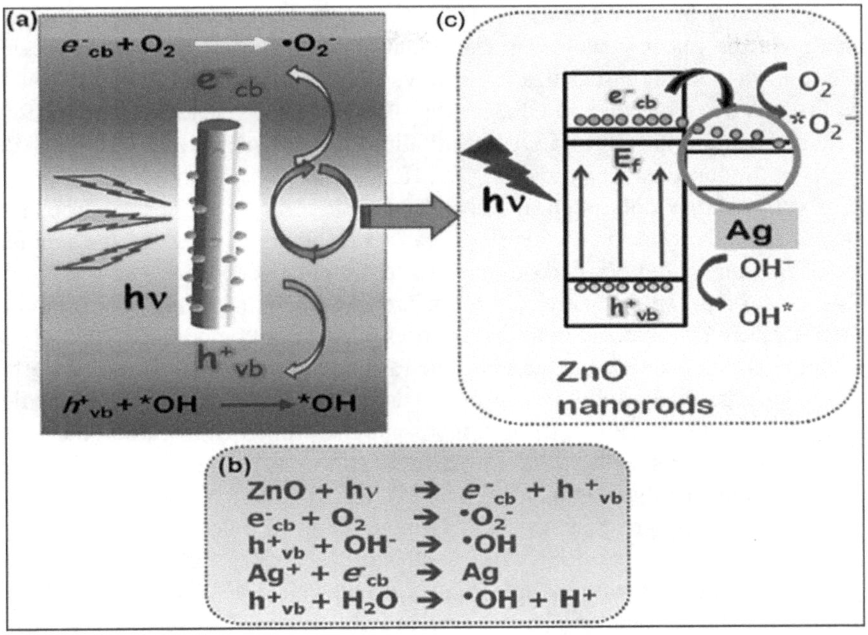

FIGURE 2.5 Schematic representation of photocatalysis mechanism for hybrid ZnO@Ag core–shell nanorods: (a) pictorial representation of silver nanoparticles deposited on the ZnO nanorods; (b) Band diagram of ZnO@Ag core-shell nanorods showing the transfer of electrons between energy levels of ZnO and Ag; (c) Equations showing the stepwise photo reaction mechanism.

accordingly. The Ag^+ doped TiO_2 was used to degrade the dyes from fabric dyeing [91]. The results indicated that Ag^+ doped TiO_2 could degrade 98% of dye in five times diluted real textile wastewater after UV irradiation for 420 minutes.

2.3.5 Quantum Dots

Generally, quantum dots (QDs) are the size of a few nanometers and have distinct semiconductor properties than their bulk materials due to the quantum confinement effect. Moreover, QDs can acquire unique optical and electronic properties and, therefore, are utilized in the field of photovoltaic, medicine, catalyst, biosensors, and bioimaging due to their small size, chemical stability, high surface area, and low toxicity. The applications of several types of QDs (graphene quantum dots (GQDs), TiO_2 QDs, perovskite QDs, carbon QDs, etc.) in the photocatalytic degradation of dyes have been studied owing to efficient visible light absorption and suitable band gap. Roushani et al. [92] have prepared GQDs via pyrolyzing of citric acid and applied to degrade a cationic dye (New Fuchsin) under visible light irradiation. There were two pathways demonstrated: photocatalytic and photosensitization. Mechanistically, GQD absorbed visible light, and consequently, electrons excited to the CB from the VB, generating electron–hole pairs. The electrons quickly reduce the O_2 molecule at the interface into the $O_2^{\cdot-}$ and HOO. species. While holes at the VB can directly oxidize the New Fuchsin dye molecules adsorbed on GQDs and generate the HO$^{\cdot}$ radicals via the reaction with water which in turn mineralize the dye molecules. Moreover, the self-photosensitization pathway involves the adsorption of light by New Fuchsin dye molecules and the transfer of a few photo-generated electrons from the excited state to the CB of GQDs facilitating oxidizing/degrading dye molecules using photo-induced oxygen radicals ($O_2^{-\cdot}$, HOO$^{\cdot}$, and $^{\cdot}$OH) (Figure 2.6).

Carbon quantum dots (CQDs) are comparatively easy to prepare and can be prepared in bulk by using low-cost or waste precursors. CQDs are the combination of sp^2 and sp^3 hybrids carbons and create discrete energy levels demonstrating unique electron-accepting and electron-transporting capabilities, and photo-stability. Moreover, the electronic and optical properties can be easily modified by modifying the chemical composition via surface functionalization or doing. These properties make them a promising photoactive material for dye degradation in water bodies. N-doping is quite common to impart photocatalytic properties in carbon materials. In this regard, various methods have been reported to synthesize N-doped CQD and their application for dye degradation. The extract of *Cucurbita pepo* was successfully utilized for the green synthesis of N-modified carbon dots (NCQDs) through the hydrothermal method [93]. The synthesized NCQDs exhibited excitation-dependent PL emission with a fluorescence quantum yield of 12.19%. Accordingly, the photoactivity was explored under visible light taking CV dye in the presence of hydrogen peroxide and resulted in 99.9% dye degradation in 180 minutes. The higher activity was attributed to the efficient visible light absorption, electron transfer properties of NCQD, and generation of semiconducting localized states as a result of surface functionalities. The trapping studies revealed that $^{\cdot}$OH radicals played a key role during the photocatalytic reduction process. It is well known that the electronic and optical properties of the QDs depend on their size and thus can significantly affect photocatalytic activity. Zhou et al. [94] have synthesized QDs with three different sizes and tested their photocatalytic activity towards the degradation of RhB and MB dyes. In this method, CDs with different sizes were prepared through a microwave-mediated method and separated by size exclusion chromatography. Electronic studies revealed that the light absorption and band gap were found to change with the size of CDs. However, no correlation was established between the size and PL emission of CDs indicating a quantum-sized independent PL mechanism. Separated fractions of CDs were individually evaluated for the photocatalytic degradation of organic dyes using a sunlight simulator. Experimental results confirmed that photocatalytic activity was dependent on the size of the particles. The smaller the size, the better the degradation of dyes (RhB and MB). Based on the scavenger studies, holes and superoxide radicals were the main active species implicated in the visible-light-driven photocatalytic degradation process. Moreover, CDs displayed high stability under multiple cycles and showed comparable activity to the metal-based photocatalyst. These results clearly demonstrated the role of QD size in determining their electronic properties which in turn can significantly affect photocatalytic activity. In addition to the CQDs, inorganic QDs (TiO_2, CdS, ZnS, etc.) have also been explored for their photocatalytic activity. ZnS QDs with the lowest average crystallite size in the range of 4.2–29.6 nm were prepared via co-precipitation

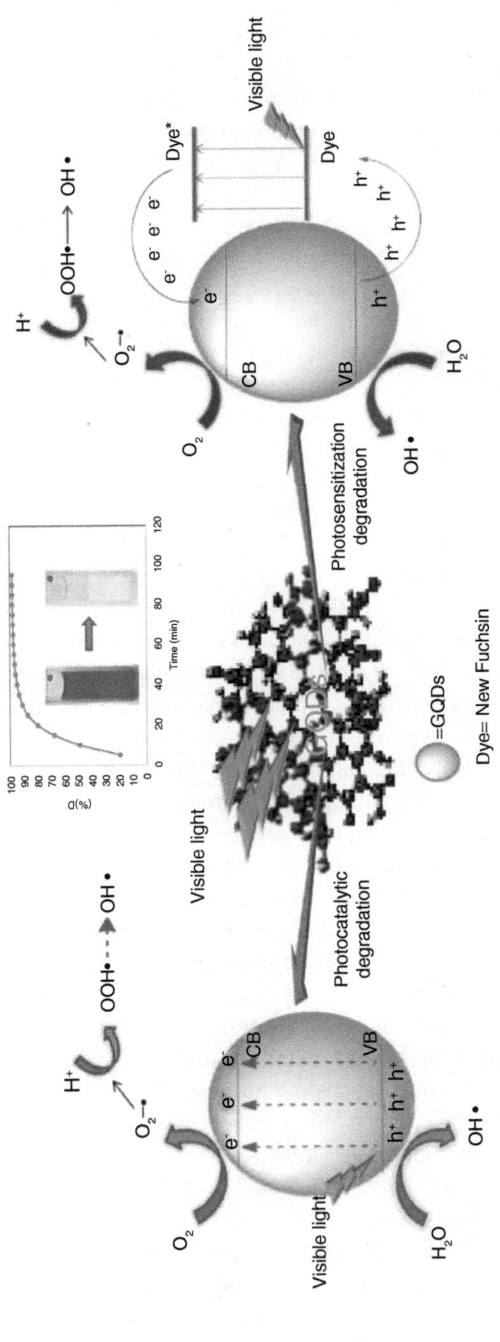

FIGURE 2.6 Schematic representation for photocatalytic and photosensitization mechanism for degradation of New Fuchsin dye under visible light irradiation.

method using 2-mercaptoethanol as a capping agent [95]. Experimental data showed that the capping agent influenced the light absorption suggesting direct interaction with ZnS. Moreover, thermogravimetry analysis revealed high thermal stability of ZnS QDs. ZnS QD was found active for the visible-light-driven degradation of MB. In another report, Bhattacharjee et al. [96] developed a method based on microwave heating for producing SnO_2 QDs with an average diameter of 4.0 nm using serine amino acid. A clear blue shift was monitored in the band gap energy (~4.5 eV) due to the quantum confinement effect. The synthesized SnO_2 QDs were employed for the solar light-driven photodegradation of eosin Y dye. Further, in situ synthesis of highly stable CdS QDs in aqueous media was reported procuring $Na_2S_2O_3$ (precursor) and thioglycolic acid (catalyst and capping agent) [97]. The synthesized CdS QDs had comparatively cubic crystalline structures with smaller sizes (2.65–2.93 nm) and good optical properties and thus examined for degradation of industrial dyes (Mordant red, Alizarin, acid violet, and Thymol blue) in the presence of visible light. Kaur et al. [98] prepared well crystalline ZnS QDs having a cubic phase of zinc blende structure in high yield via co-precipitation method utilizing as stabilizing agent (sodium dodecyl sulfate). The synthesized QDs possessed good optical properties and were consequently tested for the solar light-assisted photocatalytic degradation of brilliant green dye. 88% dye degradation was achieved, and the reaction followed a pseudo-first-order kinetic model. Moreover, a probable mechanism for the dye degradation was also presented. ZnS irradiated by sunlight generated the holes and electrons in the VB and CB, respectively. Generally, the photoreduction of dye can proceed via three different pathways. First, photo-generated holes can oxidize the dye molecules forming cation radicals, which in turn react with oxygen, giving the end product. Second, holes can react with water molecules and form hydroxyl radicals that oxidize the dye molecules. Third, superoxide anions form because of the oxidation of dissolved oxygen by electrons that can mineralize the dye molecules. In this method, oxidizing species directly participated in the photodegradation process. Moreover, highly crystalline and TiO_2 QDs with sizes in the range of 5–8 nm have been prepared through the sol–gel method, excluding any capping or chelating agents [99]. The photocatalytic performance of synthesized material was explored for the degradation of indigo carmine dye. Excellent photocatalytic behavior was observed under UV light irradiation affording 95% indigo carmine dye degradation in 60 minutes. The effect of pH, initial dye concentration and catalyst dose, reaction temperature were also examined and found that a catalyst dose of 0.75 g/L and 5–10 mg/L dye concentration in acidic pH at 25°C optimized reaction parameters.

Among the various QDs photocatalysts, perovskite QDs have also been utilized as a promising photocatalyst due to their photocatalytic efficiency, tailored electronic properties, and simple structure. Generally, perovskite has a chemical formula of ABX_3 where B is a divalent metal ion (A and B: organic/inorganic cations and X: halogen anion). Spherical-shaped $CsPbX_3$ (X: Cl and Br) QDs were constructed at room temperature via emulsion fabrication and de-emulsion method and investigated the dye degradation under visible light [100]. Reasonably monodispersed $CsPbCl_3$ and $CsPbBr_3$ QDs demonstrated higher photocatalytic activity by decomposing 90% and 89% of methyl orange within 100 minutes, respectively. ESI-MS results indicated the dissociation of methyl orange dye molecules into smaller and relatively nontoxic fragments. Moreover, radical trapping studies found that $^{\cdot}O_2^-$ species were more active than h^+ and $^{\cdot}OH$ species.

2.4 CONCLUSIONS AND FUTURE PROSPECTIVES

Heterogeneous photocatalysts assisted degradation of dye molecules in aqueous media via an advanced oxidation process is one of the well-accepted approaches in the scientific world. This approach involves various materials including metal oxides, MOF, plasmonic nanoparticles, and their composites. These nanostructured materials can be modified in terms of morphology, electronic and surface properties, and crystalline and chemical nature to impart photoactivity for dye degradation via different reductive pathways. Doping (metal and non-metals) and coupled semiconductor approaches are generally utilized for tailoring electronic properties such as band gap modulation and visible light harvesting. The applicability of these nanomaterials and their heterostructures for the reduction of dyes under light irradiation into harmless products have gained a lot of interest in the recent past due to their efficiency and easy recyclability. However, implementation of photocatalytic degradation of dyes technologies at the industry level is still lacking due to the challenges related to bulk synthesis, low efficiency, unsustainable approaches, and no direct use of sunlight. Therefore, the synthesis of new materials with the aim of reducing the cost of the process avoiding the energy-intensive steps and harmful precursors is required. Materials with high surface area and the possibility of tuning their electronic properties via economically and environmentally friendly approaches are highly desirable. Moreover, the stability of the photocatalyst in terms of recyclability is also an important parameter to assess its applicability at the industrial level. In this regard, recycling, and regeneration of the photocatalysts must maintain the sustainability of the process while managing the waste and their disposal. Photocatalysis is a low-cost, nontoxic, and sustainable way to degrade industrial dyes. In this regard, several nanostructured materials (metal oxides, organic polymer composites, doped carbon materials) including their heterostructures have been developed. However, the stability of photocatalysts against photo-corrosion is a major concern that needs to be addressed besides the rapid recombination rate of electrons and holes to enhance their efficiency. In the chapter, we have discussed the strategies to develop diverse photocatalysts by tailoring the morphology, doping (metal and nonmetal), and hybridizing suitable nanostructures. Generally, hybrid and doped porous materials exhibited better photocatalytic activity due to the easy accessibility of active sites and diminished the recombination rate of charge carriers by generating mid-energy states. The active sites in the form of defects and doped elements (metals and nonmetals) participate in the formation of oxygenated active species (superoxide radicals) which react with dye molecules. Although there are significant advancements in improving photocatalytic efficiency, challenges related to the photocatalyst stability and degradation mechanism (kinetics and thermodynamics) of dyes are still a matter of concern. Moreover, complex synthesis processes for catalyst and dye degradation are also not desirable for the applicability of developed technology at the industrial level. Furthermore, the use of actual industrial wastewater containing industrial dyes needs to be used for evaluating the photocatalytic activity of the developed photocatalyst under natural sunlight. Studies based on real industrial wastewater and natural sunlight would provide reliable and practical data to develop effective technologies and therefore, should be encouraged.

REFERENCES

1. Sabnis, R. Manufacture of Dye Intermediates, Dyes, and Their Industrial Applications. In: *Handbook of Industrial Chemistry and Biotechnology*, Springer, Cham, 581–676 (2017).
2. Mani, S.; Chowdhary, P. Dyes: Industrial Applications and Toxicity Profile. In: *Contaminants and Clean Technologies*, CRC Press, 137–148 (2020).
3. Hassaan, M. A.; El Nemr, A.; Hassaan, A. Health and Environmental Impacts of Dyes: Mini Review. *American Journal of Environmental Science and Engineering*, 1(3), 64–67 (2017). DOI:10.11648/j.ajese.20170103.11.
4. Singha, K.; Pandit, P.; Maity, S.; Sharma, S. R. Harmful Environmental Effects for Textile Chemical Dyeing Practice. In: *Green Chemistry for Sustainable Textiles*; Ibrahim, N., Hussain, C. M. (Eds.), Woodhead Publishing, Elsevier, 153–164 (2021). DOI: 10.1016/B978-0-323-85204-3.00005-1.
5. Verma, S.; Gupta, G. Natural Dyes and Its Applications: A Brief Review. *International Journal of Research and Analytical Reviews*. 4(4), 57–60 (2017).
6. Shahid, M.; Mohammad, F. Recent Advancements in Natural Dye Applications: A Review. *Journal of Cleaner Production*. 53, 310–331 (2013). DOI: 10.1016/j.jclepro.2013.03.031.
7. Saxena, S.; Raja, A. Natural Dyes: Sources, Chemistry, Application and Sustainability Issues. In: *Roadmap to Sustainable Textiles and Clothing. Eco-Friendly Raw Materials Technologies and Processing Methods*, Springer, Singapore, 37–80 (2014). DOI:10.1007/978-981-287-065-0_2.
8. Katheresan, V.; Kansedo, J.; Lau, S. Y. Efficiency of Various Recent Wastewater Dye Removal Methods: A Review. *Journal of Environmental Chemical Engineering*. 6(4), 4676–4697 (2018). DOI: 10.1016/j.jece.2018.06.060.
9. Shindhal, T.; Rakholiya, P.; Varjani, S.; Pandey, A.; Ngo, H. H.; Guo, W.; Ng, H. Y.; Taherzadeh, M. J. A critical review on advances in the practices and perspectives for the treatment of dye industry wastewater. *Bioengineered*, 12(1), 70–87 (2020). DOI: 10.1080/21655979.2020.1863034.
10. Hai, F. I.; Yamamoto, K.; Fukushi, K. Hybrid Treatment Systems for Dye Wastewater. *Critical Reviews in Environmental Science and Technology*. 37(4), 315–377 (2007). DOI: 10.1080/10643380601174723.
11. Su, C. X.-H.; Low, L. W.; Teng, T. T.; Wong, Y. S. Combination and Hybridisation of Treatments in Dye Wastewater Treatment: A Review. *Journal of Environmental Chemical Engineering*. 4(3), 3618–3631 (2016). DOI: 10.1016/j.jece.2016.07.026.
12. Anandan, S.; Ponnusamy, V. K.; Ashokkumar, M. A Review on Hybrid Techniques for the Degradation of Organic Pollutants in Aqueous Environment. *Ultrasonic Sonochemistry*. 67, 105130 (2020). DOI: 10.1016/j.ultsonch.2020.105130.
13. Gogate, P. R.; Pandit, A. B. A Review of Imperative Technologies for Wastewater Treatment II: Hybrid Methods. *Advances in Environmental Research*. 8(3–4), 553–597 (2004). DOI: 10.1016/S1093-0191(03)00031-5.

14. Bhatia, D.; Sharma, N. R.; Singh, J.; Kanwar, R. S. Biological Methods for Textile Dye Removal from Wastewater: A Review. *Critical Reviews in Environmental Science and Technology*. 47(19), 1836–1876 (2017). DOI: 10.1080/10643389.2017.1393263.
15. Donkadokula, N. Y.; Kola, A. K.; Naz, I.; Saroj, D. A Review on Advanced Physico-Chemical and Biological Textile Dye Wastewater Treatment Techniques. *Reviews in Environmental Science and Bio/Technology*. 19, 543–560 (2020). DOI: 10.1007/s11157-020-09543-z.
16. Tan, B. H.; Teng, T. T.; Omar, A. M. Removal of Dyes and Industrial Dye Wastes by Magnesium Chloride. *Water Research*. 34(2), 597–601 (2000). DOI: 10.1016/S0043-1354(99)00151-7.
17. Bagotia, N.; Sharma, A. K.; Kumar, S. A Review on Modified Sugarcane Bagasse Biosorbent for Removal of Dyes. *Chemosphere*. 268, 129309 (2021). DOI: 10.1016/j.chemosphere.2020.129309.
18. Vakili, M.; Rafatullah, M.; Salamatinia, B.; Abdullah, A. Z.; Ibrahim, M. H.; Tan, K. B.; Gholami, Z.; Amouzgar, P. Application of Chitosan and Its Derivatives as Adsorbents for Dye Removal from Water and Wastewater: A Review. *Carbohydrate Polymers*. 113, 115–130 (2014). DOI: 10.1016/j.carbpol.2014.07.007.
19. Piaskowski, K.; Świderska-Dąbrowska, R.; Zarzycki, P. K. Dye Removal from Water and Wastewater Using Various Physical, Chemical, and Biological Processes. *Journal of AOAC International*. 101(5), 1371–1384 (2018). DOI: 10.5740/jaoacint.18-0051.
20. Bal, G.; Thakur, A. Distinct Approaches of Removal of Dyes from Wastewater: A Review. *Materials Today: Proceedings*. 50, 1575–1579 (2022).
21. Forgacs, E.; Cserháti, T.; Oros, G. Removal of Synthetic Dyes from Wastewaters: A Review. *Environment International*. 30(7), 953–971 (2004).
22. Sharma, S.; Kaur, A. Various Methods for Removal of Dyes from Industrial Effluents – a Review. *Indian Journal of Science and Technology*. 11(1) (2018).
23. Ahmad, A.; Mohd-Setapar, S. H.; Chuong, C. S.; Khatoon, A.; Wani, W. A.; Kumar, R.; Rafatullah, M. Recent Advances in New Generation Dye Removal Technologies: Novel Search for Approaches to Reprocess Wastewater. *RSC Advance*. 5(39), 30801–30818 (2015). DOI: 10.1039/C4RA16959J.
24. Krishnan, J.; Kishore, A. A.; Suresh, A.; Madhumeetha, B.; Prakash, D. G. Effect of pH, Inoculum Dose and Initial Dye Concentration on the Removal of Azo Dye Mixture under Aerobic Conditions. *International Biodeterioration & Biodegradation*. 119, 16–27 (2017).
25. Roy, D. C.; Biswas, S. K.; Saha, A. K.; Sikdar, B.; Rahman, M.; Roy, A. K.; Prodhan, Z. H.; Tang, S.-S. Biodegradation of Crystal Violet Dye by Bacteria Isolated from Textile Industry Effluents. *PeerJ*, 6, 5015 (2018). DOI: 10.7717/peerj.5015.
26. Masarbo, R. S.; Karegoudar, T. Decolourisation of Toxic Azo Dye Fast Red E by Three Bacterial Strains: Process Optimisation and Toxicity Assessment. *International Journal of Environmental Analytical Chemistry*. 102(11), 2686–2696 (2022). DOI: 10.1080/03067319.2020.1759048.
27. Danouche, M.; El Arroussi, H.; Bahafid, W.; El Ghachtouli, N. An Overview of the Biosorption Mechanism for the Bioremediation of Synthetic Dyes Using Yeast Cells. *Environmental Technology Reviews*. 10(1) 58–76 (2021). DOI: 10.1080/21622515.2020.1869839.
28. Soh, E. Y.; Lim, S. S.; Chew, K. W.; Phuang, X. W.; Ho, V. M.; Chu, K. Y.; Wong, R. R.; Lee, L. Y.; Tiong, T. J. Valorization of Spent Brewery Yeast Biosorbent with Sonication-Assisted Adsorption for Dye Removal in Wastewater Treatment. *Environmental Research*. 204, 112385 (2022). DOI: 10.1016/j.envres.2021.112385.

29. Mahmoud, M. S. Decolorization of Certain Reactive Dye from Aqueous Solution Using Baker's Yeast (*Saccharomyces cerevisiae*) Strain. *HBRC Journal.* 12(1) 88–98 (2016). DOI: 10.1016/j.hbrcj.2014.07.005.
30. Azeez, R. A.; Al-Zuhairi, F. K. I. Biosorption of Dye by Immobilized Yeast Cells on the Surface of Magnetic Nanoparticles. *Alexandria Engineering Journal.* 61(7), 5213–5222 (2022). DOI: 10.1016/j.aej.2021.10.044.
31. Jun, L. Y.; Yon, L. S.; Mubarak, N.; Bing, C. H.; Pan, S.; Danquah, M. K.; Abdullah, E.; Khalid, M. An Overview of Immobilized Enzyme Technologies for Dye and Phenolic Removal from Wastewater. *Journal of Environmental Chemical Engineering.* 7(2), 102961 (2019). DOI: 10.1016/j.jece.2019.102961.
32. Joshni, T. C.; Subramaniam, K. Enzymatic Degradation of Azo Dyes – a Review. *International Journal of Environmental Science and Technology.* 1(6), 1250–1260 (2011). DOI: 10.1016/j.ibiod.2015.04.027.
33. Ariaeenejad, S.; Motamedi, E.; Salekdeh, G. H. Application of the Immobilized Enzyme on Magnetic Graphene Oxide Nano-Carrier as a Versatile Bi-Functional Tool for Efficient Removal of Dye from Water. *Bioresource Technology.* 319, 124228 (2021). DOI: 10.1016/j.biortech.2020.124228.
34. Chiong, T.; Lau, S. Y.; Lek, Z. H.; Koh, B. Y.; Danquah, M. K. Enzymatic Treatment of Methyl Orange Dye in Synthetic Wastewater by Plant-Based Peroxidase Enzymes. *Journal of Environmental Chemical Engineering.* 4(2), 2500–2509 (2016). DOI: 10.1016/j.jece.2016.04.030.
35. Kim, T.-H.; Park, C.; Yang, J.; Kim, S. Comparison of Disperse and Reactive Dye Removals by Chemical Coagulation and Fenton Oxidation. *Journal of Hazardous Material.* 112(1–2), 95–103 (2004). 10.1016/j.jhazmat.2004.04.008
36. Ismail, G. A.; Sakai, H. Review on Effect of Different Type of Dyes on Advanced Oxidation Processes (AOPs) for Textile Color Removal. *Chemosphere.* 291, 132906 (2022). DOI: 10.1016/j.chemosphere.2021.132906.
37. Ulson, S. M. de A. G.; Bonilla, K. A. S.; de Souza, A. A. U. Removal of COD and Color from Hydrolyzed Textile Azo Dye by Combined Ozonation and Biological Treatment. *Journal of Hazardous Materials.* 179(1–3), 35–42 (2010). DOI: 10.1016/j.jhazmat.2010.02.053.
38. Nidheesh, P. V.; Gandhimathi, R.; Ramesh, S. T. Degradation of Dyes from Aqueous Solution by Fenton Processes: A Review. *Environmental Science and Pollution Research.* 20, 2099–2132 (2013). DOI: 10.1007/s11356-012-1385-z.
39. Natarajan, S.; Bajaj, H. C.; Tayade, R. J. Recent Advances Based on the Synergetic Effect of Adsorption for Removal of Dyes from Waste Water Using Photocatalytic Process. *Journal Environmental Science.* 65, 201–222 (2018). DOI: 10.1016/j.jes.2017.03.011
40. Singh, S.; Lo, S. L.; Srivastava, V. C.; Hiwarkar, A. D. Comparative Study of Electrochemical Oxidation for Dye Degradation: Parametric Optimization and Mechanism Identification. *Journal of Environmental Sciences.* 4(3), 2911–2921 (2016). DOI: 10.1016/j.jece.2016.05.036.
41. Abdi, J.; Vossoughi, M.; Mahmoodi, N. M.; Alemzadeh, I. Synthesis of Amine-Modified Zeolitic Imidazolate Framework-8, Ultrasound-Assisted Dye Removal and Modeling. *Ultrasonics Sonochemistry.* 39, 550–564 (2017). DOI: 10.1016/j.ultsonch.2017.04.030.
42. Iervolino, G.; Vaiano, V.; Palma, V. Enhanced Azo Dye Removal in Aqueous Solution by H_2O_2 Assisted Non-Thermal Plasma Technology. *Environmental Technology and Innovation.* 19, 100969 (2020). DOI: 10.1016/j.eti.2020.100969.

43. Karam, A.; Bakhoum, E. S.; Zaher, K. Coagulation/Flocculation Process for Textile Mill Effluent Treatment: Experimental and Numerical Perspectives. *International Journal of Sustainable Engineering*. 14(5), 983–995 (2021). DOI: 10.1080/19397038.2020.1842547.
44. Zhou, Y.; Lu, J.; Zhou, Y.; Liu, Y. Recent Advances for Dyes Removal Using Novel Adsorbents: A Review. *Environmental Pollution*. 252, 352–365 (2019). DOI: 10.1016/j.envpol.2019.05.072.
45. Lan, D.; Zhu, H.; Zhang, J.; Li, S.; Chen, Q.; Wang, C.; Wu, T.; Xu, M. Adsorptive Removal of Organic Dyes via Porous Materials for Wastewater Treatment in Recent Decades: *A Review on Species, Mechanisms and Perspectives. Chemosphere*. 293, 133464 (2022). DOI: 10.1016/j.chemosphere.2021.133464.
46. Essekri, A.; Hsini, A.; Naciri, Y.; Laabd, M.; Ajmal, Z.; El Ouardi, M.; AitAddi, A.; Albourine, A. Novel Citric Acid-Functionalized Brown Algae with a High Removal Efficiency of Crystal Violet Dye from Colored Wastewaters: Insights into Equilibrium, Adsorption Mechanism, and Reusability. *International Journal of Phytoremediation*. 23(4), 336–346 (2021). DOI: 10.1080/15226514.2020.1813686.
47. Cao, X. T.; Kim, D. W.; Showkat, A. M.; Jeong, Y. T.; Lim, K. T. Enhancing Adsorption of Multi-Walled Carbon Nanotubes for Dye Removal. *Science of Advanced Materials*. 8(2), 322–326 (2016). DOI: 10.1166/sam.2016.2487.
48. Dutta, S.; Gupta, B.; Srivastava, S. K.; Gupta, A. K. Recent Advances on the Removal of Dyes from Wastewater Using Various Adsorbents: A Critical Review. *Materials Advances*. 2(14), 4497–4531 (2021). DOI: 10.1039/D1MA00354B.
49. Cao, X. T.; Vo, T. K.; An, T. N. M.; Nguyen, T. D.; Kabtamu, D. M.; Kumar, S. Enhanced Dye Adsorption of Mixed-Matrix Membrane by Covalent Incorporation of Metal-Organic Framework with Poly (Styrene-alt-maleic Anhydride). *Chemistry Select*. 6(19), 4689–4697 (2021). DOI: 10.1002/slct.202100615.
50. Moosavi, S.; Lai, C. W.; Gan, S.; Zamiri, G.; AkbarzadehPivehzhani, O.; Johan, M. R. Application of Efficient Magnetic Particles and Activated Carbon for Dye Removal from Wastewater. *ACS Omega*. 5(33), 20684–20697 (2020). DOI: 10.1021/acsomega.0c01905.
51. Ali, S.; Abbas, Y.; Zuhra, Z.; Butler, I. S. Synthesis of γ-Alumina (Al_2O_3) Nanoparticles and Their Potential for Use as an Adsorbent in the Removal of Methylene Blue Dye from Industrial Wastewater. *Nanoscale Advances*. 1(1), 213–218 (2019). DOI: 10.1039/C8NA00014J.
52. Zhang, Y.; Xia, K.; Liu, X.; Chen, Z.; Du, H.; Zhang, X. Synthesis of Cationic-Modified Silica Gel and Its Adsorption Properties for Anionic Dyes. *Journal of the Taiwan Institute of Chemical Engineers*. 102, 1–8 (2019). DOI: 10.1016/j.jtice.2019.05.005.
53. Kubra, K. T.; Salman, M. S.; Hasan, M. N. Enhanced Toxic Dye Removal from Wastewater Using Biodegradable Polymeric Natural Adsorbent. *Journal of Molecular Liquids*. 328, 115468 (2021). DOI: 10.1016/j.molliq.2021.115468.
54. Yagub, M. T.; Sen, T. K.; Afroze, S.; Ang, H. M. Dye and Its Removal from Aqueous Solution by Adsorption: A Review. *Advances in Colloid and Interface Science*. 209, 172–184 (2014). DOI: https://doi.org/10.1016/j.cis.2014.04.002.
55. Hube, S.; Eskafi, M.; Hrafnkelsdóttir, K. F.; Bjarnadóttir, B.; Bjarnadóttir, M. Á.; Axelsdóttir, S.; Wu, B. Direct Membrane Filtration for Wastewater Treatment and Resource Recovery: A Review. *Science of the Total Environment.* 710, 136375 (2020). DOI: 10.1016/j.scitotenv.2019.136375.
56. Rashidi, H. R.; Sulaiman, N. M. N.; Hashim, N. A.; Hassan, C. R. C.; Ramli, M. R. Synthetic Reactive Dye Wastewater Treatment by Using Nano-Membrane

Filtration. *Desalination and Water Treatment.* 55(1), 86–95 (2015). DOI: 10.1080/19443994.2014.912964.

57. Joseph, J.; Radhakrishnan, R. C.; Johnson, J. K.; Joy, S. P.; Thomas, J. Ion-Exchange Mediated Removal of Cationic Dye-Stuffs from Water Using Ammonium Phosphomolybdate. *Materials Chemistry and Physics.* 242, 122488 (2020). DOI: 10.1016/j.matchemphys.2019.122488.
58. Bandala, E. R.; Peláez, M. A.; García-López, A. J.; Salgado, M. de J.; Moeller, G. Photocatalytic Decolourisation of Synthetic and Real Textile Wastewater Containing Benzidine-Based Azo Dyes. *Chemical Engineering and Processing: Process Intensification.* 47(2), 169–176 (2008). DOI: 10.1016/j.cep.2007.02.010.
59. Zhao, C.; Zhang, Y.; Jiang, H.; Chen, J.; Liu, Y.; Liang, Q.; Zhou, M.; Li, Z.; Zhou, Y. Combined Effects of Octahedron NH_2-UiO-66 and Flowerlike $ZnIn_2S_4$ Microspheres for Photocatalytic Dye Degradation and Hydrogen Evolution under Visible Light. *Journal of Physical Chemistry C.* 123(29), 18037–18049 (2019). DOI: 10.1021/acs.jpcc.9b03807.
60. Ding, J.; Yang, Z.; He, C.; Tong, X.; Li, Y.; Niu, X.; Zhang, H. UiO-66 (Zr) Coupled with Bi_2MoO_6 as Photocatalyst for Visible-Light Promoted Dye Degradation. *Journal of Colloid and Interface Science.* 497, 126–133 (2017). DOI: 10.1016/j.jcis.2017.02.060.
61. Lakshmi Prasanna, V., Rajagopalan, V. A New Synergetic Nanocomposite for Dye Degradation in Dark and Light. *Scientific Reports.* 6(1), 1–10 (2016). DOI: 10.1038/srep38606.
62. Rosu, M.-C.; Coros, M.; Pogacean, F.; Magerusan, L.; Socaci, C.; Turza, A.; Pruneanu, S. Azo Dyes Degradation Using TiO_2-Pt/Graphene Oxide and TiO_2-Pt/Reduced Graphene Oxide Photocatalysts under UV and Natural Sunlight Irradiation. *Solid State Sciences.* 70, 13–20 (2017). DOI: 10.1016/j.solidstatesciences.2017.05.013.
63. Lan, M.; Fan, G.; Yang, L.; Li, F. Enhanced Visible-Light-Induced Photocatalytic Performance of a Novel Ternary Semiconductor Coupling System Based on Hybrid Zn–In Mixed Metal Oxide/gC_3N_4 Composites. *RSC Advances.* 5(8), 5725–5734 (2015). DOI: 10.1039/C4RA07073A.
64. Zalfani, M.; Hu, Z.-Y.; Yu, W.-B.; Mahdouani, M.; Bourguiga, R.; Wu, M.; Li, Y.; Van Tendeloo, G.; Djaoued, Y.; Su, B.-L. $BiVO_4/_3$DOM TiO_2 Nanocomposites: Effect of $BiVO_4$ as Highly Efficient Visible Light Sensitizer for Highly Improved Visible Light Photocatalytic Activity in the Degradation of Dye Pollutants. *Applied Catalysis B: Environmental.* 205, 121–132 (2017). DOI: 10.1016/j.apcatb.2016.12.019.
65. Yan, M.; Wu, Y.; Yan, Y.; Yan, X.; Zhu, F.; Hua, Y.; Shi, W. Synthesis and Characterization of Novel $BiVO_4/Ag_3VO_4$ Heterojunction with Enhanced Visible-Light-Driven Photocatalytic Degradation of Dyes. *ACS Sustainable Chemistry & Engineering.* 4(3), 757–766 (2016). DOI: 10.1021/acssuschemeng.5b00690.
66. Mohini, R.; Lakshminarasimhan, N. Coupled Semiconductor Nanocomposite G-C_3N_4/TiO_2 with Enhanced Visible Light Photocatalytic Activity. *Materials Research Bulletin.* 76, 370–375 (2016). 10.1016/j.materresbull.2015.12.034.
67. Singla, S.; Sharma, S.; Basu, S. MoS_2/WO_3 Heterojunction with the Intensified Photocatalytic Performance for Decomposition of Organic Pollutants under the Broad Array of Solar Light. *Journal of Cleaner Production.* 324, 129290 (2021). DOI: 10.1016/j.jclepro.2021.129290.
68. Ara, B.; Malik, S.; Saba, H.; Khan, H.; Amir, S.; Zia, T. U. H.; Taube, P. S.; Gul, K. Photocatalytic Degradation of Textile Dyes Laden Industrial Wastewater Using Fabricated Bismuth Ferrite Coated Nickel/Nickel Oxide Foam. *Eitschrift Fur Physikalische Chemie.* (2023). DOI: 10.1515/zpch-2023-0297.

69. Alamgir.; Talha, K.; Wang, Y.-J.; Ullah, R.; Wang, B.; Wang, L.; Wu, W.; Chen, S.; Xie, L.-H.; Li, J.-R. Construction of a Mixed Ligand MOF as "Green Catalyst" for the Photocatalytic Degradation of Organic Dye in Aqueous Media. *RSC Advances*. 11(38), 23838–23845 (2021). DOI: 10.1039/D1RA02994K.
70. Zhang, M.; Wang, L.; Zeng, T.; Shang, Q.; Zhou, H.; Pan, Z.; Cheng, Q. Two Pure MOF-Photocatalysts Readily Prepared for the Degradation of Methylene Blue Dye under Visible Light. *Dalton Transactions*. 47(12), 4251–4258 (2018). DOI: 10.1039/C8DT00156A.
71. Chen, X.-H.; Zhang, Y.-S.; Li, W.-B.; Guan, X.-W.; Ye, J.-W.; Chen, L.; Wang, H.-P.; Bai, J.; Mo, Z.-W.; Chen, X.-M. A Porphyrin-Based Metal–Organic Framework with Highly Efficient Adsorption and Photocatalytic Degradation Performances for Organic Dyes. *Inorganic Chemistry Frontiers*. 9(10), 2328–2335 (2022). DOI: 10.1039/D2QI00091A.
72. Liu, C.; Zhang, W.; Wang, N.; Guo, P.; Muhler, M.; Wang, Y.; Lin, S.; Chen, Z.; Yang, G. Highly Efficient Photocatalytic Degradation of Dyes by a Copper–Triazolate Metal–Organic Framework. *Chemistry – A European Journal*. 24(63), 16804–16813 (2018). DOI: 10.1002/chem.201803306.
73. Sarkar, A.; Adhikary, A.; Mandal, A.; Chakraborty, T.; Das, D. Zn-BTC MOF as an Adsorbent for Iodine Uptake and Organic Dye Degradation. *Crystal Growth & Design*. 20(12), 7833–7839 (2020). DOI: 10.1021/acs.cgd.0c01015.
74. Dong, J.-P.; Shi, Z.-Z.; Li, B.; Wang, L.-Y. Synthesis of a Novel 2D Zinc (II) Metal–Organic Framework for Photocatalytic Degradation of Organic Dyes in Water. *Dalton Transactions*. 48(47), 17626–17632 (2019). DOI: 10.1039/C9DT03727F.
75. Yu, L.; Ning, K.; Chunmei, W.; Kai, Y.; Jinghua, L.; Chunxiao, W.; Baibin, Z. A Hybrid Borotungstate-Coated Metal–Organic Framework with Supercapacitance, Photocatalytic Dye Degradation and H_2O_2 Sensing Properties. *Dalton Transactions*. 51(19), 7613–7621 (2022). DOI: 10.1039/D2DT00976E.
76. Priyanka; Srivastava, V. C. Photocatalytic Oxidation of Dye Bearing Wastewater by Iron Doped Zinc Oxide. *Industrial & Engineering Chemistry Research*. 52(50), 17790–17799 (2013). DOI: 10.1021/ie401973r.
77. Alam, U.; Khan, A.; Raza, W.; Khan, A.; Bahnemann, D.; Muneer, M. Highly Efficient Y and V Co-Doped ZnO Photocatalyst with Enhanced Dye Sensitized Visible Light Photocatalytic Activity. *Catalysis Today*. 284, 169–178 (2017). DOI: 10.1016/j.cattod.2016.11.037.
78. Kuvarega, A. T.; Krause, R. W.; Mamba, B. B. Nitrogen/Palladium-Codoped TiO_2 for Efficient Visible Light Photocatalytic Dye Degradation. *Journal of Physical Chemistry C*. 115(45), 22110–22120 (2011). DOI: 10.1021/jp203754j.
79. Han, F.; Li, H.; Fu, L.; Yang, J.; Liu, Z. Synthesis of S-Doped WO_3 Nanowires with Enhanced Photocatalytic Performance towards Dye Degradation. *Chemical Physics Letters*. 651, 183–187 (2016). DOI: 10.1016/j.cplett.2016.03.017.
80. Sudrajat, H.; Babel, S.; Sakai, H.; Takizawa, S. Rapid Enhanced Photocatalytic Degradation of Dyes Using Novel N-Doped ZrO_2. *Journal of Environmental Management*. 165, 224–234 (2016). DOI: 10.1016/j.jenvman.2015.09.036.
81. Shah, J. H.; Fiaz, M.; Athar, M.; Ali, J.; Rubab, M.; Mehmood, R.; Jamil, S. U. U.; Djellabi, R. Facile Synthesis of N/B-Double-Doped Mn_2O_3 and WO_3 Nanoparticles for Dye Degradation under Visible Light. *Environmental Technology*. (2019). DOI: 10.1080/09593330.2019.1567604.
82. Ikram, M.; Inayat, T.; Haider, A.; Ul-Hamid, A.; Haider, J.; Nabgan, W.; Saeed, A.; Shahbaz, A.; Hayat, S.; Ul-Ain, K. Graphene Oxide-Doped MgO Nanostructures

for Highly Efficient Dye Degradation and Bactericidal Action. *Nanoscale Research Letters*. 16, 1–11 (2021). DOI: 10.1186/s11671-021-03516-z.

83. Singh, J.; Dhaliwal, A. Plasmon-Induced Photocatalytic Degradation of Methylene Blue Dye Using Biosynthesized Silver Nanoparticles as Photocatalyst. *Environmental Technology*. (2018). DOI: 10.1080/09593330.2018.1540663.
84. Mehata, M. S. Green Route Synthesis of Silver Nanoparticles Using Plants/Ginger Extracts with Enhanced Surface Plasmon Resonance and Degradation of Textile Dye. *Materials Science and Engineering B*. 273, 115418 (2021). DOI: 10.1016/j.mseb.2021.115418.
85. Devi, T. A.; Sivaraman, R. M.; Thavamani, S. S.; Amaladhas, T. P.; AlSalhi, M. S.; Devanesan, S.; Kannan, M. M. Green Synthesis of Plasmonic Nanoparticles Using Sargassum Ilicifolium and Application in Photocatalytic Degradation of Cationic Dyes. *Environmental Research*. 208, 112642 (2022). DOI: 10.1016/j.envres.2021.112642.
86. Xu, D.; Shi, W.; Song, C.; Chen, M.; Yang, S.; Fan, W.; Chen, B. In-Situ Synthesis and Enhanced Photocatalytic Activity of Visible-Light-Driven Plasmonic Ag/AgCl/$NaTaO_3$ Nanocubes Photocatalysts. *Applied Catalysis B: Environmental*. 191, 228–234 (2016). DOI: 10.1016/j.apcatb.2016.03.036.
87. Pattappan, D.; Kavya, K.; Varghese, S.; Kumar, R. R.; Haldorai, Y. Plasmonic Effect and Charge Separation-Induced Photocatalytic Degradation of Organic Dyes Utilizing Au/$ZnFe_2O_4$@rGO Ternary Composite. *Applied Physics A*. 126, 1–9 (2020). DOI: 10.1007/s00339-020-03974-9.
88. Dinesh, V.; Biji, P.; Ashok, A.; Dhara, S.; Kamruddin, M.; Tyagi, A.; Raj, B. Plasmon-Mediated, Highly Enhanced Photocatalytic Degradation of Industrial Textile Dyes Using Hybrid ZnO@ Ag Core–Shell Nanorods. *RSC Advances*. 4(103), 58930–58940 (2014). DOI: 10.1039/C4RA09405K.
89. Xu, S.; Guo, L.; Sun, Q.; Wang, Z. L. Piezotronic Effect Enhanced Plasmonic Photocatalysis by AuNPs/$BaTiO_3$ Heterostructures. *Advanced Functional Materials*. 29(13), 1808737 (2019). DOI: 10.1002/adfm.201808737.
90. D'amato, C.; Giovannetti, R.; Zannotti, M.; Rommozzi, E.; Ferraro, S.; Seghetti, C.; Minicucci, M.; Gunnella, R.; Di Cicco, A. Enhancement of Visible-Light Photoactivity by Polypropylene Coated Plasmonic Au/TiO_2 for Dye Degradation in Water Solution. *Applied Surface Science*. 441, 575–587 (2018). DOI: 10.1016/j.apsusc.2018.01.290.
91. Sahoo, C.; Gupta, A. K.; SasidharanPillai, I. M. Photocatalytic Degradation of Methylene Blue Dye from Aqueous Solution Using Silver Ion-Doped TiO_2 and Its Application to the Degradation of Real Textile Wastewater. *Journal of Environmental Science and Health, Part A*. 47(10), 1428–1438 (2012). DOI: 10.1080/10934529.2012.672387.
92. Roushani, M.; Mavaei, M.; Rajabi, H. R. Graphene Quantum Dots as Novel and Green Nano-Materials for the Visible-Light-Driven Photocatalytic Degradation of Cationic Dye. *Journal of Molecular Catalysis*. 409, 102–109, (2015). DOI: 10.1016/j.molcata.2015.08.011.
93. Smrithi, S.; Kottam, N.; Vergis, B. R. Heteroatom Modified Hybrid Carbon Quantum Dots Derived from CucurbitaPepo for the Visible Light Driven Photocatalytic Dye Degradation. *Topics in Catalysis*. 1–12 (2022). DOI: 10.1007/s11244-022-01581-x.
94. Zhou, Y.; Zahran, E. M.; Quiroga, B. A.; Perez, J.; Mintz, K. J.; Peng, Z.; Liyanage, P. Y.; Pandey, R. R.; Chusuei, C. C.; Leblanc, R. M. Size-Dependent Photocatalytic Activity of Carbon Dots with Surface-State Determined Photoluminescence.

Applied Catalysis B: Environmental. 248, 157–166 (2019). DOI: 10.1016/j.apcatb.2019.02.019.

95. Rafiq, A.; Imran, M.; Ikram, M.; Naz, M.; Aqeel, M.; Majeed, H.; Hussain, S.; Ali, S. Photocatalytic and Catalytic Degradation of Organic Dye by Uncapped and Capped ZnS Quantum Dots. *Materials Research Express*. 6(5), 055801 (2019). DOI:10.1088/2053-1591/aaff8e.
96. Bhattacharjee, A.; Ahmaruzzaman, M. Facile Synthesis of SnO_2 Quantum Dots and Its Photocatalytic Activity in the Degradation of Eosin Y Dye: A Green Approach. *Materials Letters*. 139, 418–421 (2015). DOI: 10.1016/j.matlet.2014.10.121.
97. Samadi-Maybodi, A.; Sadeghi-Maleki, M.-R. In-Situ Synthesis of High Stable CdS Quantum Dots and Their Application for Photocatalytic Degradation of Dyes. *Spectrochimica Acta, Part A: Molecular and Biomolecular Spectroscopy*. 152, 156–164 (2016). DOI: 10.1016/j.saa.2015.07.052.
98. Kaur, S.; Sharma, S.; Umar, A.; Singh, S.; Mehta, S.; Kansal, S. K. Solar Light Driven Enhanced Photocatalytic Degradation of Brilliant Green Dye Based on ZnS Quantum Dots. *Superlattices and Microstructures*. 103, 365–375 (2017). DOI: 10.1016/j.spmi.2016.10.046.
99. Sood, S.; Kumar, S.; Umar, A.; Kaur, A.; Mehta, S. K.; Kansal, S. K. TiO_2 Quantum Dots for the Photocatalytic Degradation of Indigo Carmine Dye. *Journal of Alloys and Compounds*. 650, 193–198 (2015). DOI 10.1016/j.jallcom.2015.07.164.
100. Gao, G.; Xi, Q.; Zhou, H.; Zhao, Y.; Wu, C.; Wang, L.; Guo, P.; Xu, J. Novel Inorganic Perovskite Quantum Dots for Photocatalysis. *Nanoscale*. 9(33), 12032–12038 (2017). DOI: 10.1039/C7NR04421F.

3 Micellar Catalysis for Dye Degradation

Shanta Raj Lakshmi†, Dhruvi Chaudhari†, and Kushan Parikh

3.1 INTRODUCTION

3.1.1 Dye

Dye is a natural or artificial material used to give and/or modify color. Dyes are essentially chemical substances that may attach to surfaces or textiles to impart color. The bulk of dyes are complex chemical compounds that need to be resistant to a variety of factors. Synthetic dyes are widely employed in many domains of sophisticatedt echnology [1]. Additionally, synthetic dyes are used in the following applications: groundwater tracing [2], measuring the specific surface area of activated sludge [3], sewage [4], and wastewater treatment [5]. Dyes have a wide range of applications, including textiles, paper, paints, coatings, plastics, construction, cosmetics, food, glass, automotive, and printing inks [6].

Various types of dyes (Table 3.1), such as acid dyes, basic dyes, disperse dyes, reactive dyes, vat dyes, and sulfur dyes, are discussed in Figure 3.1.

Acid dyes are organic sulfonic acids; typically, sodium salts, with strong water solubility, are the forms that are commercially accessible [7]. Basic dyes with a positive charge, sometimes referred to as cationic dyes, typically have an ammonium cation as a source. Basic dyes can be dissolved in water and produce colorful cations when dissolved [8]. To color cellulosic fibers, sulfur dyes are employed. When applied to the substrate, they are reduced using a sodium sulfide solution from their insoluble state in water to the water-soluble leuco form. Following that, chemical or atmospheric oxidation produces the sulfur dye itself within the fiber pores [9]. Reactive dyes are distinct from other types of dyes because their molecules contain one or more reactive groups that can create a covalent connection with a fiber group [10]. Disperse dyes are primarily water-insoluble colors with substantiality for one or more hydrophobic fibers including nylon, cellulose, cellulose acetate, and acrylic fibers. They are often applied from fine aqueous dispersion. Disperse dyes typically include azo, anthraquinone, and nitro groups [11]. The majority of dyes are direct dyes, which are water-soluble colors that may be easily applied to cellulose fibers [12].

† Deceased.

DOI: 10.1201/9781003441083-3

TABLE 3.1
Different types of dyes

Types	Dyes
Acid dye	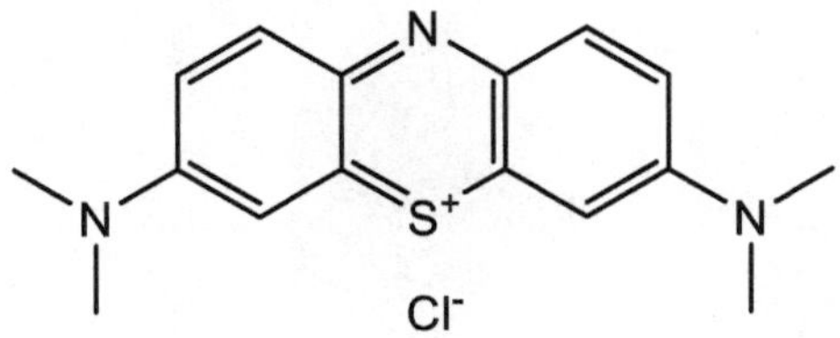 methylene blue
Basic dye	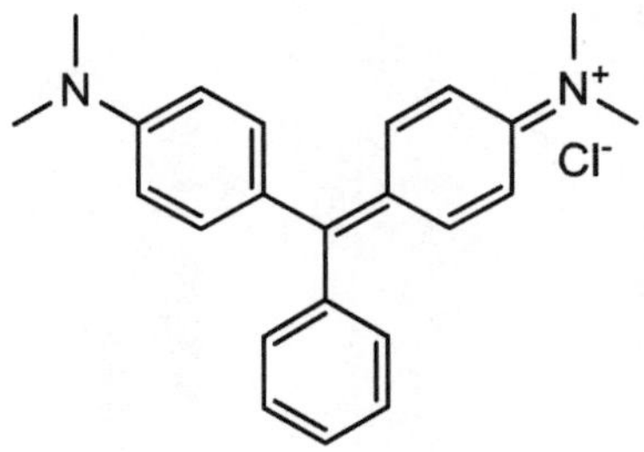 malachite green
Disperse dye	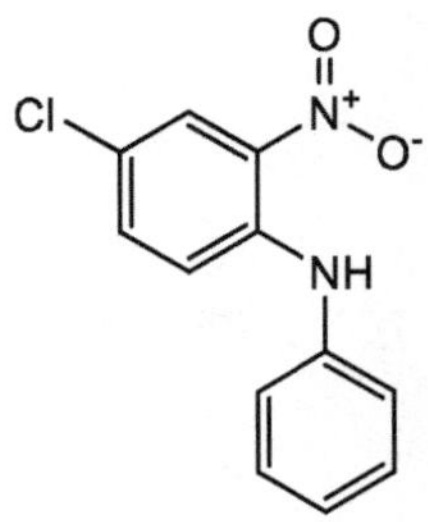 Disperse Yellow 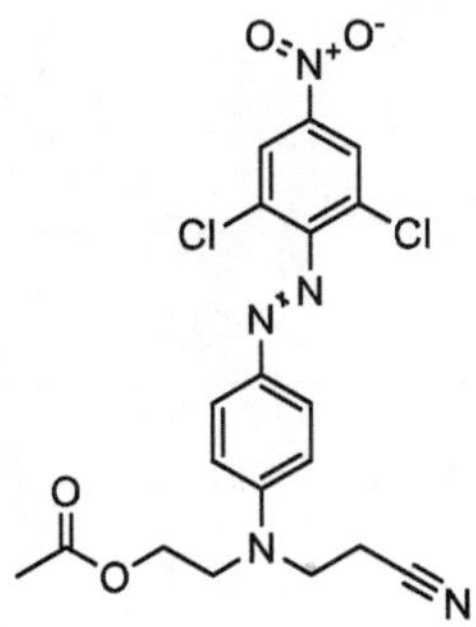 Disperse Orange
Direct dye	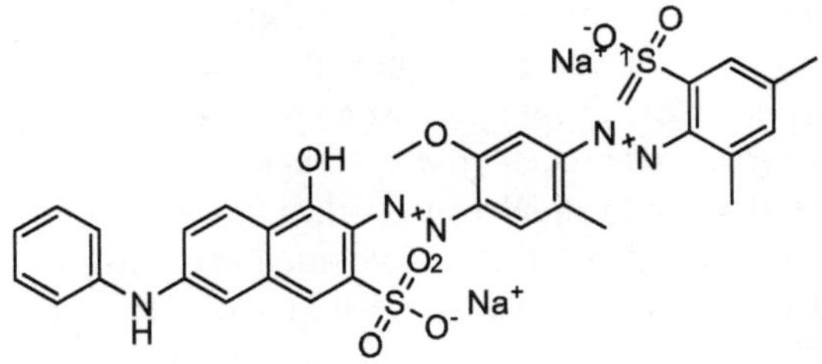 Direct Violet

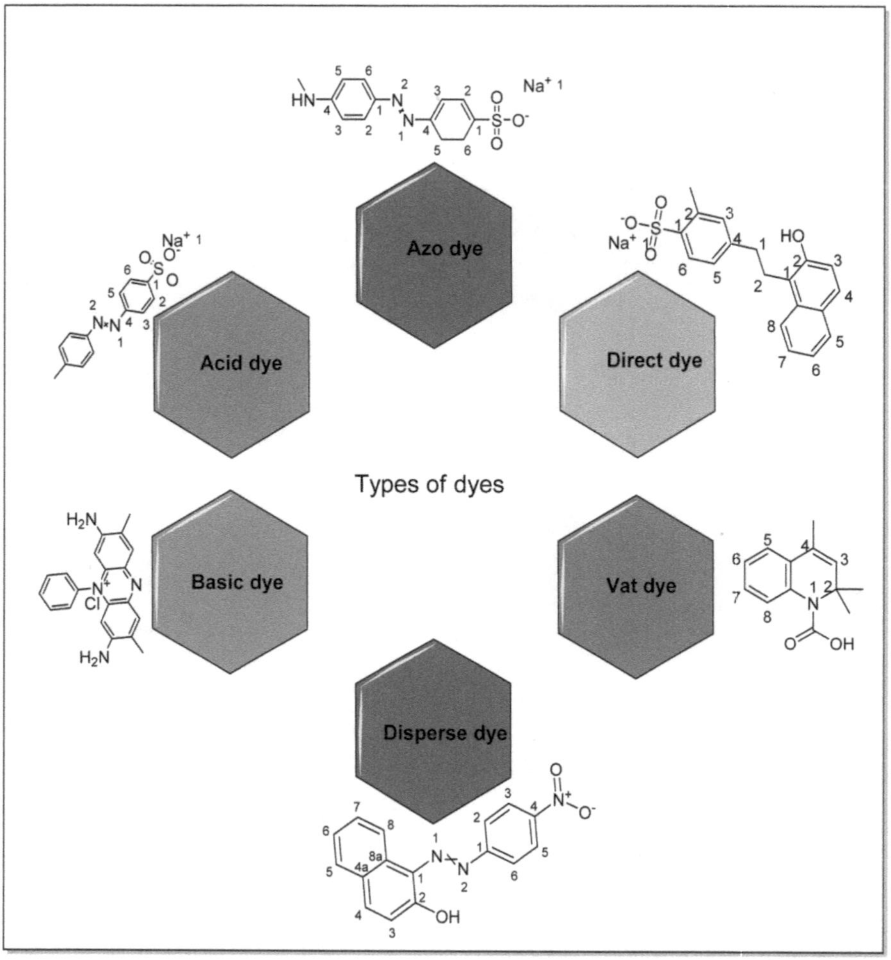

FIGURE 3.1 Different types of dyes.

3.1.2 Dye Degradation Process: Types and Classification

Dyes are subjected to various factors, such as light, heat, chemicals, and biological agents, and they may lose their color and/or effectiveness. This process is known as "dye degradation." The use of natural and synthetic dyes in biomedical imaging, inkjet printing, and textile dyeing are just a few instances where this could occur. As a result of the degradation process, the dye's chemical structure may change, causing the dye to break down into smaller molecules, lose its chromophore or auxochrome groups, lose its reactive sites, or undergo oxidation or reduction reactions.

Dye degradation comes in a variety of forms. A catalyst that produces radicals in the presence of light is present during photodegradation. Photo-generated radicals degrade the target pollutant by attacking it [13]. The capacity of biodegradation, an environmentally benign method of removing leftover colors from wastewater and

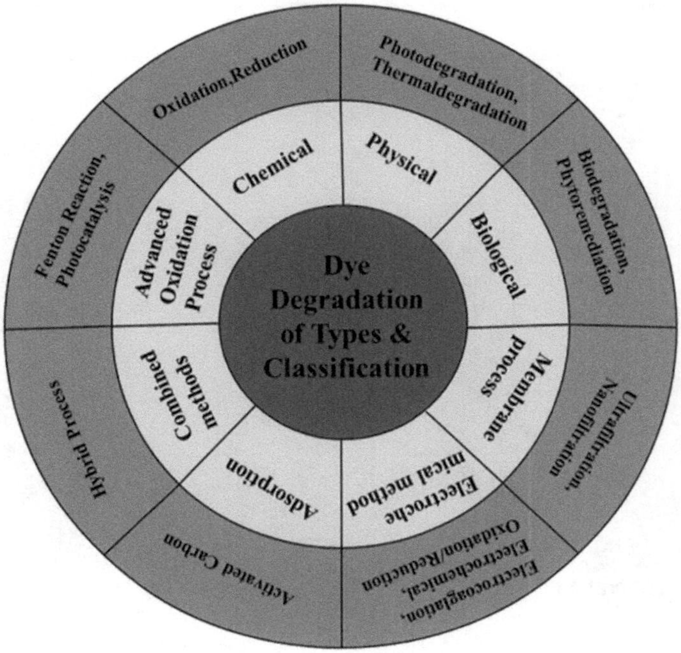

FIGURE 3.2 Dye degradation of types and classification.

degrading hazardous pollutants, is dependent on the enzyme activity, adaption of the targeted microbes, and the growing circumstances of the microorganisms, such as algae, bacteria, yeast, and fungi. While fresh and sustainable techniques to break down various colors are being developed using microorganisms isolated from the environment [14], advanced oxidation techniques (AOPs) are thought to be an effective method for removing organic contaminants that are difficult to remove, such as dyes [15]. Adsorption is the word used to describe the build-up of a material at the boundary between two phases (Figure 3.2) [16–18].

3.1.3 Dye–Surfactant Interaction

In both dyeing theory and dyeing technique, interactions between dyes and surfactants in aqueous solutions are important [19, 20]. The interaction between dye and surfactant is important because it plays a crucial role in the dyeing process and dye removal. The nature and method of dye–surfactant interaction employing various dyes and surfactants in diverse media (Figure 3.3) [21–24]. A surfactant's cationic, anionic, or nonionic nature; its absorption and/or fluorescence behavior below and above the critical micelle concentration (CMC); ion-association processes; and the impact of additives on these processes are just a few of the variables that can affect how forces that cause the binding of dye molecules with surfactant aggregates behave [20]. When the dying process actively works onto the textile fibers, dye–surfactant interactions should have a significant role in many effective steps, such as improving dye leveling,

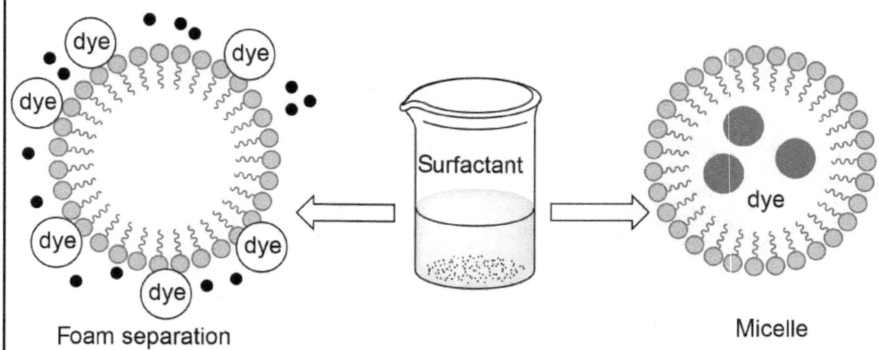

FIGURE 3.3 Different mechanisms of dye–surfactant interactions.

encouraging fiber wetting and penetration, improving color fastness, and raising dye exhaustion [25, 26].

3.1.4 Role of Surfactants

Surfactants are organic compounds that include at least one lyophilic ("solvent-loving") group and one lyophobic ("solvent-fearing") group. The phrases "hydrophilic" and "hydrophobic" are utilized if the surfactant is to be employed in a water- or aqueous-based solvent. A surfactant, in its most basic form, consists of at least one polar (or ionic) group and one non-polar group. Surfactant molecules in an aqueous solution can form micelles at a specific concentration known as critical micelle concentration (CMC), and this micelle formation.

Different types of surfactant are usually recognized by a change in the physical properties of the solution [27, 28]. Because of the structure of the molecules, they are made of surfactants that behave like conventional electrolytes when added to a

TABLE 3.2
Different types of surfactants

Cationic surfactant	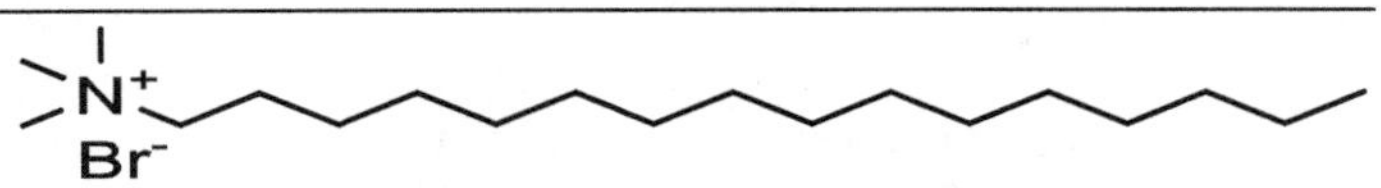 N, N, N -trimethylhexadecan-1-aminium bromide
	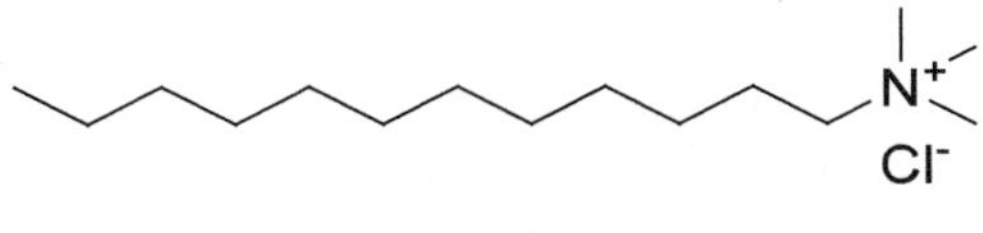 Dodecyltrimethylammonium chloride
Anionic surfactant	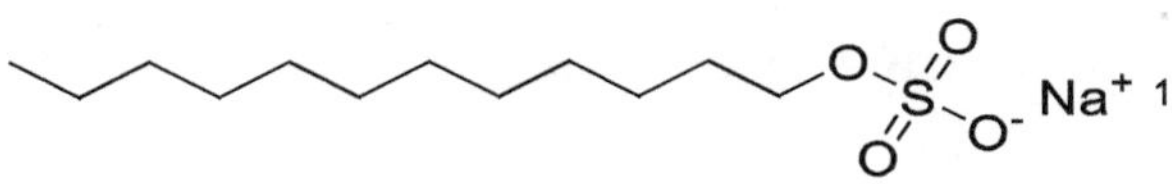 Sodium dodecyl sulfate
Gemini surfactant	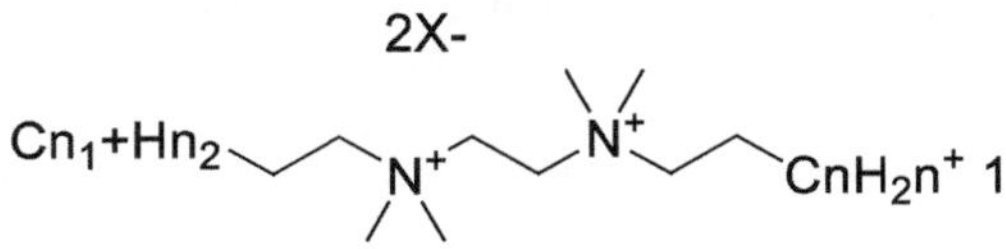 Gemini surfactant

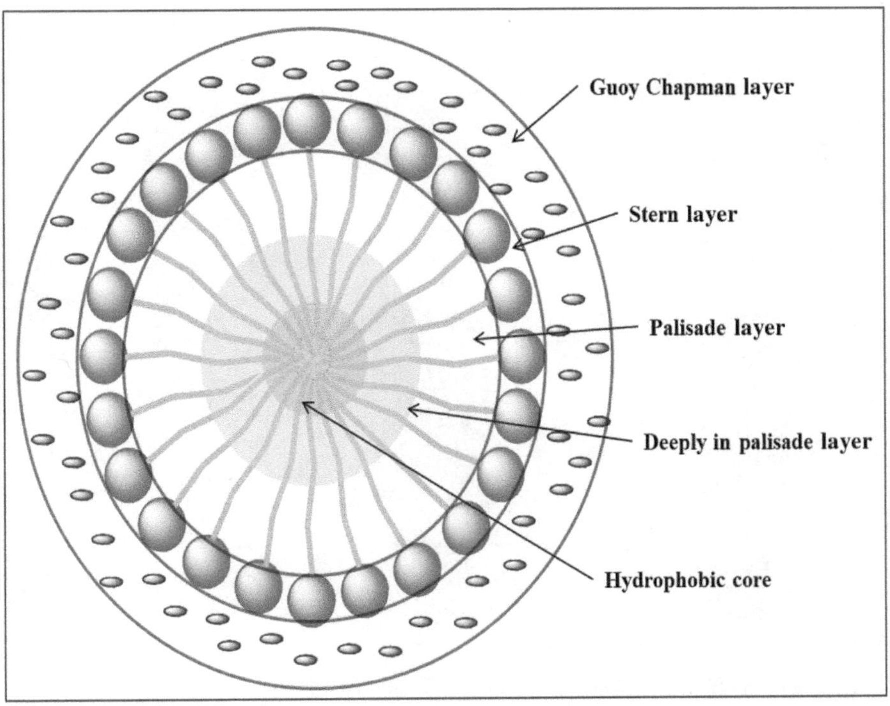

FIGURE 3.4 Various solubilization sites of the normal micelle.

solution in tiny amounts. However, when applied in sufficient quantities, they act substantially differently after reaching a limit, sometimes referred to as the CMC, by creating an aggregation of many molecules known as a micelle (Figure 3.4) [29]. Surfactants are primarily categorized based on the type of electrical charge (positive or negative) on the polar head group (hydrophilic) that they possess [30]. Gemini surfactant (also known as dimeric) is a name that implies twins or two, much like the sign of the zodiac [31]. Due to their superior physicochemical qualities over single-tailed and other classes of surfactants in terms of both commercial uses and academic points of view, they are now being used as a second-generation surfactant in surface chemistry (Figure 3.5) [32]. Gemini and conventional surfactants (Table 3.3) have gained a lot of interest recently due to their numerous uses as wetting agents, stabilizers for suspensions and emulsions, and particularly agents for bio-applications [33].

3.2 DYE INTERACTION BY MICELLAR SOLUTION

Malachite green, crystal violet, and other triphenylmethyl dyes were particularly susceptible to micellar modulation during the degradative processes of synthetic dyes in alkaline environments, although indigoid colors like indigo carmine were less likely to experience it [34–36]. The presentation includes information on how

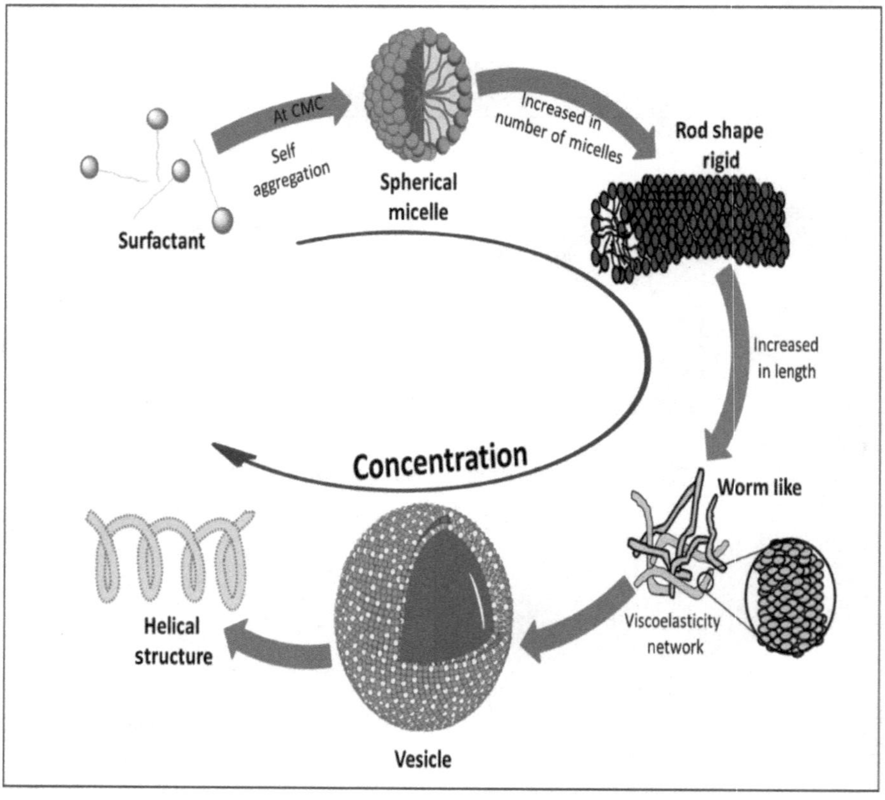

FIGURE 3.5 Different surfactant morphologies with increase in concentration.

TABLE 3.3
Interaction of dye–surfactant

Method	Surfactant (Types)	Mechanism of Dye Removal
Micelle formation	Anionic surfactants	Hydrophobic dye molecules can be solubilized and trapped in micelles' hydrophobic cores, removing them from solution.
	Cationic surfactants	Electrostatic forces between cationic surfactant micelles and negatively charged dye molecules generate insoluble complexes that are removed from the solution.
	Nonionic surfactants	Encapsulating hydrophobic dye molecules in nonionic surfactant micelles helps remove them from aqueous solutions.
	Amphoteric surfactants	In dye removal, amphoteric surfactants can interact with many dyes via electrostatic and hydrophobic interactions.
	Bio surfactants	Equilibration, solubilization, and surface adsorption by biosurfactant micelles can remove dyes.
	Polymeric surfactants	Polymeric surfactant micelles remove dye molecules by electrostatic and hydrophobic interactions.

the photochemical characteristics of the azo dye methyl orange are affected by its interaction with cationic micelles [37]. The impact of different surfactant types on the spectral characteristics of crystal violet as a function of surfactant concentration, spanning from below to above the critical micelle concentration (CMC). [38]. Sodium dodecyl sulfate (SDS) micelles caused curcumin to deteriorate quickly; however, cetyltrimethylammonium bromide (CTAB) or dodecyltrimethylammonium bromide (DTAB) micelles caused just 10% of the curcumin to decay. The interactions of curcumin with cationic single-chain surfactants were compared to those with cationic Gemini surfactant micelles (Figure 3.6) [39].

When dye micelles interact, electrostatic contact is a key factor in the process [40]. Due to its essential role in the dyeing process and dye removal, the interaction between dye and surfactant is interesting. Using different dyes and surfactant types in diverse media, multiple researchers have explored the nature and mechanism of dye–surfactant interaction because the structures of surfactants and dyes might vary greatly [41–45]. The cationic, anionic, or nonionic nature of a surfactant, absorption and/or fluorescence behavior below and above the CMC, ion-association processes, the impact of additives on these processes, etc., all play a significant role in the nature of the forces that cause dye molecules to bind with surfactant aggregates [46]. At various

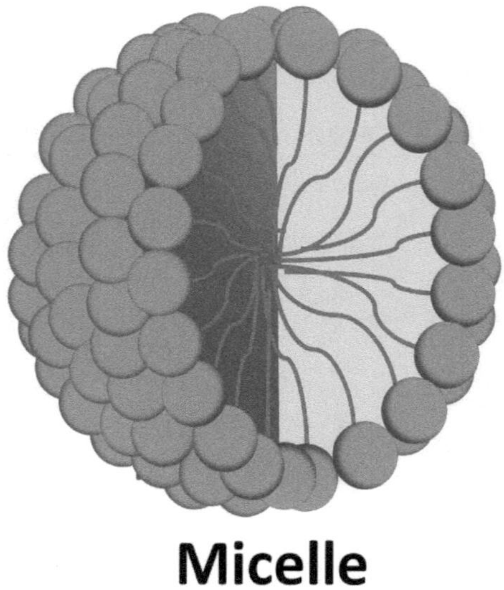

FIGURE 3.6 Structure of micelle.

surfactant concentrations, several equilibria are seen between surfactant monomers, micelles, dye aggregates, dye–surfactant pre-micellar complex, and dye particles absorbed into the micelles (Figure 3.7) [47]. Electrostatic repulsion forces are strong when a dye and a surfactant have the same charge, and the values of the complex formation constants are two to three orders smaller than they are in systems with dyes and surfactants that are charged in opposition to one another [42]. The negatively charged groups in the dye cause electrostatic contact between the surface of cationic surfactant micelles and anionic dyes [50]. This might be due to participation of van der Waals interactions (between neighboring surfactant chains and the dye organic moiety), hydration of the hydrophilic –SO; (or $-COO^-$) group, solvation of the aromatic ring of the dye by the $-CH_n$ group, and hydration of the hydrophilic –SO; (or $-COO^-$) group. According to the electronic characteristics for aromatic substituents [51], a –SO group interacts with the aromatic system less favorably than a $-COO^-$ group. The cationic end of the surfactant will tend to interact electrostatically less with the –COO group than with the –SO group in the latter instance because the negative charge is delocalized and dispersed throughout the terminal $-COO^-$ group and the aromatic ring [52]. Through the negatively charged groups of the dye, anionic dyes interact electrostatically with the surface of cationic surfactant micelles. The group's involvement is in the dye's aromatic ring's solvation and the dye's organic moiety's engagement in van der Waals interactions with nearby surfactant chains. The ionization of readily dissociable groups in the dye is caused by the ionic interaction of charged micelles with an aromatic dye through the group, which encourages electron withdrawal from the aromatic rings along the conjugated n-system [20]. van der Waals forces and hydrophobic interactions between identically charged dye particles are affected by the creation of the dye–surfactant complex, which also reduces the repulsion forces [28]. Strong electrostatic repulsion forces existed, and complex formation constant values were two to three orders lower than in systems containing

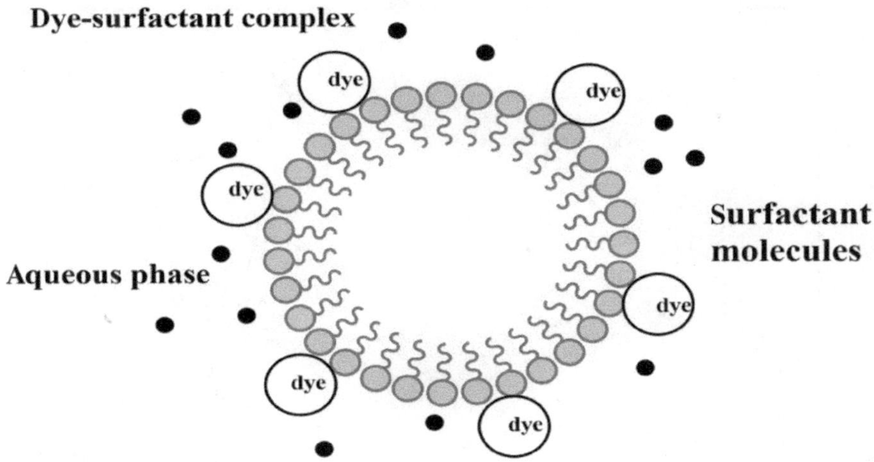

FIGURE 3.7 Structure of dye–micelle.

dyes and surfactants that were negatively and positively charged in opposition [28]. An interaction between surfactant dye molecule plays a significant role in the degradation process. In the case of Gemini surfactant, as surfactant concentration increases, intensity increases, but once it reaches its CMC, it remains constant. If the dye is in a polar environment below the CMC, due to high electrostatic contact, the dye intensity increases quickly as the concentration of Gemini does. This mechanism will be enhanced by changing the charge and nature of the Gemini molecules and dye molecules, respectively [53]. Micellar catalysis results from a difference in the rate of reaction of the substrate in the bulk solution and the micellar phase, as well as the distribution of the substrate between these two phases. Electrostatic and hydrophobic interactions between the micellar phase and the reactants, transition state, and products might be the cause of the shift in rate. In rare instances, it may also result from the structure of the water nearby [54–56].

3.3 DYE DEGRADATION BY MICELLAR SOLUTION

The conventional surfactant will interact with the dye molecule and make a premicellar structure by forming dimers and minimizing the mutual repulsive forces. This is verified by various analytical techniques [57–59]. The charge of the surfactant also plays a significant role in the gradual degradation of the dye molecules (Figure 3.8).

In a cationic micellar solution, the dye is solubilized in the hydrophobic core of the micelle and gradually degrades. The purpose of this study is to increase the solubility qualities of curcumin by using aggregates of mixed double- and single-chained cationic surfactants (Figure 3.9). Compared to single surfactant systems, they offer a more hydrophobic environment, have charges on the surface as well as in the center of the mixed vesicles, and are more stable in aggregation. A succession of double-chained surfactants with progressively longer chains is used to accomplish this. A series of competitive dynamic association–dissociation equilibriums, which may be

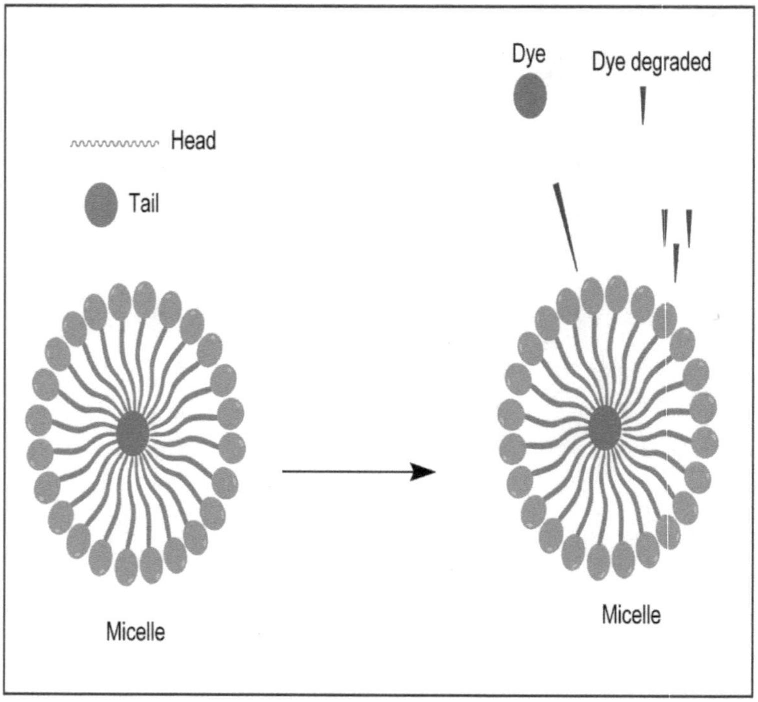

FIGURE 3.8 Schematic diagram of dye degradation.

thought of as global processes for the production of micelles, regulate the distribution of surfactant between various states of aggregation. The following process describes how the reaction takes place both in solution and micelles. Many studies have looked at how dye dissolves in surfactant micelles and degrades in alkaline environments. Dye occurs in the neutral state in the pH range of 1–7; when pH increases, the dye is deprotonated [62]. Studies on the solubilization and stability of dye in the presence of cationic surfactant tetradecyl trimethylammonium bromide (TTAB), nonionic surfactant Triton X-100, and anionic surfactant SDS were conducted in the pH range of 5–8. The findings indicated that SDS and Triton X-100 micelles were extremely effective in stabilizing the dye [63], This effect was generally not observed in the case of cationic surfactants CTAB and DTAB, while in anionic surfactant SDS, it was present generally by raising the alkalinity up to pH 13. Although just 10% of the dye degrades in the presence of either CTAB or DTAB micelles, the dye degrades quickly in the SDS micelles [64]. The greater electrostatic interaction between Cur3 and the Gemini micelle allowed the Gemini surfactant to maintain the dye more effectively [65]. Our knowledge of how dye degrades in the presence of these surfactants at varied amounts is improved by this study's additional understanding of the issue. It is discovered that a factor affecting the effectiveness of photodegradation is the solubility of the dye molecules. The photodegradation can be accelerated by a variety of nonionic surfactants, which can also increase dye degradation. When using cationic Gemini surfactant, the intensity increases with surfactant concentration and stays steady till it

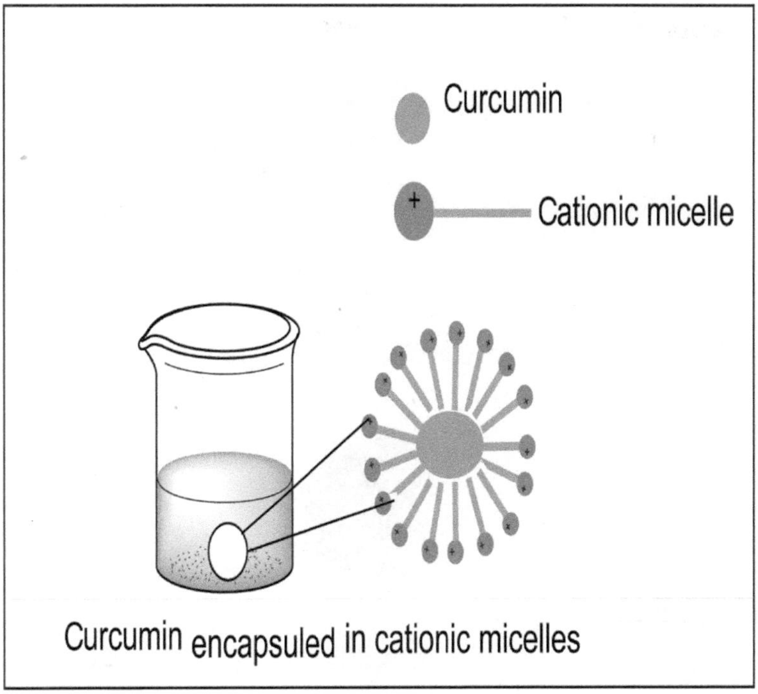

FIGURE 3.9 Dye degradation of curcumin in cationic micelles.

reaches CMC. Below the CMC, the dye is in a polar environment; when the surfactant concentration increases, the dye intensity increases quickly as a result of strong electrostatic contact, showing that the dye detects a more hydrophobic environment and is soluble in micellar medium (Figure 3.10) [65].

In an anionic micellar solution, dye molecules form strong bonds with sulfate or sulfonic ions. Due to their rigid and complex structure, nonionic surfactants form stable excited complexes with dye molecules. The cationic charge when the dye is deprotonated in an alkaline environment and the density of the surfactant head group play a significant role in electrostatic contact, preventing further degradation [60]. The rate of degradation was lowest (%) when cationic surfactants were present. Surfactant micelles, which also protect them from degeneration, can accommodate and dissolve curcumin molecules. Cationic micelles offer significantly more protection for curcumin than anionic or nonionic surfactants. The cationic head groups of the micelles stabilize the ionized curcumin by electrostatic forces. The higher charge density per surfactant molecule stabilizes curcmin, preventing its degradation in an alkaline environment much more effectively than DTAB. The ionized curcumin will be found in the head group region of the cationic micelle. Anionic and nonionic surfactants do not exhibit these desirable interactions, which increase solubilization and reduce degradation under alkaline conditions. In the case of Gemini surfactant, as surfactant concentration increases, intensity increases, but once it reaches its CMC, it remains constant. If the dye is in a polar environment below the CMC, due to

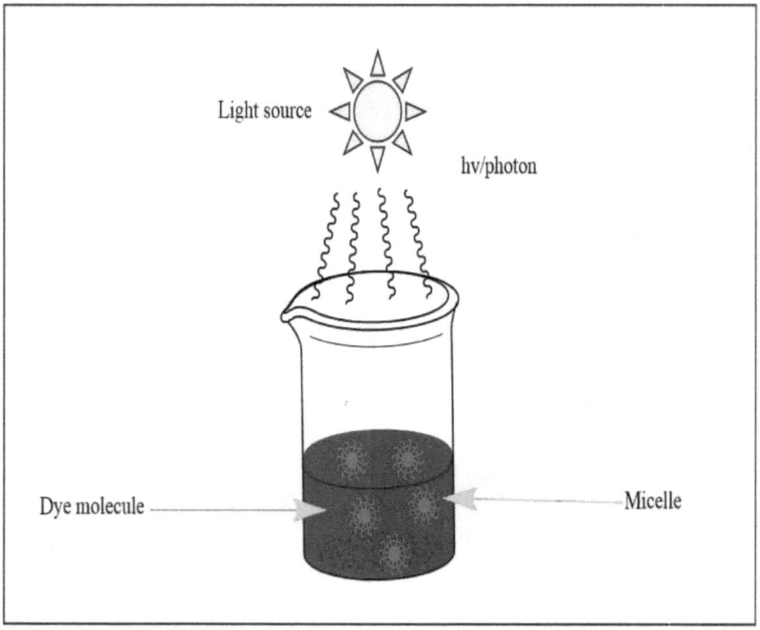

FIGURE 3.10 Dye degradation in aqueous micellar solution by external stimuli (light source).

high electrostatic contact, the dye intensity increases quickly as the concentration of Gemini does. This mechanism will be enhanced by changing the charge and nature of the Gemini and dye molecules, respectively. The degradation rate is influenced by surfactant (SDS) content. The target dye is degrading at about the CMC of SDS, and throughout the observed period, the degradation progressed to 94%. In comparison to the other two surfactants, SDS has a much higher micellar concentration, suggesting that the micelles generated are more than the dye molecules that need to be solubilized by the available micelles. We can assume that each micelle solubilizes one dye molecule; however, as more micelles are available, fewer dye molecules are encapsulated in each micelle than anticipated [61]. The structure of the tween 80 micelle is loose enough to allow the production of OH inside the micelle, but at a relatively slower rate, when OH is available outside or near the surface of the micelle. Nonionic surfactant is relatively wetter, so we can imagine a situation where Rhodamine B (RhB) is moving into and out of the micelles, which may allow the OH radical to oxidize the RhB molecules. It was discovered that there was no change in the spectra after examining the effects of CTAB and CPC on the absorption spectra of dye in areas of pre-micellar and micellar concentration. The repulsive interaction keeps dye in the bulk phase and prevents it from evaporating into CTAB or CPC micelles. This is due to the cationic dye's phenyl rings' electrostatic attraction and hydrophobic contact with the TTAB alkyl chain (tetradecyl trimethyl ammonium ion) as a result of dye solubilization in the micelle's hydrophobic center. DTAB intensity decreases with increasing surfactant content and pace, if another hydrogen source or sensitizer is present in the solution.

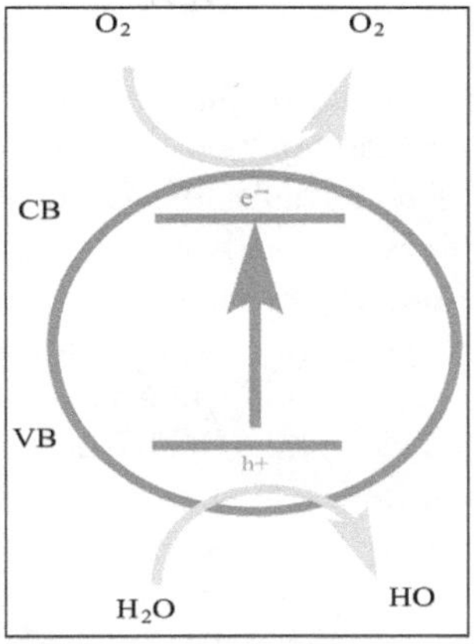

FIGURE 3.11 Schematic diagram of dye degradation mechanism.

Photodegradation of the dye might be further increased. The dye's color was purportedly eliminated along with the dye's photodegradation. The effectiveness of photodegradation is shown to be significantly influenced by the dye molecules' solubility. Numerous nonionic surfactants can accelerate photodegradation while simultaneously improving the solubility of dye (Figure 3.11). Conjugated chains or rings that absorb specific wavelength ranges give dye their color. Most organic dyes' chromophores are made up of C=C bonds, N=N bonds, aromatic rings, and heterocyclic rings with oxygen, nitrogen, or sulfur [62]. The cationic and nonionic surfactants' micellar environment considerably improved the rate of dye decolorization. All three surfactants, especially cationic micelles, had the strongest promoting activity when it came to increasing the decolorization of dye under micellar applications. A series of competitive dynamic association–dissociation equilibriums, which may be thought of as global processes for the production of micelles, regulate the distribution of surfactant between various states of aggregation. The following equations (Equations 3.1–3.3) describe how the reaction takes place both in solution and micelles [61].

$$\mathrm{nS + D} \xleftrightarrow{\mathrm{km}} \mathrm{SnD} \tag{3.1}$$

$$\mathrm{SnD} \xrightarrow{\mathrm{km[ox]}} \mathrm{Products} \tag{3.2}$$

$$\mathrm{D} \xrightarrow{\mathrm{km[ox]}} \mathrm{Products} \tag{3.3}$$

Here, S is the surfactant, D is the dye, n represents the number of surfactant molecules involved in the catalytic act, K_m is the dissociation constant of the catalytic micelle SnD, km[ox] is the rate constant in the micellar phase, in the aqueous medium. The rate is influenced by the K_m and the hydrogen-generating potential of the chosen surfactant. The degradation processes in micellar catalysis, research on reaction kinetics, intermediate species, and reaction mechanisms are essential.

3.4 FUTURE ASPECTS

The majority of studies on dye–surfactant interactions, according to a review of recent literature, have focused on the separation of dye molecules from wastewater utilizing anionic or cationic dyes and the molecules of their opposingly charged surfactants. Nonionic dyes, such as vat dyes, sulfur dyes, and dispersion dyes, which are frequently used to color both natural and synthetic colors, have not yet been the subject of any scientific studies on removal [63]. The discovery and development of new micellar catalysts with improved stability and catalytic activity may be the primary field of study. This could include creating catalytic nanoparticles or adding other cutting-edge elements to the micellar systems. Exploring the use of photocatalysis with micellar catalysis for dye degradation will be the key aspect for researchers. Photocatalytic micellar systems might use sun energy to increase the efficiency of degradation. To explore more, ecologically friendly and sustainable micellar catalytic methods will make use of biodegradable micellar systems and renewable surfactants. Using electrochemical dye degradation with micellar catalysis has advantages in terms of energy efficiency and controllability. This system can enhance dye degradation with interaction in an eco-friendly way to not release toxic molecules in the environment compared to photocatalytic degradation.

ABBREVIATIONS

AOPs advanced oxidation techniques
CMC critical micelle concentration
CTAB cetyltrimethylammonium bromide
DTAB dodecyltrimethylammonium bromide
RhB Rhodamine B
SDS sodium dodecyl sulfate
TTAB tetradecyl trimethylammonium bromide

REFERENCES

1. Sokolowska-Gajda, J., Freeman, H. S., and Reife, A. Synthetic dyes based on environmental considerations. Part 2: iron complexes formazan dyes. *Dyes and Pigments.* 30(1), 1–20, (1996). DOI: 10.1016/0143-7208(95)00048-8.
2. Field, M. S., Wilhelm, R. G., Quinlan, J. F., and Aley, T. J. An assessment of the potential adverse properties of fluorescent tracer dyes used for groundwater tracing. *Environmental Monitoring and Assessment.* 38(1), 75–96, (1995). DOI: 10.1007/bf00547128.
3. He, L. M., and Tebo B. M. Surface charge properties of and Cu (II) adsorption by spores of the marine *Bacillus* sp. strain SG-1. *Applied and Environmental Microbiology*, 64(3), 1123–1129, (1998). DOI: 10.1128/aem.64.3.1123-1129.1998.
4. Morgan-Sagastume J. M., Jimenez B., and Noyola A. Tracer studies in a laboratory and pilot scale UASB reactor. *Environmental Technology*, 18(8), 817–825, (1997). DOI: 10.1080/09593331808616600.
5. Hsu, T., and Chiang C. Activated sludge treatment of dispersed dye factory wastewater. *Journal of Environmental Science and Health. Part A: Environmental*

Science and Engineering and Toxicology, 32(7), 1921–1932, (1997). DOI: 10.1080/10934529709376655.

6. Głowacki, E. D., Voss, G., Leonat, L., Irimia-Vladu, M., Bauer S., and Sarıciftci, N. S. Indigo and tyrian purple – from ancient natural dyes to modern organic semiconductors. *Israel Journal of Chemistry*, 52, 1–12, (2015). DOI: 10.1002/ijch.201100130.
7. Ayad, M. M., and El-Nasr, A. A. Anionic dye (acid green 25) adsorption from water by using polyaniline nanotubes salt/silica composite. *Journal of Nanostructure Chemistry*, 3(3), 2–9, (2012). DOI: 10.1186/2193-8865-3-3.
8. Hunger, K. *Industrial Dyes: Chemistry, Properties, Applications. Wiley-VCH, Weinheim*, 47, (2003).
9. Pereira, L. and Alves, M. Dyes-environmental impact and remediation. In: Malik, A. and Grohmann, E. (Eds.), *Environmental Protection Strategies for Sustainable Development, Strategies for Sustainability*. Springer, New York. 111–162, (2012). DOI: 10.1007/978-94-007-1591-2_4.
10. Gupta, V. K., Suhas, M., and Burkinshaw, S. M. *Physico-chemical Aspects of Textile Coloration*. John Wiley & Sons, Hoboken. 2313–2342, (2009).
11. Considine, D. M. *Van Nostrand's Scientific Encyclopaedia*. Springer, New York, USA, (1995). DOI: 10.1007/978-3-319-33892-7.
12. Muthu, S. S. and Khadir, A. *Advanced Removal Techniques for Dye-containing Wastewaters*. Springer, (2021). DOI: 10.1007/978-981-16-3164-1.
13. Dabrowski A. Adsorption – from theory to practice. Azo dye in water using H_2O_2/UV photo Fenton treatment. *Journal of Hazardous Materials*. 174, 352–356, (2010).
14. Gul S. and Ozcan Yildlrln O. Degradation of reactive red 194 and reactive yellow 145 azo dyes by O_3 and H_2O_2/UV-C process. *Chemical Engineering Journal,* 155, 684–690, (2009).
15. Al-Hamedi F. H., Rauf M. A., and Asraf S. S. Degradation of Rhodamine B in the presence of UV/H_2O_2. *Desalination*, 239, 159–166, (2009). DOI: 10.1016/j.desal.2008.03.016.
16. Anacker, E. W. J. Modeling dye–surfactant interactions. *Colloid Interface Science*, 164(1), 54–62, (1994). DOI: 10.1006/jcis.1994.1143.
17. Liang, K., Law, K.-Y., and Whitten D. G. Multiple aggregation of surfactant squaraines in Langmuir–Blodgett films and in DMSO-water mixtures G. *Journal of Physical Chemistry*, 98, 13379–13384, (1994). DOI: 10.1021/j100101a043.
18. Tanaka, F., Harada, Y., Ikeda, N., Aratono, M., and Motomura, K., Bull. Interaction of acid dyes with sodium dodecyl sulfate in adsorbed film and micelle. *Chemical Society of Japan*, 36, 2367–2378, (1994). DOI: 10.5650/jos1956.43.704.
19. Tanaka, F., Harada, Y., Todoroki, N., Aratono, M., and Motomura, K. Bull. Interaction of sodium 4′-(butylamino)azobenzene-4-sulfonate with 2-(octylsulfinyl) ethanol in adsorbed film and micelle. *Chemical Society of Japan*, 66(7), 1929–1933, (1993). DOI: 10.1246/bcsj.66.1929.
20. Span, J., Simoni, B., Forte, P., and Brarko, S. A study of dye-surfactant interactions. Part 1. Effect of chemical structure of acid dyes and surfactants on the complex formation. *Dyes and Pigments*, 36(1), 1–14, (1995). DOI: 10.1016/S0143-7208(97)00001-6.
21. Bielska, M., Sobczynska, A., and Prochaska, K. Dye–surfactant interaction in aqueous solutions. *Dyes and Pigments*, 80(2), 201–205, (2009). DOI: 10.1016/j.dyepig.2008.05.009.

22. Chandravanshi, S., and Upadhyay, S. K. Natural dye-surfactant interactions: thermodynamic and surface parameters. *Coloration Technology*, 128, 300–305, (2012). DOI: 10.1111/j.1478-4408.2012.00380.x.
23. Ortona, O., Vitagliano, V., and Robinson, B. H. Dye interactions with surfactants in colloidal dispersions. *Journal of Colloid and Interface Science*, 125, 271–278, (1988). DOI: 10.1016/0021-9797(88)90075-6.
24. Simoncic, B., and Kert, M. A study of anionic dye–cationic surfactant interactions in mixtures of cationic and nonionic surfactants. *Dyes and Pigments*, 54, 221–237, (2002). DOI: 10.1016/S0143-7208(02)00046-3.
25. Garcia, M. E. D. and Sanz-Medel, A. Dye–surfactant interactions: a review. *Talanta*, 33(3), 255–264, (1986). DOI: 10.1016/0039-9140(86)80060-1.
26. Rashid T. U., Kabir, S. F. M., Biswas, M. C., and Bhuiyan, M. A. R. Sustainable wastewater treatment via dye surfactant interaction: a critical review. *Industrial and Engineering Chemistry Research*, 59(21), 9719–9745, (2020). DOI: 10.1021/acs.iecr.0c00676.
27. Gokturk, S., and Tuncay, M., Dye-surfactant interaction in the premicellar region. *Journal of Surfactants and Detergents*, 6, 325–330, (2003). DOI: 10.1007/s11743-003-0277-y.
28. Mouxiou, E., Eleftheriadis, I., Nikolaidis, N., and Tsatsaroni, E. Reactive dyeing of cellulosic fibers: use of cationic surfactants and their interaction with reactive dyes. *Journal of Applied Polymer Science*, 108, 1209–1215, (2008). DOI: 10.1002/app.27705.
29. Moulik, S. P. and Ghosh, S. Interfacial and micellization behaviors of binary and ternary mixtures of amphiphiles (tween-20, Brij-35, and sodium dodecyl sulfate) in aqueous medium. *Journal Molecular Liquids*, 208, 357–366, (1997). DOI: 10.1006/jcis.1998.5752.
30. Ghosh, S. Surface chemical and micellar properties of binary and ternary surfactant mixtures (cetyl pyridinium chloride, tween-40, and brij-56) in an aqueous medium. *Journal of Colloid Interface Science*, 244, 128–138, (2001). DOI: 10.1006/jcis.2001.7855.
31. Chakraborty, T., Chakraborty, I., and Ghosh, S. The methods of determination of critical micellar concentrations of the amphiphilic systems in aqueous medium. *Arabian Journal of Chemistry*, 4, 265–270, (2011). DOI: 10.1016/j.arabjc.2010.06.045.
32. Fendler, J. *Catalysis in Micellar and Macromoleular Systems*. Elsevier, New York, 2012.
33. Garcia-Rio, L. Hervella, P., Mejuto, J. C., and Parajo, M. Spectroscopic and kinetic investigation of the interaction between crystal violet and sodium dodecylsulfate. *Chemical Physics*, 335(2–3), 164–176, (2007). DOI: 10.1016/j.chemphys.2007.04.006.
34. Tadros, T. F. *Applied Surfactants: Principle, Applications*. Wiley, Morlenbach, 13, 2005.
35. Rempp, P. F. and Franta, E. (1984). Macromonomers: synthesis, characterization and applications. In: *Polymerization Reactions. Advances in Polymer Science*. Springer, Berlin, Heidelberg, 58. DOI: 10.1007/3-540-12793-3_6.
36. Astray, G., Cid, A., Manso, J. A., Mejuto, J. C., Moldes, O. A., and Morales, J. Alkaline fading of triarylmethyl carbocations in self-assembly micro heterogeneous media. *Progress in Reaction Kinetics and Mechanism*, 36(2), 139–165, (2011). DOI: 10.3184/146867811X12984793755693.
37. Dasmandal, S., Mandal, H. K., Kundu, A., and Mahapatra, A. Kinetic investigations on alkaline fading of malachite green in the presence of micelles and reverse

micelles. *Journal of Molecular Liquid*, 193, 123–131, (2014). DOI: 10.1016/j.molliq.2013.12.017.
38. Zhang, Y., Li, X., Liu, J., and Zeng, J. Micellar catalysis of composite reactions – The effect of SDS micelles and premicelles on the alkaline fading of crystal violet and malachite green. *Journal of Dispersion Science Technology*, 23, 473–48, (2002). DOI: 10.1081/DIS-120014015.
39. Gehlen, M. G., Ferreira, M., and Neumann, M. G. Interaction of methyl orange with cationic micelles and its effect on dye photochemistry. *Journal of Photochemistry and Photobiology A: Chemistry*, 87, 55–60, (1995). DOI: 10.1016/1010-6030(94)03956-U.
40. Ghosh, S., Mondal, S., Das. S., and Biswas, R. Spectroscopic investigation of interaction between crystal violet and various surfactants (cationic, anionic, nonionic and gemini) in aqueous solution. *Fluid Phase Equilibria*, 332, 1–6, (2012). DOI: 10.1016/j.fluid.2012.06.019.
41. Leung, M. H., Colangelo, H., and Kee, T. W. Encapsulation of curcumin in cationic micelles suppresses alkaline hydrolysis. *Langmuir*, 24, 5672–5675, (2008). DOI: 10.1021/la800780w.
42. Shah, S. S., Ahmed, R., Shah, S. W. H., Asif, K. M., and Naeem K. Synthesis of cationic hemi cyanine dyes and their interactions with ionic surfactants. *Colloids and Surfaces A: Physicochemical and Engineering Aspects*, 137, 301–305, (1998). DOI: 10.1016/S0927-7757(97)00384-1.
43. Candravanshi, S. and Upadhyay, S. K. Natural dye–surfactant interactions: thermodynamic and surface parameters. *Coloration Technology*, 128, 300–305, (2012). DOI: 10.1111/j.1478-4408.2012.00380.x.
44. Rashidi-Alavijeh, M., Javadian, S., Gharibi, H., Moradi, M., Tehrani-Bagha, A. R., Shahir, A. A. Intermolecular interactions between a dye and cationic surfactants: effects of alkyl chain, head group, and counterion. *Colloids and Surfaces A: Physicochemical and Engineering Aspects,* 380, 119–127,(2011). DOI: 10.1016/j.colsurfa.2011.02.011
45. Ramadan, M. Sh., El-Mallah, N. M., Nabil, G. M., Abd-Elmenem, S. M. Hydrophobic effect for anionic dye–cationic surfactant interaction in aqueous and mixed solvent. *Journal of Dispersion Science and Technology,* 40, 1110–1120, (2018).DOI:10.1080/01932691.2018.1496837.
46. Pereira, R. V. and Gehlen, M. H. Fluorescence of acridinic dyes in anionic surfactant solution. *Spectrochimica Acta Part A: Molecular and Biomolecular Spectroscopy*, 61, 2926–2932, (2005). DOI: 10.1016/j.saa.2004.11.009.
47. Gokturk, S. and Tunçay, M. Spectral studies of Safranin-O in different surfactant solutions. *Spectrochimica Acta Part A: Molecular and Biomolecular Spectroscopy*, 59, 1857–1866, (2003). DOI: 10.1016/S1386-1425(02)00418-3.
48. Savvin, S. B., Marov, I. N., Chernova, R. K., Shtykov, S. N., and Sokolov, A. B. Electrostatic and hydrophobic effect in the formation of associates of organic reagents with cationic surfactants *Journal of Analytical Chemistry*. 36(5), 850, (1981).
49. Gracia, M. D., Sanz-Medel, A. Dye-surfactant interaction: a review. *Advances in Drug Research,* 33, (1979).
50. Bailey B. W., Chester J. E., Dagnall R. M., and West T. S. Analytical applications of ternary complexes-VII1: elucidation of mode of formation of sensitized metal-chelate systems and determination of molybdenum and antimony. *Talanta*, 15, 1359–1369, (1968). DOI: 10.1016/0039-9140(68)80195-X.
51. Moulik, S. P., Ghosh, S., and Das, A. R. Interaction of acridine orange monohydrochloride dye with sodium dodecylsulfate (SDS), cetyltrimethylammonium

bromide (CTAB) and p-tert-octylphenoxypolyoxyethanol (Triton X-100). *Colloid and Polymer Science*, 257, 645-655, (1979). DOI: https://doi.org/10.1007/BF01548834.

52. Cordes, E. H. and Gittler, H. Reaction kinetics in the presence of micelle forming surfactant. *Progress in Bioorganic Chemistry,* 25, 1–10, (1973).
53. Sharma, S., and Kaur, A. Various methods for removal of dyes from industrial effluents – a review. *Indian Journal of Science and Technology*, 11, (2018). DOI: 10.17485/ijst/2018/v11i12/120847.
54. Duxbury D. -F. The photochemistry and photophysics of triphenylmethane dyes in solid and liquid media. *Chemical Reviews*, 93, 381–433, (1993). DOI: 10.1021/cr00017a018.
55. Henderson, B. W. and Dougherty, T. J. (Eds.). Basic principles and clinical applications. *Photodynamic Therapy*, 480, (1992). DOI: 10.1201/9781003066897.
56. Sarkar, M. and Poddar, S. Studies on the interaction of surfactants with cationic dye by absorption spectroscopy. *Journal of Colloid Interface Science*, 221, 181–185, (2000). DOI: 10.1006/jcis.1999.657.
57. Sharma, R., Kamal, A., Mahajan, R. K. Detailed study of interactions between eosin yellow and gemini pyridinium surfactants. *RSC advances*, 6(75), 71692-71704, (2016). DOI: 10.1039/C6RA12056C
58. Aboudiab, B., Ali, R. T.-B., and Patra, D. Curcumin degradation kinetics in micellar solutions: enhanced stability in the presence of cationic surfactants. *Colloids and Surfaces A: Physicochemical and Engineering Aspects*, 592, 124, (2020). DOI: 10.1016/j.colsurfa.2020.124602.
59. Carriere, J., Jones, J. P., and Broadbent, A. D. Decolorization of textile wastewaters by ozonation. In: *Photodegradation Mechanism and Rate Improvement of Chlorinated Aromatic Dye in Non-ionic Surfactant Solutions*. 35, 232, (1991).
60. Kinugasa, T., Ohta, A., and Nishii, Y. Removal and recovery of acid azo dyes by solvent extraction using cetyltrimethylammonium chloride. *Separation Science and Technology*, 50, 1369–1376, (2015). DOI: 10.1080/01496395.2014.967776.
61. Bunton C. A. The dependence of micellar rate effects upon reaction mechanism. *Advances in Colloid Interface Science*, 123–126, 333–343, (2006). DOI: 10.1016/j.cis.2006.05.008.
62. Lee, W. H., Loo, C. Y., Bebawy, M., Luk, F., Mason, R. S., and Rohanizadeh, R. Curcumin and its derivatives: their application in neuropharmacology and neuroscience in the 21st century. *Current Neuropharmacology*, 11, 338–378, (2013). DOI: 10.2174/1570159X11311040002.
63. Tønnesen, H. H. Solubility, chemical and photochemical stability of curcumin in surfactant solutions. Studies of curcumin and curcuminoids, XXVIII. *Die Pharmazie*, 57, 820–824, (2002).
64. Wan, Z., Ke, D., Hong, J., Ran, Q., Wang, X., Chen, Z., An, X., and Shen, W. Comparative study on the interactions of cationic Gemini and single-chain surfactant micelles with curcumin. *Colloids and Surfaces A: Physicochemical and Engineering Aspects*, 414, 267–273, (2012). DOI: 10.1016/j.colsurfa.2012.08.046.
65. Soumen, G., Mondal, S., Das, S., and Biswas, R. Spectroscopic investigation of interaction between crystal violet and various surfactants (cationic, anionic, nonionic and Gemini) in aqueous solution. *Fluid Phase Equilibria*, 332, 1–6, (2012). DOI: 10.1016/j.fluid.2012.06.019.

4 Electrocatalysis for Dye Degradation

Podilapu Atchutha Rao, Anil Kumar Behera, Preeti Nanda Sahu, Ravi Kumar Ganta, Rahul Shukla, Harihara Padhy, and Anik Sen

4.1 INTRODUCTION

4.1.1 Background

A challenging issue has been the degradation of dyes and other organic contaminants. Only 45–47% of dyes have been recognized as organic colors that can be easily dissolved in water and biodegrade. The remaining hues are hazardous, and there is currently discussion over their continued existence in wastewater [1]. Azo and anthraquinone dyes, which account for 70% and 15% of all color groups, are the most widely used dyes in the textile industry. Approximately 900,000 tonnes of dye are produced annually, with approximately 15% of synthetic dyes being released as effluents during production. Several adverse health consequences, such as immunological suppression, respiratory difficulties, deviations of the central nervous system (CNS), behavioral disorders, allergic reactions, tissue necrosis, and eye infections, can be brought on by using polluted water. Dye degradation in wastewater has consequently grown to be an important problem in the fight against pollution [2–4]. Dyes are organic compounds that impart color to various substrates such as textiles, paper, leather, and plastics. They have been used for centuries to add color to textiles and have become essential in various industries, including fashion, printing, and painting. Dyes are divided into several categories based on their origin, solubility, and application [5].

4.1.2 Significance of Dye Degradation

Dye degradation is of significant importance due to its environmental implications and the need for sustainable solutions in various industries. The degradation of dyes plays a crucial role in the treatment of wastewater from textile, paper, and dye manufacturing industries, as well as in the remediation of contaminated sites. Here are some key points highlighting the significance of dye degradation:

Environmental impact: Dyes, especially synthetic ones, are a major source of water pollution. They can have adverse effects on aquatic ecosystems by reducing light penetration, depleting dissolved oxygen, and disrupting the balance of

DOI: 10.1201/9781003441083-4

flora and fauna. Dye degradation processes help mitigate these harmful effects by breaking down dyes into less toxic compounds.

Wastewater treatment: Dye-containing wastewater is often discharged from textile, paper, and dye manufacturing industries. Treating such wastewater before it is released into the environment is crucial for maintaining water quality standards. Dye degradation methods, such as photocatalysis, biological degradation, and advanced oxidation processes, aid in the removal of dyes and their by-products, making the treated water safer for the environment [6].

Resource conservation: The degradation of dyes allows for the recovery and reuse of valuable resources. Some dyes are derived from non-renewable sources, making their extraction unsustainable. By degrading dyes and recovering their components, such as organic compounds or metals, the recycling and reuse of these resources become feasible, reducing the demand for virgin materials [7].

Remediation of contaminated sites: Dyes and their breakdown products can persist in the environment for long periods, leading to soil and groundwater contamination. Dye degradation technologies can be employed in the remediation of contaminated sites, facilitating the breakdown of dyes, and reducing their environmental impact [8].

4.1.3 Challenges in Dye Degradation

Dye molecules are known for their complex nature, which arises from their intricate chemical structures. These molecules are designed to possess vibrant colors and high stability, enabling them to withstand various environmental conditions and chemical treatments. However, this complexity also contributes to the difficulty in their complete degradation. Here are some key factors that highlight the challenges associated with the degradation of dye molecules:

Chemical diversity: Dye molecules encompass a wide range of chemical structures, including aromatic compounds, azo dyes, anthraquinones, and phthalocyanines, among others. Each type of dye possesses unique molecular arrangements and functional groups, making their degradation pathways diverse and complex [9].

Stability: Dyes are designed to exhibit excellent color fastness and stability, which means they resist fading and maintain their vibrant hues even in the presence of light, heat, and chemical agents. These stability features are a result of the structural modifications and chemical bonds present in dye molecules, which render them resistant to degradation [10].

High chromophore density: Dyes typically contain multiple chromophores, which are responsible for their coloration. Chromophores are conjugated systems of alternating single and double bonds or contain extended electron delocalization. The high density of chromophores in dye molecules enhances their color intensity but also makes them more resistant to degradation [11].

Complex molecular structures: Dye molecules often possess large, complex structures with multiple branches, substituents, and functional groups. These features make it challenging for enzymes or chemical agents to access and break down the dye molecules effectively. Additionally, the presence of various functional groups can lead to the formation of stable dye intermediates during degradation, further complicating the process [12].

Synthetic dye variants: Synthetic dyes, widely used in industries such as textiles, printing, and cosmetics, are often designed to be resistant to fading and chemical degradation. Many of these synthetic dyes are derived from petrochemical sources and incorporate complex synthetic routes to achieve the desired colors and properties. These synthetic variants often lack natural degradation pathways, making their complete breakdown more difficult [13].

Environmental persistence: Dye molecules are frequently released into the environment through industrial effluents or consumer products. Due to their stability and resistance to degradation, dyes can persist in water bodies, soil, and sediments for extended periods, leading to environmental pollution and potential harm to ecosystems [14].

Toxicity concerns: Some dye molecules, especially those containing heavy metals or aromatic amines, can pose environmental and health risks due to their toxic properties. The incomplete degradation of these dyes can lead to the release of harmful intermediates or by-products, further emphasizing the need for effective and complete degradation methods [15].

Addressing the complete degradation of dye molecules remains a significant challenge. Researchers are actively exploring various approaches, including advanced oxidation processes, enzymatic treatments, photocatalysis, and bioremediation, to develop efficient and sustainable methods for the degradation and removal of dyes from the environment.

4.1.4 Role of Electrocatalysis

Electrocatalysis, the process of using an electric current to drive chemical reactions, holds promise as a potential solution for enhancing the degradation efficiency of dyes. By employing electrocatalysis, the degradation of dye molecules can be accelerated, and their complete breakdown can be achieved more effectively. Here's how electrocatalysis offers a potential solution in the context of dye degradation:

Generation of reactive species: Electrocatalysis can generate reactive species, such as hydroxyl radicals ($^{\bullet}OH$) and oxygen species ($O2^{\bullet -}$), through electrochemical reactions. These reactive species are highly oxidizing and can effectively attack and degrade dye molecules. The electrochemical oxidation process enables the production of these species directly at the electrode surface, providing a localized and controlled environment for efficient degradation [16].

Enhanced mass transport: Electrochemical systems can facilitate enhanced mass transport of the reactants to the electrode surface. By applying an electric potential, the convection and diffusion of dye molecules towards the electrode can be increased, ensuring a higher concentration of dyes in the vicinity of the catalytic surface. This improved mass transport enables more frequent collisions between the dye molecules and reactive species, enhancing the degradation efficiency [17].

Surface reactions and adsorption: Electrodes used in electrocatalysis often possess specific surface properties, such as high surface area, tailored surface chemistry, or the presence of active sites. These surface characteristics facilitate the adsorption of dye molecules onto the electrode surface, providing a proximity for degradation reactions. The surface reactions between the adsorbed dye molecules and the generated reactive species contribute to the enhanced degradation efficiency.

Tuneable electrochemical parameters: Electrocatalysis offers the advantage of tunable electrochemical parameters, such as electrode potential and current density. These parameters can be optimized to maximize the degradation efficiency based on the specific dye molecules and electrocatalytic materials used. By adjusting the applied potential and current, the electrochemical system can be fine-tuned to promote efficient degradation without causing unwanted side reactions [18].

Catalyst design: Electrodes and catalyst materials can be specifically designed to enhance the electrocatalytic activity toward dye degradation. Various catalysts, including metal oxides, carbon-based materials, and modified electrodes, have shown promising catalytic properties for dye degradation. These catalysts can be tailored to provide high surface area, improved charge transfer kinetics, and catalytic sites to facilitate the electrochemical oxidation of dye molecules [19].

Potential for continuous operation: Electrocatalysis can be implemented in continuous flow systems, allowing for continuous dye degradation. This feature is particularly advantageous for industrial-scale applications, where a steady and efficient dye removal process is required. Continuous electrocatalytic systems can be integrated into wastewater treatment plants or industrial processes, providing a sustainable and scalable solution for dye degradation [20].

While electrocatalysis shows promise for enhancing the degradation efficiency of dyes, further research and development are needed to optimize the electrocatalytic materials, operating conditions, and system design for different dye molecules and application scenarios. Nonetheless, electrocatalysis represents a potential solution that combines the advantages of efficient dye degradation, controllable process parameters, and scalability for addressing the challenges associated with dye pollution.

4.2 ELECTROCATALYSIS

Electrolysis is a promising technique for the degradation of dye pollutants in wastewater. Dyes are widely used in various industries, such as textiles, paper, and leather, and are notorious for their resistance to biodegradation and their toxicity to aquatic organisms. Electrolysis, also known as electrochemical oxidation, is an advanced oxidation process that utilizes an electrical current to generate reactive species such as hydroxyl radicals, which can oxidize organic pollutants including dyes. Several studies have reported successful degradation of various dye pollutants using electrolysis, and the process has shown to be effective even for complex dye mixtures. Furthermore, electrolysis can be performed at ambient temperature and pressure, making it a cost-effective and environmentally friendly approach for dye removal. In this context, this chapter will review the recent advances in the application of electrolysis for dye degradation in wastewater. The chapter will cover the types of dyes, the basic principles of the electrolysis process, the factors affecting the performance of electrolysis, and the challenges and opportunities associated with the implementation of electrolysis in industrial settings.

4.2.1 Electrochemical Principles

Any process that is either brought on or accompanied by the flow of an electric current and often involves the transfer of electrons between two substances, one of which is a solid and the other a liquid, is known as an electrochemical reaction. There are many chemical reactions that, when allowed to proceed in contact with two electronic conductors, separated by conducting lines, liberate what is known as electrical energy, resulting in the generation of an electric current. Under normal circumstances, a chemical reaction is accompanied by the liberation or absorption of heat and not any other form of energy. On the other hand, many chemical processes that do not happen naturally may be induced by the energy of an electric current. When properly organized, a process that directly converts chemical energy into electrical energy is referred to as an electrical cell. An electrolytic process is one in which electrical energy is instantly transformed into chemical energy.

There are many chemical reactions that, when allowed to proceed in contact with two electronic conductors, separated by conducting lines, liberate what is known as electrical energy, resulting in the generation of an electric current. Under normal circumstances, a chemical reaction is accompanied by the liberation or absorption of heat and not any other form of energy. On the other hand, many chemical processes that do not happen naturally may be induced by the energy of an electric current. When properly organized, a process that directly converts chemical energy into electrical energy is referred to as an electrical cell. An electrolytic process is one in which electrical energy is instantly transformed into chemical energy. A significant percentage of the electrical energy used in the electrolysis may be recovered if this reverse reaction is permitted to take place under the right circumstances. The process of electrolysis used to charge an accumulator results in a chemical change due to the electric current flowing through it. The accumulator functions as a cell that generates an electric current during the discharge of the cell when the opposite chemical reaction takes place.

4.2.2 Electrocatalysis Concepts

Electrocatalysis is a process that involves the use of a catalyst to facilitate electrochemical reactions. It plays a crucial role in various electrochemical systems, including dye degradation reactions. Dye degradation refers to the process of breaking down organic dyes into simpler and less harmful compounds, typically through oxidation reactions.

In the context of dye degradation, electrocatalysis utilizes a catalyst to enhance the rate of the electrochemical oxidation of dye molecules. The catalyst acts as a mediator, facilitating the transfer of electrons between the electrode and the dye molecules, thus promoting their degradation. It lowers the activation energy required for the reaction, allowing it to proceed more rapidly and efficiently [20]. Electrocatalysts used in dye degradation reactions are typically materials with high electrical conductivity and high catalytic activity. Commonly used electrocatalysts include metal oxides, metal chalcogenides, metallo-porphyrins, carbon-based materials (such as carbon nanotubes and graphene), and various composite materials [21]. The electrocatalytic process involves several steps. First, the dye molecules are adsorbed onto the surface of the electrode. Then, under the influence of an applied electric potential, the catalyst facilitates the transfer of electrons from the electrode to the dye molecules, leading to their oxidation. The oxidized dye molecules subsequently undergo further reactions, such as fragmentation or mineralization, resulting in the degradation of the dye [22]. Electrocatalysis offers several advantages for dye degradation reactions compared to other conventional methods. It provides a more selective and controlled degradation process, allowing for efficient removal of dyes from wastewater. Additionally, electrocatalysis can be performed under milder conditions, such as ambient temperature and pressure, reducing energy consumption and operational costs. It also offers the potential for the regeneration and reuse of the catalyst, making it a more sustainable approach [23].

4.2.3 Classification of Electrocatalysts

Electrocatalysts used in various electrochemical reactions can be classified into different types based on their composition and properties. Here are some commonly encountered types of electrocatalysts:

Metal-based electrocatalysts: These electrocatalysts are composed of metals or metal alloys. They possess excellent electrical conductivity and often exhibit high catalytic activity. Examples include platinum (Pt), palladium (Pd), gold (Au), silver (Ag), and their alloys. Metal-based electrocatalysts are widely used in fuel cells, water splitting, and various other electrochemical processes [24].

Metal oxide electrocatalysts: These electrocatalysts are composed of metal oxides and are often used in a wide range of electrochemical reactions. Metal oxides, such as iridium oxide (IrO_x), ruthenium oxide (RuO_x), and manganese oxide (MnO_x), exhibit high catalytic activity, stability, and resistance to corrosion. They find applications in water oxidation, oxygen evolution reaction (OER), and other redox processes [25].

Carbon-based electrocatalysts: Carbon-based materials, including carbon nanotubes (CNTs), graphene, and carbon nanofibers, are widely studied electrocatalysts. They possess high electrical conductivity, large surface area, and excellent chemical stability. Carbon-based electrocatalysts are used in various reactions such as oxygen reduction reaction (ORR), hydrogen evolution reaction (HER), and organic molecule oxidation [26, 27].

Composite electrocatalysts: Composite electrocatalysts are composed of multiple materials combined to achieve synergistic effects and enhanced catalytic performance. For example, metal nanoparticles (NPs) supported on carbon or metal oxides, such as Pt/C or Pt-TiO_x, exhibit improved catalytic activity and stability compared to individual components [28, 29].

4.2.4 Selection Criteria for Electrocatalysts

Dye degradation methods are employed to remove synthetic dyes from wastewater, which can be harmful to the environment if not properly treated. Various methods for dye degradation exist, including physical, chemical, and biological methods. Some commonly used methods, along with their references, are as follows [30, 31].

4.2.4.1 Physical Methods

Physical methods such as adsorption, filtration, and photodegradation are used to remove dyes from wastewater. Adsorption involves the use of materials like activated carbon, clay, and zeolites to adsorb dyes from wastewater. Filtration involves the use of membranes or filters to remove dyes from wastewater. Photodegradation uses UV or visible light to break down the dye molecules into simpler compounds.

4.2.4.2 Chemical Methods

Chemical methods, such as oxidation, reduction, electrocatalysis, advanced oxidation process, and chemical coagulation, are used to degrade dyes from wastewater. Oxidation involves the use of chemicals like hydrogen peroxide, ozone, and persulphate to oxidize dyes. Reduction involves the use of chemicals like sodium sulfite or sodium bisulfite to reduce dyes. Electrocatalysis involves the release of hydroxyl radicles to degrade the dyes. Chemical coagulation involves the use of chemicals like alum or ferric chloride to coagulate the dyes, which can be easily removed.

4.2.4.3 Biological Methods

Biological methods involve the use of microorganisms, such as bacteria, fungi, and algae, to degrade dyes from wastewater. These microorganisms use the dyes as a source of carbon and energy. Biodegradation can occur under aerobic or anaerobic conditions, depending on the microorganism involved.

Among all, electrocatalysis is a promising method for the degradation of dyes in wastewater due to its high efficiency, selectivity, and sustainability. Electrocatalysis uses an electrode to catalyze a reaction that can degrade the dye molecules into simpler, non-toxic compounds. Here are some reasons why electrocatalysis is a good method for dye degradation [32–34].

4.2.4.4 High Efficiency

Electrocatalysis is a highly efficient method for dye degradation, as it can achieve a high degree of dye removal in a short time. The electrochemical process can also operate at room temperature and atmospheric pressure, making it more energy-efficient than other methods.

4.2.4.5 Selectivity

Electrocatalysis is a selective method that can target specific dyes for degradation. By selecting the appropriate electrode and electrocatalyst, it is possible to achieve selective degradation of specific dye molecules while leaving other pollutants intact.

4.2.4.6 Sustainability

Electrocatalysis is a sustainable method for dye degradation, as it does not produce any secondary pollutants or waste. The process is also compatible with renewable energy sources, such as solar and wind power, making it an environmentally friendly option.

4.2.5 Electrocatalysis (Advanced Oxidation Process)

Electrochemical approaches have attracted particular attention for wastewater clean-up during the past ten years [35, 36]. Electrocoagulation, electrochemical reduction, electrochemical oxidation, indirect electrooxidation with strong oxidants (electrooxidation with active chlorine, electro-Fenton), and photo-assisted electrochemical techniques (photo electro-Fenton, photo electrocatalysis) are some of the electrochemical techniques used to remove the dye [37]. Additionally, they provide benefits including easy operation, reduced operating temperatures, and the usage of basic equipment. It is noteworthy to note that with good use of energy resources, greater amounts of contaminating compounds may be eliminated with the use of less energy and more dye. According to the generalized process described below, when an electric current initiates a redox reaction on an electrode's surface, the organic molecules are transformed and destroyed and completely oxidized to CO_2 and H_2O [38].

Any one of the following methods can be used to conduct electrochemical oxidation (EO) of dyes in an electrochemical cell.

1. Direct anodic oxidation results in extremely poor decontamination as the redox reaction occurs during the cyclic process (at anode oxidation and cathode reduction reaction).
2. Chemical process where water discharge at the anode produces OH and the reaction occurs through the electrogenerated species. For instance, "active oxygen" that is chemically adsorbed (oxygen in the lattice of a metal oxide (MO) anode) or physically adsorbed (hydroxyl radical ($^{\cdot}OH$)). The OH radical has a high standard electrode potential (E_0 = 2.80 V vs. SHE) and is the second-strongest oxidant known after fluorine.

Organic dyes are selectively transformed into biodegradable compounds usually carboxylic acids by chemisorbed "active oxygen" in the form of metal oxides, whereas organics are completely oxidized to CO_2 and inorganic ions by physisorbed OH (electrochemical combustion or electrochemical incineration method) [39].

4.2.5.1 Platinum (Pt)

Platinum is an exceptionally valuable and frequently utilized precious metal in a variety of applications, including electrochemistry and catalysis. Its high catalytic capabilities make it an excellent choice for many electrochemical applications, particularly electrocatalytic dye degradation. This chapter will investigate the special properties of platinum electrodes and their applications in the efficient degradation of dyes by electrocatalysis.

4.2.5.1.1 Platinum Electrodes Catalytic Properties

Platinum has exceptional catalytic characteristics, making it extremely useful in a variety of electrochemical reactions. The following characteristics contribute to its extraordinary catalytic activity. Platinum electrodes with a large surface area may be manufactured, resulting in more active sites accessible for catalysis; these are exceptionally stable and lasting due to their non-corrosiveness and resistance to deterioration. Another characteristic is that it has a low overpotential, which means it uses less energy during the electrocatalytic dye degradation process and has a speedy kinetic reaction owing to the rapid electron transfer during the electrochemical process [40–42]. In electrochemistry research, Pt is a prominent electrode material [43]. Due to its remarkable electrical conductivity and chemical stability, platinum has a long history as an anode material for the oxidation of organic pollutants, which occurs in a quick, uncontrolled reaction of hydroxyl radicals generating oxygen [44].

The authors Comninellis and Pulgarin [45], developed Pt electrodes for the first time for the degradation of phenol in wastewater treatment, achieving 60% removal efficiency by electrochemical oxidation approach due to its superior electrical conductivity, strong corrosion resistance, and catalytic activity. Furthermore, platinum anodes have low oxygen evolution overpotential (1.6 V vs. SHE in 0.5 M H_2SO_4) and may convert organic pollutants selectively with poor current efficiency [46]. Ammar et al. [47] achieved a minimal degradation efficiency of 34% after 5 hours at a current density of 150 mA/cm^2. The Pt electrode, which acts as an "active" anode, has a high percentage of decolorization, but the low degree of decontamination caused by the Pt anode results in a lower yield of hydroxyl radicals. The Pt–Pd model achieved 98% decolorization of the RG15 dyes in an alkaline medium (pH 9.0) after 60 minutes and 12 V power [48]. The electrochemical degradation of metanil yellow is an irreversible process that is regulated by diffusion; the electrochemical degradation process reduces COD by nearly 91.7% [49].

4.2.5.2 Gold (Au)

Gold is often used as ornamental and is assumed to be inert [50]. Nonetheless, gold offers unique nanoscale optoelectronic characteristics and has found applications in catalysis, sensing, electronics, biological diagnostics, drug delivery, and medicine

[51]. AuNPs stabilized with various monolayers are well-known for their superior electrocatalytic properties [52]. The electrochemical behavior of MB molecules in the aqueous medium using gold electrodes depends on several influential factors such as the surface area of two electrodes 0.1156 and 0.1530 cm^2, pH of 7.90, temperature 221°C, electrolyte concentration (KNO_3 and NaF) was 1 M, and electric current density at constant potential in the range of (EG = −0.286 V) at the CV of = 50 mV/s. The lowering of MB at the gold/aqueous electrolyte interface causes considerable decolorization [53]. Kim et al. [54] reported on Rhodamine B and MB electrocatalytic degradation employing porous Gold (PAu) electrodes, attaining 100% and 95% degradation efficiencies with low energy consumption and high durability.

4.2.5.3 Palladium (Pd)

Palladium NPs have been extensively researched as catalysts in recent years due to their unique properties and applications. Energy generation, hydrogenation/dehydrogenation processes, drug administration, and pollution treatment catalysts are some examples [55a–55g]. Popli et al. [56] reported on Palladium (Pd0 4 mM) used as a cathode material for the electrochemical reduction method, which decolorized > 98% of the Reactive Black 5 (50 mg/L) dye in less than 30 minutes and 99% of a mono-azo dye methyl orange (50 mg/L) in about 30 minutes at current density 20 mA/cm^2 [56].

4.2.5.4 Ruthenium (RuO_2)

Nonetheless, the first basic study on the characteristics of RuO_2, the key component of dimensionality stable anodes (DSAs), was published in the free domain in 1971. Many studies have shown that Ru is the more efficient metal for electrocatalysis, owing to its high surface area, chemical stability, and a wide range of accessible oxidation states; these properties make it an excellent choice for a variety of electrochemical applications, including electrocatalytic dye degradation [57, 58]. Acridine orange (AO) is eliminated more quickly in a Ruthenium-doped Pt electrode than in a platinum electrode alone, with anodic oxidation accounting for 98% of the degradation [59, 60]. Shilpa et al. [61] reported on acridine orange dye degradation utilizing Ru thin film doped graphite as anode and Pt as cathode, achieving 95% COD degradation.

4.2.5.5 Titanium Oxide (TiO_2)

TiO_2 has a large bandgap, which allows for effective charge separation and stimulates redox processes at the surface. TiO_2 also works as an electron acceptor, capturing and transferring electrons produced by the electrode to the adsorbed dye molecules. This mechanism causes redox reactions, which cause the dye molecules to degrade into simpler and less toxic chemicals [62–64]. Gomathi et al. [65] presented a titanium-doped-stainless steel electrode, which degraded 94% of scarlet red from the solution after 50 minutes at a current density of 0.4 mA/cm^2. Chang et al. [66] reported that Rhodamine B degradation obtained 63.57% TiO_2/activated semi-coke by electrocatalysis in 60 minutes at 16 V current density.

4.2.5.5.1 Photocatalytic Properties of TiO_2

Titanium oxide has photocatalytic activity because of its tendency to create electron–hole pairs in the presence of light. When photons with energies greater than the bandgap are absorbed, electrons in the valence band are stimulated to the conduction band, leaving positively charged holes behind. These electron–hole pairs are involved in redox reactions that result in the breakdown of organic contaminants or other photocatalytic activities. Titanium oxide photocatalysis is commonly used to degrade organic contaminants such as dyes, insecticides, and volatile organic compounds (VOCs). The photocatalytic process includes the adsorption of contaminants onto the TiO_2 surface [67]). Prominent hydrogen generation [68], dye-sensitized solar cells (DSSCs), work as an electron acceptor, assisting in the transit of electrons created by light absorption in the dye [69]. Photocatalytic breakdown of pollutants [70] is commonly utilized for the breakdown of organic pollutants such as dyes, insecticides, and VOCs.

4.2.5.6 Tin Dioxide (SnO_2)

Tin dioxide (SnO_2) is a semiconductor with remarkable electrocatalytic characteristics that make it valuable in a variety of electrochemical applications. SnO_2 exhibits excellent catalytic activity toward the HER, which is critical for hydrogen production and fuel cell applications. This is due to its unique electronic structure, surface properties, and redox reactions such as the OER [71, 72]. SnO_2 catalyst for electrocatalytic carbon dioxide reduction (CO_2RR), a potential technique for reducing CO_2 into valuable fuels and chemicals such as HCOOH and methanol [73, 74]. The OER using Ag-embedded SnO_2 thin film involves the electrochemical creation of oxygen gas from water, as well as the generation of surface intermediates such as OOH* and O [75]. SnO_2 has demonstrated remarkable electrocatalytic activity for the oxidation of methanol. It can promote methanol oxidation by enabling the adsorption and activation of methanol molecules, as well as subsequent electrochemical reactions by carbon-supported Pt–Sn NPs [76].

4.2.5.7 Iron Oxide

Iron oxide occurs naturally in a variety of forms, including hematite (Fe_2O_3), magnetite (Fe_3O_4), and goethite (FeO(OH)) [77–79], and it has tunable qualities such as magnetic properties, stability, density, and a variety of colors in different oxidation states [80]. By electrocatalytic degradation of textile dye C. I. Direct Red 80 (DR80), iron oxide was utilized as an anode, and practically complete color loss between 83 and 99 was obtained at pH neutral and basic medium. At 1 V applied potential, 50% COD elimination was accomplished [81]. Muthukumar et al. [82] reported on the almost complete removal of CI Acid orange 10 dye by electrocoagulation at two different current densities (8, 16 mA/cm^2), with 61% TOC removal achieved and subsequently transformed into value-added products aniline and 1-amino-2-naphthol-6,8-disulfonic acid. After 60 minutes of treatment with KCl as an electrolyte at a current density of 155.0 mA/cm^2, an iron oxide nanoflower-based electrode exhibited a notable degradation efficiency of 99% in 30 minutes, with a reduction in TOC value of roughly 20% [83].

4.2.5.8 Manganese Dioxide (MnO_2)

MnO_2 has recently been widely employed in environmental purification due to its inexpensive cost, high environmental compatibility, high purification activity, and low toxicity. In addition, Density Functional Theory (DFT) calculations show that MnO_2 has a significant Gibbs free energy barrier in OERs [84, 85]. As reported by Sun et al. [86], a carbon, cloth-supported MnS/MnO_2 heterostructure was employed in this work for the removal of methylene blue in wastewater by electrochemical advanced oxidation processes (EAOPs) removal efficiency (100%) and TOC removed efficiency (73.6%) in 30 minutes. Furthermore, the anode catalyst exhibits a greater high mineralization current efficiency (MCE) (73.2%), reduced energy consumption (23.4 kWh/kg TOC), and desired stability. The electrode titanium-supported manganese oxide thin films (Ti@MnO_2) absorbed the Reactive Violet 5 (RV5) azo dye and delivered 100% decolorization in less than 90 minutes in this investigation. This conclusion is especially intriguing given that the electrolysis was performed under modest operating conditions. Color fading varied from 80% to 90% in the absence of chlorides at a constant current of 200 A/m^2 and ambient temperature [87, 88].

4.3 CONDUCTIVE POLYMER ELECTROCATALYSTS

4.3.1 Polyaniline (PANI)

Polyaniline is most likely the most often used conducting polymer [89]. Because of its environmental stability, simplicity of synthesis, and antistatic or anticorrosion properties, PANI is one of the most intriguing conducting polymers [90]. Although the conducting polymers are insoluble in aqueous settings, when added to an organic dye solution, the optical absorption reduces as the dye concentration falls [91]. In the absence of a dye, the average conductivity of PANI in the synthesis of PANI was (4.50 ± 1.76) S/cm. The average conductivity (3.90 ± 1.83) S/cm corresponds to colorless PANI [92]. A coral-like PANI/Sunset yellow (SY) was produced as a consequence of the chemical oxidative polymerization of aniline in the presence of Sunset yellow as a dopant and surfactant. The findings showed that SY could control the development and morphology of PANI by adjusting the feeding molar ratio of SY to aniline. The results demonstrated outstanding conductivity, a significant specific capacitance, and fine electrochemical stability. After 1000 cycles, coral-like PANI/SY exhibited the highest specific capacitance of 467 F/g at 2 A/g, the best capacitance retention of 82.2%, and the highest maximum conductivity of 15.0 S/cm [93]. Another study on Acid Red 27-crosslinked PANI (ARCP) by chemical oxidative polymerization found that as the feeding molar ratio of AR-27 to aniline increased, the diameter of ARCP nanofiber decreased from 300 to 60 nm, exhibiting a large specific capacitance of 463 F/g at 2 A/g and great electrochemical cycling stability with specific capacitance retention of 85.5% after 1000 cycles [94]. The MB can be eliminated from an aqueous solution using the deprotonated Chitosan/PANI hybrid (CH/PANI). 100 mL of 3.6 mg/L of MB cationic dye was employed in combination with 50 mg of deprotonated CH/PANI hybrid at pH 11. Within 60 minutes, the CH/PANI combination exhibits excellent removal effectiveness of 98% [95]. Gao et al. [96] reported that binder-free anthraquinone (AQS)/PANI) modified carbon felt (CF) cathode (AQS/PANI@CF) has an efficient electrode for the degradation of the dye molecule (Rhodamine B) in aqueous media due to the high conductivity of PANI, which contributed to the reaction and resulted in up to 98.8% degradation efficiency at pH 2.0, and TOC removal efficiency of Rh.B. reached nearly 70% within 4 hours, with a rate constant at 0.0714/min.

4.3.2 Polypyrrole (PPy)

PPy is unique in that it is gaining commercial attention due to its high stability, greater conductivity, and ease of homopolymer and composite synthesis. When doped with halogenic electron acceptors such as bromine or iodine, PPy is an insulator in its undoped virgin state and has a constant conductivity of 10^{-5} s/m. PPy is a conducting polymer with electrocatalytic properties, making it a potential material for a variety of electrochemical applications such as dye degradation [97–100]. Lopes et al. reported on the 100% electrochemical removal of the textile dye C. I. Direct Red 80 (DR80) by electrochemical degradation over 70 hours at a reduced energy consumption of 5.46 kW·h/m^3 [81]. Zhang et al. reported on the H_2O_2 electro generation on the anthraquinone monosulfonate/polypyrrole (AQS/PPy) composite modified cathode with heterogeneous CuO/–Al_2O_3 catalyst and found that the oxygen flow rate (VO_2) = 0.4 mL/min, cathode potential (Eca) = 0.4 V, and pH 4.30 were achieved [101].

4.3.3 Other Conductive Polymers

4.3.3.1 Polythiophene (PTh)

Due to their unique electrical behavior, strong environmental stability, low optical band gap, stability in doped/neutral states, and, most importantly, their ease of production, PTh and its nanocomposites have been proposed as potential electrocatalytic and photocatalytic candidates [102, 103]. Cobalt-based species anchored on PTh (Co@PTh), proposed by Xing et al. [104], demonstrated strong OER performance in an alkaline electrolyte, demonstrating an overpotential of 338 mV versus reversible hydrogen electrode (RHE) at a current density of 10 mA/cm^2 and a Tafel slope of 52 mV/dec. Bora et al. [105] reported on the electrical conductivity of PTh and PTh/graphene oxide (GO) nanocomposite. When compared to pure PTh (5.8×10^5 S/cm) at room temperature, the PTh/GO composite demonstrated noticeably improved thermal stability and electrical conductivity (2.7×10^4 S/cm) and specific capacitance was (99 F/g) which is considerably less than the PTh/GO composite. Due to the sheet-like shape of GO and its ability to provide more active surfaces for simple oxidation–reduction reactions, increasing the GO concentration enhances the specific capacitance.

4.3.3.2 Poly(3,4-Ethylenedioxythiophene) (PEDOT)

As a result, PEDOT can be produced easily from the monomer 3,4-ethylenedioxythiophene (EDOT) at low electrochemical potential and has exceptional stability and electrical conductivity, it has been regarded as one of the most promising conducting polymers [106, 107]. PEDOT has several uses in a variety of industries, including transistors and solar energy. PEDOT has strong electrical conductivity, outstanding stability, flexible shape, and visibility [108, 109]. PEDOT is frequently employed as a hole-conducting material in pseudo-capacitors [110], sensors [111], photovoltaic devices [112], and catalysis [113] because of its outstanding characteristics. The PEDOT doped with nanocrystalline cellulose utilized for electrochemical catalysis was the subject of a paper by Fan et al. [107]. The nanocomposite displayed extremely low electrochemical impedance, a high charge storage capacity, and good electrocatalytic activity. The charge storage capacity retention of the PEDOT/NCC modified electrode was found to be around 78% after 1500 CV cycles, respectively, and 95% of the steady-state current was reached within 3 seconds, according to the research. As the ORR current density increased from 0.13 mA/cm^2 for bare CC to 1.1 mA/cm^2 on the surface of modified CC electrode associated with lower overpotentials, and current density increased from j = 0.13–0.45 mA/cm^2 compared to bare CC electrode, which is due to the enhancement of o, the ZIF-8/PEDOT/carbon cloth electrode exhibits remarkable electrocatalytic activity towards ORR [114].

4.3.4 Hybrid Electrocatalysts

To produce hybrid electrocatalysts, several materials are combined to make a composite material with improved catalytic activity for electrochemical processes. These substances are made to increase the effectiveness and performance of a variety of electrochemical devices, including electrocatalysts [115], fuel cells [116], electrolyzers [117], and batteries [118]. To improve the electrode, Liu et al. [119] reported on the manufacture and degradation of Eosin Y using the reverse microemulsion method to create the nanostructured BiOCl/TiO_2 composites. Finally, 50% hybrid BiOCl/TiO_2 material was used as an electrode for effective electrocatalytic dye degradation. After 120 minutes of treatment in an acidic medium (pH 4.0), the color removal efficiency was 93.6%, and the TOC removal efficiency was 68.3%. Pahra et al. [120] demonstrated how a single-step flame combustion process was used to synthesize the interconnected carbon NPs of candle soot, covered with nickel foam substrate and placed above the flame tip to form a novel hybrid electrocatalyst (CSn@NF) for electrocatalytic hydrogen generation and wastewater treatment using methylene blue textile dye. At a current density of 425 mA/cm^2 at 1.25V (vs. RHE) and a lowered overpotential (117 mV at 10 mA/cm^2), the catalyst degraded the dye by roughly 62% in 90 minutes. Hydrothermally, a new hybrid material, CdS@NiCo-LDH hybrid photoelectrocatalyst, was synthesized. It has a high degradation capacity and a lengthy lifespan. The dye molecule Alluric acid was treated in wastewater by a synthesized hybrid catalyst, which eliminated 98% of the dye molecule's azo groups within 60 minutes at pH 11, with a bias voltage of 2 V at an atmospheric temperature [121].

4.3.5 Comparative Analysis of Electrode Materials

During the electrochemical degradation process, the major operating cost is associated with electrical energy consumption (E). PAu electrodes in the presence of KCl as supporting electrolytes have high removal efficiency due to their well-porous structure, high electrochemical activity, fast kinetics, very low energy consumption (0.315 kWh/m), and high durability. After 10 repeats for electrochemical degradation of RhB over 60 minutes, the performance of the PAu electrode demonstrated high repeatability and maintained a degradation rate and efficiency of about 95%. Their cost, however, is very expensive, limiting their scalability for large-scale applications [54]. It has exceptional electrocatalytic degradation efficiency on methyl orange, reaching 100% complete removal of the dye molecule, and the kinetic rate constant is 0.179/min. The TOC removed efficiency on OV-MnS/MnO_2-CC was 73.6% over 30 minutes with a lower Ec (23.4 kWh/kg TOC) and to check the stability of the anode by conducting recycling tests under acidic and nematic conditions. In an acidic environment, the removal rate declined from 100% to 95.6% after 30 minutes, but the methyl orange removal rate was 92% over 120 minutes in a neutral medium. Metal oxides are less expensive than noble metals, making them more economically feasible for large-scale applications [86]. The cyclic voltammetric electrodeposition approach was used to create an anthraquinone (AQS)/polyaniline (PANI) modified carbon felt (CF) (AQS/PANI@CF) cathode. It has a good active surface area of 7.4/cm^2 and charge transfer resistance (Ω), which results in a good degrading efficiency of 98.8% during 60 minutes. Over 240 minutes, the TOC removal rate was about 70%, and the reaction rate-constant was 0.0714/min. The reaction sweep rate was 50 mV/s. After the sixth cycle, the cathode exhibited nearly the same degrading efficiency of 98.1%, indicating that the binder-free manufactured cathode (AQS/PANI@CF) retained superior consistency. Carbon-based polymer materials are generally inexpensive and commercially available, which increases their scalability. Their electrocatalytic performance, however, may be inferior to that of other materials, and modifications or combinations with other metal oxide catalysts may be required to improve their catalytic activity [96].

4.4 MECHANISMS OF DYE DEGRADATION

4.4.1 Direct Electron Transfer

Direct electron transfer refers to the process in which electrons are transferred directly from the electrode surface to the dye molecule, resulting in its degradation (Figure 4.1). This mechanism is commonly observed in systems such as DSSCs, where dyes are adsorbed onto semiconductor electrodes. When a dye molecule is adsorbed onto the electrode surface, it can undergo an electron transfer process. The dye molecule absorbs light and enters an excited state, where an electron is promoted to a higher energy level. This excited state electron can be injected into the conduction band of the semiconductor electrode, leading to the formation of a reduced dye molecule. The energy level alignment between the dye and the electrode facilitates the electron transfer reaction. The direct electron transfer mechanism offers an efficient pathway for dye degradation as it bypasses the need for intermediate reactive species [122]. The transferred electron can react directly with the dye molecule, resulting in its degradation or decolorization. This process can involve the breaking of chemical bonds within the dye molecule, leading to the formation of smaller, less colored, or colorless products [123].

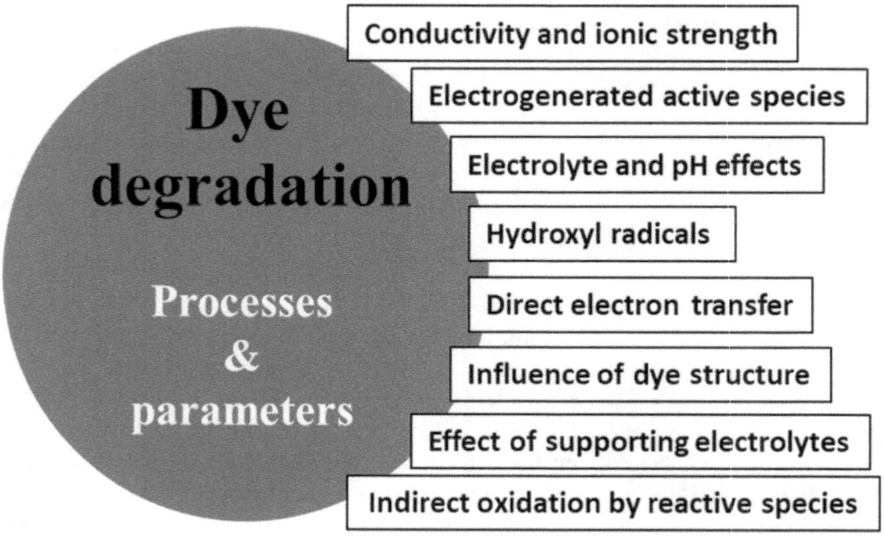

FIGURE 4.1 Different processes for dye degradations.

When a dye molecule is adsorbed onto the electrode surface, it can undergo an electron transfer process. The electron from the excited state of the dye can be injected into the conduction band of the semiconductor electrode, leading to the formation of a reduced dye molecule. The energy level alignment between the dye and the electrode facilitates this electron transfer reaction.

The direct electron transfer mechanism offers an efficient pathway for dye degradation as it bypasses the need for intermediate reactive species. This process can result in the conversion of the dye molecule into its reduced form, ultimately leading to its degradation or decolorization. The efficiency of direct electron transfer depends on various factors such as the redox potential of the dye, the energy level alignment with the electrode, and the surface properties of the electrode material [124].

Dye degradation is an essential process in various applications, including wastewater treatment and DSSCs. Understanding the mechanisms involved in dye degradation is crucial for optimizing degradation strategies and improving the efficiency of these processes. One of the mechanisms through which dye degradation occurs is direct electron transfer, where electrons are transferred directly from the electrode to the dye molecule. This chapter aims to explain the direct transfer of electrons and its role in the degradation of dyes.

4.4.2 Electrogenerated Active Species

Electrogenerated active species play a significant role in the degradation of dyes [125]. During electrolysis or electrooxidation, anodic reactions can lead to the production of reactive species. The specific reactions depend on the nature of the electrode material, the applied potential, and the electrolyte composition.

One of the primary sources of electrogenerated active species, including hydroxyl radicals, is water electrolysis. At the anode, water molecules can undergo oxidation reactions, resulting in the generation of hydroxyl radicals [126]. The following reaction illustrates the formation of hydroxyl radicals during water electrolysis:

$$2H_2O \rightarrow O_2 + 4H^+ + 4e^-$$

$$H_2O + O\cdot \rightarrow HO\cdot + H^+$$

In this reaction, hydroxyl radicals ($\cdot OH$) are formed by the reaction of water molecules with oxygen radicals ($O^\cdot$). These hydroxyl radicals are highly reactive and can readily participate in oxidation reactions.

4.4.2.1 Role of Hydroxyl Radicals in Dye Degradation

Hydroxyl radicals play a crucial role in the degradation of dyes due to their strong oxidative nature. These radicals can attack and oxidize the dye molecules, leading to their degradation and eventual mineralization [127]. The degradation of dyes by hydroxyl radicals follows a complex series of reactions, involving the breaking of chemical bonds and the formation of intermediate products.

Upon reaction with hydroxyl radicals, the dye molecules undergo various degradation pathways, depending on their chemical structure and functional groups. Hydroxyl radicals can initiate the oxidation of aromatic systems, such as azo groups or aromatic rings, present in many dyes. This oxidation leads to the breaking of chemical bonds and the formation of smaller, less colored, or colorless degradation products [128].

4.4.2.2 Factors Influencing the Generation of Hydroxyl Radicals and Dye Degradation

The generation of hydroxyl radicals and subsequent dye degradation is influenced by several factors, including the applied potential, electrode material, and electrolyte composition. The choice of electrode material can affect the redox potential of the system and the generation of electrogenerated active species [129, 130]. Certain electrode materials, such as metal oxides, exhibit enhanced catalytic properties for the formation of reactive oxygen species, including hydroxyl radicals. For example, titanium dioxide (TiO_2) is widely used in photocatalytic and electrochemical systems due to its ability to generate hydroxyl radicals upon irradiation or electrochemical excitation [131].

The electrolyte composition also plays a significant role in the generation of electrogenerated active species. The presence of certain salts, such as chloride or sulfate ions, can enhance the degradation efficiency by facilitating the formation of hydroxyl radicals. Additionally, the pH of the electrolyte can influence the stability of the dye molecules and the reactivity of the generated hydroxyl radicals [129].

In acidic conditions, the electrochemical processes may generate a higher concentration of hydroxyl radicals due to the easier oxidation of water. However, the acidic environment can also lead to the protonation of dye molecules, affecting their adsorption and degradation processes.

4.4.3 Indirect Oxidation by Reactive Species

In addition to the direct electron transfer and the generation of electrogenerated active species, indirect oxidation plays a crucial role in the degradation of dyes. In this mechanism, reactive species are generated through electrochemical reactions and subsequently participate in the oxidation of dye molecules.

Indirect oxidation commonly occurs through the formation of reactive oxygen species, such as hydrogen peroxide (H_2O^2), superoxide radicals ($O_2^{\cdot -}$), and peroxyl radicals ($ROO^{\cdot}$). These reactive species can be generated either by electrochemical reactions or by the reaction of electrogenerated active species with oxygen [132].

Once these reactive species are formed, they can diffuse away from the electrode surface and react with dye molecules, leading to their degradation. Oxidation reactions can involve the breaking of chemical bonds within the dye molecule, resulting in the formation of smaller, less colored, or colorless products [123].

The specific reaction pathways and degradation products formed during the indirect oxidation of dyes depend on the nature of the dye molecule, the reactive species involved, and the reaction conditions.

4.4.4 Influence of Dye Structure on Degradation Mechanisms

The molecular structure of dyes plays a significant role in determining the degradation mechanisms and reaction pathways. Different dye classes and functional groups exhibit varying susceptibilities to degradation processes. For example, dyes containing aromatic systems, such as azo dyes, are often more prone to degradation due to the presence of easily oxidizable double bonds [133, 134].

The presence of electron-donating or electron-withdrawing groups in the dye molecule can also influence its degradation behavior. Electron-donating groups can stabilize the dye molecule, making it less susceptible to oxidation. On the other hand, electron-withdrawing groups can enhance the susceptibility of the dye to degradation by facilitating electron transfer processes.

Furthermore, the solubility and adsorption characteristics of dyes on the electrode surface can impact their degradation mechanisms. Dyes that strongly adsorb onto the electrode surface may undergo direct electron transfer reactions more readily, while dyes with weaker adsorption may rely more on indirect oxidation mechanisms. Understanding the influence of dye structure on degradation mechanisms is crucial for the design and development of efficient degradation strategies for various dye pollutants [135, 136].

4.5 ELECTROLYTE AND PH EFFECTS

The electrolyte composition and pH have significant effects on the degradation mechanisms of dyes during electrochemical processes. The choice of electrolyte can influence the redox potential of the system and the generation of electrogenerated active species. For example, the presence of certain salts, such as chloride or sulfate ions, in the electrolyte can enhance the degradation efficiency by facilitating the formation of reactive species. Additionally, the pH of the electrolyte can affect the stability of the dye molecules and the reactivity of the generated species.

In acidic conditions, the electrochemical processes may generate a higher concentration of reactive species, such as hydroxyl radicals, due to the easier oxidation of water. However, the acidic environment can also lead to the protonation of dye molecules, affecting their adsorption and degradation processes.

Conversely, in alkaline conditions, the generation of reactive species may be limited, but certain dye molecules can exhibit enhanced stability and slower degradation rates. Therefore, the choice of electrolyte composition and pH conditions should be carefully considered to optimize the degradation efficiency and selectivity for specific dye pollutants [137, 138].

4.5.1 Role of Electrolytes

Electrolytes play a crucial role in electrochemical processes, including the degradation of dyes. They not only provide a conductive medium for the flow of current but also influence the electrocatalytic activity and degradation efficiency. This section will discuss the key roles of electrolytes in enhancing electrocatalytic activity and degradation efficiency during dye degradation [139].

4.5.1.1 Facilitating Electron Transfer

Electrolytes provide ions that can participate in the redox reactions occurring at the electrode surface. These ions act as charge carriers, facilitating the transfer of electrons between the electrode and the dye molecules. The presence of mobile ions in the electrolyte allows for efficient charge transport, minimizing the ohmic resistance and ensuring a high current density. This promotes direct electron transfer and enhances the overall electrocatalytic activity for dye degradation [134].

4.5.1.2 Adjusting Redox Potentials

The choice of electrolyte composition can influence the redox potentials of the system. By selecting appropriate electrolytes, the redox potentials can be tuned to match the energy levels of the dye molecules, facilitating electron transfer processes. This ensures efficient oxidation or reduction reactions at the electrode surface, leading to enhanced degradation efficiency. For example, the addition of supporting electrolytes, such as chloride or sulfate ions, can shift the redox potential and improve the electrocatalytic activity for dye degradation [140].

4.5.1.3 Generation of Reactive Species

Certain electrolytes can play a crucial role in the generation of reactive species that actively participate in the degradation of dyes. Electrolysis of water in the presence of chloride ions can lead to the formation of highly reactive chlorine species, such as hypochlorous acid ($HOCl$) and hypochlorite ions (OCl^-). These species possess strong oxidizing capabilities and can effectively degrade dye molecules [141]. Similarly, the presence of other reactive ions, such as persulfate ($S_2O_8^{2-}$), can enhance the generation of sulfate radicals ($SO_4^{\cdot-}$) through electrochemical reactions, further promoting the degradation efficiency [142].

4.5.1.4 pH Control

Electrolytes also influence the pH of the electrolyte solution, which can have a significant impact on the degradation efficiency. The pH affects the stability of dye molecules, their adsorption onto the electrode surface, and the reactivity of the generated reactive species. For example, acidic conditions can enhance the generation of hydroxyl radicals (·OH), which are highly reactive and contribute to efficient dye degradation [143]. On the other hand, alkaline conditions can promote the stability of certain dye molecules, reducing their degradation rates [144]. Therefore, the choice of electrolyte composition and pH conditions should be carefully optimized to achieve the desired degradation efficiency for specific dye pollutants.

4.5.1.5 Electrode Protection

Electrolytes can also play a role in protecting the electrode surface from undesired side reactions or fouling. Some electrolytes contain additives or surfactants that can form protective layers on the electrode surface, preventing the adsorption of unwanted species or minimizing electrode passivation. This ensures sustained electrocatalytic activity and extends the lifetime of the electrode during continuous dye degradation processes [145].

4.5.2 Influence of pH on Dye Degradation

The pH of the electrolyte solution has a profound impact on the ionization of dyes and their electrochemical behavior during degradation. pH affects the protonation and deprotonation of functional groups present in the dye molecules, thereby influencing their reactivity and adsorption properties [146].

In acidic conditions, the concentration of protons (H^+) increases, leading to the protonation of functional groups within the dye molecules. Protonation can affect the charge distribution, solubility, and adsorption characteristics of dyes on the electrode surface. It may also influence the electron transfer processes and the formation of reactive species.

Conversely, in alkaline conditions, the concentration of hydroxide ions (OH^-) increases, which can lead to deprotonation of functional groups. Deprotonation affects the molecular structure and electrochemical properties of dyes. It can impact the adsorption behavior on the electrode surface and the reactivity of the generated species [147].

The choice of pH can be critical for optimizing the degradation efficiency of specific dye pollutants. The ionization state of the dye molecules, their adsorption behavior, and the generation of reactive species can vary significantly with pH [148]. Therefore, understanding the pH dependence of dye degradation is essential for designing efficient degradation strategies [149].

4.5.3 Effect of Supporting Electrolytes

The addition of supporting electrolytes can have a significant effect on dye degradation processes by enhancing the generation of reactive species and improving degradation efficiency.

The choice of supporting electrolytes in electrochemical processes can significantly impact the efficiency and effectiveness of various electrochemical reactions, including the degradation of dyes. Supporting electrolytes provide the necessary ions for charge transfer between the electrode and the species involved in the electrochemical reactions. They influence the redox potential, conductivity, pH, and stability of the electrolyte system, thus affecting the degradation mechanisms and overall performance. In this section, we will discuss the effect of supporting electrolytes on the degradation of dyes, highlighting their influence on reaction kinetics, degradation efficiency, and selectivity [150].

Furthermore, supporting electrolytes can influence the generation of reactive species during the electrochemical process [151]. Certain ions present in the electrolyte can participate in the formation of reactive species, such as hydroxyl radicals, through electrochemical reactions. These reactive species play a crucial role in the degradation of dyes by facilitating oxidation processes [152].

The choice of supporting electrolytes should be made considering their compatibility with the system, their redox potential, and their impact on the stability of the reactive species and dye molecules. Careful selection of supporting electrolytes can improve the efficiency of dye degradation by promoting the generation of reactive species and enhancing the overall electrochemical performance [153].

4.5.3.1 Influence on Redox Potential

Supporting electrolytes can influence the redox potential of the system, which in turn affects the electron transfer processes during dye degradation. Different electrolytes have varying redox potentials, which can shift the energy levels and electron transfer rates between the electrode and the dye molecules. For instance, the use of halide salts as supporting electrolytes can enhance the degradation efficiency by providing higher redox potentials, promoting the generation of reactive species, and facilitating electron transfer reactions. Conversely, electrolytes with lower redox potentials may hinder the degradation process [154].

4.5.3.2 Conductivity and Ionic Strength

The conductivity and ionic strength of the electrolyte solution play a crucial role in the electrochemical reactions and the transport of species to and from the electrode surface. Higher conductivity and ionic strength can enhance the mass transport of reactants and products, improving the overall reaction kinetics. Electrolytes with higher conductivity, such as certain salts or ionic liquids, can facilitate the movement of ions and enhance the degradation efficiency. Additionally, an appropriate ionic strength can optimize the adsorption of dye molecules on the electrode surface, promoting direct electron transfer or reactive species generation [155].

4.5.3.3 pH and Buffering Capacity

Supporting electrolytes can affect the pH of the solution and its buffering capacity. The pH of the electrolyte influences the stability and reactivity of both the dye molecules and the reactive species involved in the degradation process. Acidic conditions can promote the generation of reactive species, such as hydroxyl radicals, through easier water oxidation. However, highly acidic environments can also lead to the protonation of dye molecules, affecting their adsorption and degradation. On the other hand, alkaline conditions may limit the generation of reactive species but can provide stability to certain dye molecules, slowing down the degradation kinetics. Buffering agents can control the pH and maintain it within a desired range, optimizing the degradation efficiency and selectivity.

4.5.3.4 Electrolyte Stability

The stability of the supporting electrolyte is crucial for the longevity and reliability of the electrochemical system. Certain electrolytes may undergo side reactions or decomposition under specific conditions, leading to the generation of unwanted by-products or interfering species. The stability of the electrolyte can be influenced by factors such as temperature, applied potential, and the presence of impurities. It is important to choose electrolytes that are chemically stable under operating conditions to ensure consistent and efficient dye degradation.

The effect of supporting electrolytes on dye degradation has been extensively studied in recent years. Researchers have investigated the use of various salts, such as chloride, sulfate, nitrate, and phosphate, as supporting electrolytes in different electrochemical systems. They have also explored the use of ionic liquids and other specialized electrolytes to enhance degradation efficiency and selectivity. The choice of supporting electrolyte depends on the specific dye pollutants, the electrode material, and the desired degradation mechanism.

4.5.4 Electrolyte Optimization Strategies

To maximize dye degradation efficiency, it is essential to optimize the electrolyte composition and pH [156]. Several strategies can be employed to achieve this optimization.

4.5.4.1 Selection of Appropriate Electrolytes

The choice of electrolyte components can have a significant impact on the degradation efficiency of dyes. Certain salts and additives can facilitate the generation of reactive species, enhance electron transfer processes, and improve the overall degradation kinetics. Some strategies for optimizing the electrolyte composition include:

4.5.4.2 Supporting Electrolytes

The addition of supporting electrolytes, such as sodium chloride (NaCl) or potassium sulfate (K_2SO_4), can enhance the conductivity of the electrolyte and promote the generation of electrogenerated active species [157]. These species can participate in oxidative reactions, leading to the degradation of dyes. The concentration of supporting electrolytes should be carefully optimized to achieve the desired degradation efficiency without causing excessive side reactions or electrode fouling [158].

4.5.4.3 Redox Mediators

Redox mediators are electroactive compounds that can enhance the electron transfer processes between the electrode and the dye molecule. These mediators facilitate the regeneration of the oxidized dye and promote the degradation reactions. Examples of redox mediators include ferrocene derivatives, quinones, and metal complexes. The selection and concentration of the redox mediators should be optimized to ensure efficient electron transfer while minimizing any undesired side reactions [159].

4.5.4.4 Catalysts

Catalysts can significantly enhance the degradation efficiency of dyes by facilitating the generation of reactive species or by directly participating in oxidation reactions. For example, transition metal catalysts, such as iron or manganese-based complexes, can promote the formation of hydroxyl radicals or other reactive oxygen species. The choice of catalysts should consider their stability, reactivity, and compatibility with the electrode material and dye molecules [160].

4.5.4.5 Tuning the Electrolyte Concentration

Varying the concentration of the electrolyte can influence the conductivity of the solution, the redox potential, and the generation of reactive species. Optimal electrolyte concentrations should be determined through experimental optimization [161].

4.5.4.6 pH Adjustment

Controlling the pH of the electrolyte solution can impact the ionization state of dye molecules, their adsorption behavior, and the reactivity of reactive species. pH optimization should be carried out to achieve the most favorable conditions for dye degradation [162]. Optimizing the pH can be achieved through the following strategies.

4.5.4.7 Acidic Conditions

Acidic conditions often promote the generation of reactive species, such as hydroxyl radicals (·OH), through the oxidation of water. Acidic pH can also enhance the protonation of dye molecules, increasing their adsorption on the electrode surface and facilitating the degradation reactions. However, excessively low pH values can lead to electrode corrosion and reduced stability of the electrolyte components [163].

4.5.4.8 Alkaline Conditions

Alkaline pH can enhance the stability of certain dye molecules and slow down their degradation rates. Additionally, alkaline conditions may inhibit the formation of reactive species, reducing the overall degradation efficiency. However, for specific dye molecules, alkaline pH can promote the formation of reactive species through different electrochemical reactions. The selection of pH conditions should be based on the specific dye and the desired degradation efficiency [164].

4.5.4.9 Buffering Systems

In some cases, buffering systems can provide additional control over the pH and enhance the degradation efficiency. Buffering systems maintain the pH within a specific range, preventing drastic pH changes during the degradation process. This stability can help maintain the reactivity of the generated species and ensure consistent degradation rates. Common buffering systems include phosphate buffers, acetate buffers, and carbonate buffers. The selection of buffering systems should consider their compatibility with the dye, electrolyte components, and electrode material.

4.5.4.10 Addition of Additives

Incorporating additives or catalysts into the electrolyte solution can enhance the generation of reactive species, improve the electron transfer processes, or modify the surface properties of the electrode. Additives should be selected based on their compatibility with the system and their specific roles in enhancing degradation efficiency [165].

4.5.5 Electrode Material Considerations

The choice of electrode material can also influence the degradation efficiency and the optimization strategies for the electrolyte composition and pH. Different electrode materials exhibit varying redox potentials, reactivity toward reactive species, and adsorption properties. Strategies for electrode material optimization include the following.

4.5.5.1 Surface Modification

Surface modification techniques, such as the deposition of metal oxides or conductive polymers, can enhance the catalytic activity of the electrode material and improve the degradation efficiency. These modifications can facilitate electron transfer processes, promote the generation of reactive species, and increase the adsorption capacity for dye molecules [166].

4.5.5.2 Selection of Semiconductors

In DSSCs and related systems, the choice of semiconductor material can significantly affect the efficiency of dye degradation. Semiconductors with appropriate energy levels and band structures can facilitate efficient electron transfer from the excited dye to the conduction band, promoting degradation reactions. Optimizing the semiconductor material involves considering its energy levels, surface properties, and compatibility with the dye and electrolyte components [167].

By employing these electrolyte optimization strategies, it is possible to improve the electrocatalytic activity, increase the generation of reactive species, and maximize the dye degradation efficiency. The electrolyte composition and pH play crucial roles in the degradation of dyes during electrochemical processes. Optimizing these parameters can significantly enhance the efficiency of dye degradation. In this section, we will discuss various strategies for optimizing the electrolyte composition and pH to maximize dye degradation efficiency.

4.6 OPERATING CONDITIONS FOR EFFICIENT DYE DEGRADATION

4.6.1 Applied Potential

In electrochemical dye degradation, an applied potential drives oxidation and reduction reactions, resulting in dye molecule degradation.

The use of an applied voltage to cause oxidation or reduction processes that result in dye molecule breakdown is known as electrochemical dye degradation. The applied voltage influences the pace of dye degradation and the energy efficiency of the process via a variety of factors, including electrochemical reaction kinetics and reactive species formation [168, 169]. Within a particular range, the rate of dye degradation is frequently exactly proportional to the applied voltage. An increase in the applied voltage can boost the pace of the electrochemical reaction by providing a greater driving force for the redox reactions involved in dye degradation. This effect has been reported in a variety of electrochemical systems [170]. To accomplish effective dye degradation while avoiding these constraints, the applied potential must be optimized. The applied potential is critical in terms of energy efficiency. In general, higher applied potentials result in higher energy usage. Furthermore, the design and selection of appropriate electrode materials, electrolytes, and operating conditions can all help to improve energy efficiency [171].

4.6.2 Current Density

The relationship between dye degradation efficiency and current density is an important aspect of electrochemical dye degradation processes and is affected by several factors such as oxidative/reductive reactions, electrolyte decomposition, or dye desorption from the electrode surface. The current is delivered to the dye-sensitized electrode in these systems, which promotes the degradation of organic dyes via electrocatalytic processes [172, 173].

Degradation efficiency may be calculated by measuring the degradation rate or percentage of dye degradation over a given period. According to research, increasing the current density can considerably improve degrading efficiency [174]. Martinez-Huitle and Ferro [174] and An et al. [175] reported that increasing the current density had a positive influence on the degradation of the RB-194 dye molecule in the range 100–200 mA/cm^2, potential range from 4.2 to 5.5 V, because a higher current density leads to higher production of ·OH radicals derived from water oxidation, which increases the removal rate in the wastewater system [176]. It is crucial to note, however, that there is an ideal current density at which additional increases may not result in corresponding gains in degrading efficiency. Beyond this threshold, other variables such as limited mass transfer or secondary reactions may begin to dominate and reduce overall efficiency. To obtain optimal dye degradation, it is vital to strike a balance between current density and other factors such as dye concentration, pH, temperature, and electrode material [177, 178].

4.6.3 Temperature

Temperature plays a crucial role in the reaction kinetics and stability of electrocatalysts during dye degradation. Temperature directly influences the reaction kinetics of electrocatalytic processes. As the temperature increases, the rate of chemical reactions generally accelerates due to the increased kinetic energy of the reactant molecules. Consequently, the degradation of dyes by electrocatalysts will be more efficient at elevated/optimized temperatures [179]. The stability of electrocatalysts is a critical factor for their performance during dye degradation. High temperatures can affect catalyst stability in several ways such as thermal degradation, sintering, and catalyst poisoning at elevated temperatures the catalyst may absorb impurities or by-products onto the catalyst surface, resulting in catalyst poisoning [180–182]. As a consequence, at elevated temperatures, the degradation efficiency may be increased, which has a major influence on the kinetics of the electrochemical oxidation of Remazol Red BR (RRB) and Novacron Blue CD (NB) utilizing boron-doped diamond (BDD) anode [183].

4.6.4 Reaction Time

The ideal reaction time required for successful dye degradation varies based on the dye, the degradation mechanism, and the reaction circumstances. The reaction period should be long enough for the dye molecules to degrade significantly. A longer response time does not always imply improved degradation efficiency. The degradation rate may plateau or decrease beyond a certain point due to variables such as catalyst deactivation, side reactions, or the build-up of reaction by-products [184, 185].

Kinetic studies on the rate of disappearance of the dyes were undertaken to identify the sequence of the reaction for the electrocatalytic degradation of dyes. For the experimental results collected using Congo red dye, many orders such as zero, first, and second orders graphs were evaluated. In the case of BDD anodes, the OH radicals produced by water oxidation (Equation 4.1) can be electrochemically oxidized to dioxygen (Equation 4.2) or contribute to the full oxidation of organic molecules, in this example dyes (Equation 4.6) [186–189].

$$H_2O \rightarrow HO\cdot + H^+ + 2e^- \tag{4.1}$$

$$HO\cdot \rightarrow \frac{1}{2}O_2 + H^+ + e^- \tag{4.2}$$

$$\text{Dyes} + HO\cdot \rightarrow CO_2 + H_2O \tag{4.3}$$

4.6.5 Optimization Strategies for Operating Conditions

Provide guidelines for optimizing the applied potential, current density, temperature, and reaction time for maximum dye degradation efficiency.

It is critical to optimize the applied potential, current density, temperature, and reaction time for optimal electrocatalytic dye degradation efficiency. Following are some general rules to keep in mind.

4.6.5.1 Applied Potential

- Determine the best-applied potential by doing a series of experiments at various potentials and monitoring degradation efficiency.
- Begin with a low potential and progressively raise it until the degradation efficiency is maximized.
- It is crucial to remember that the optimal potential will differ based on the dye and electrocatalyst utilized.

4.6.5.2 Current Density

- The quantity of current per unit area is referred to as current density. It is adjustable by adjusting the applied voltage and the electrode surface area.
- In general, higher current density leads to higher deterioration efficiency. However, extremely high current densities should be avoided as they might induce electrode damage or ineffective reactions.
- Experiment with varied current densities to determine the range where degradation efficiency is maximized while guaranteeing system stability.

4.6.5.3 Temperature

- Temperature is an important factor in electrocatalytic dye degradation. Higher temperatures, in general, improve reaction kinetics and degradation efficiency.
- Run tests at various temperatures and assess deterioration efficiency to discover the best temperature.
- Avoid exceeding the temperature limitations of the catalyst or the solvent employed in the system, as this might result in degradation or decomposition.

4.6.5.4 Reaction Time

- The duration of exposure to the electrochemical treatment is determined by the reaction time.
- Experiment with different reaction times to find the ideal period that maximizes degrading efficiency.
- It is critical to find a happy medium between reaction time and energy use. Prolonging the reaction time may result in lower returns or higher energy consumption.

It is vital to note that the optimization criteria will differ based on the dye, catalyst, electrode material, electrolyte, and experimental setting (Figure 4.2).

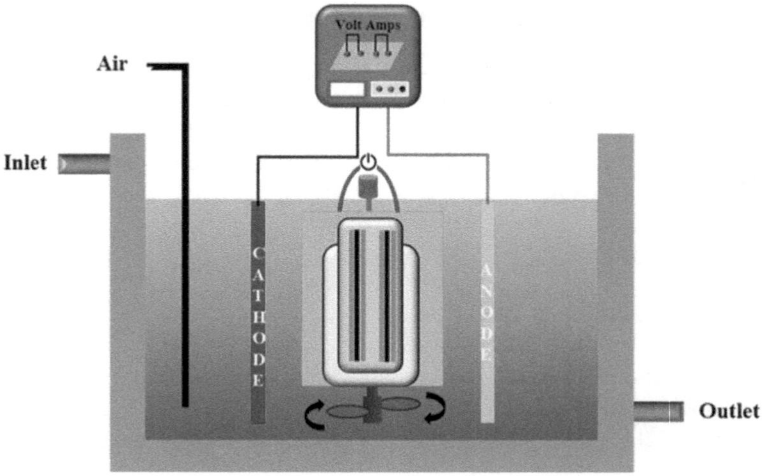

FIGURE 4.2 A schematic diagram showing the process involved in dye degradation.

4.7 ADVANCEMENTS IN ELECTROCATALYSIS FOR DYE DEGRADATION

4.7.1 Advanced Electrocatalyst Synthesis Techniques

Utilization of advanced synthesis techniques has become very important for developing efficient electrocatalysis with enhanced performance for dye degradation. Several techniques have been employed:

- *Sol–gel synthesis:* In this method, the hydrolysis and condensation of metal alkoxides form a gel, which is then calcined to obtain metal oxide or mixed-metal oxide catalysts. The advantage of the sol–gel synthesis is that it allows for precise control over composition, morphology, and structure, resulting in enhanced catalytic activity and stability [190].
- *Hydrothermal synthesis:* This method involves the reaction of metal precursors with hydrothermal solutions under high temperature and pressure conditions. This reaction condition allows for the formation of uniform and highly crystalline electrocatalysts, with improved surface area and catalytic activity. Another advantage of this method is that it can be combined with other techniques to form hybrid electrocatalysts with enhanced properties [191].
- *Electrodeposition:* Electrochemical synthesis involves the electrodeposition of metal ions onto conductive substrates, allowing precise control over morphology, composition, and structure. Electrodeposition offers high control over the electrocatalyst's properties, leading to improved catalytic activity and stability [192, 193].

4.7.2 Novel Electrode Materials

Studies have shown that the dye degradation process can also be enhanced significantly by utilizing novel electrode materials. Some of these materials include:

- *Carbon-based materials:* Carbon-based electrodes, such as graphene, carbon nanotubes, and activated carbon fall in the category of carbon-based materials. These materials are useful as they exhibit high surface area, excellent conductivity, and chemical stability. Further, these materials improve the overall electrocatalytic activity for dye degradation via efficient electron transfer and enhanced adsorption properties [194, 195].
- *Metal–organic frameworks (MOFs):* MOFs are a class of porous materials composed of metal ions coordinated with organic ligands. MOFs offer high surface area, tunable pore size, and diverse metal centers, making them suitable for adsorption and catalytic applications. Incorporating MOFs as electrode materials can enhance dye adsorption and facilitate the electrocatalytic degradation process [196].

The development of novel electrode materials provides opportunities to enhance the efficiency and effectiveness of electrocatalysis for dye degradation, leading to improved treatment outcomes.

4.7.3 Integration with Other Advanced Technologies

Combining electrocatalysis with other advanced technologies can result in synergistic effects, enhancing the efficiency and effectiveness of dye degradation processes. Two notable examples include:

- *Photocatalysis:* Integration of electrocatalysis with photocatalysis can leverage the benefits of both processes. Photocatalysis utilizes light to generate electron–hole pairs, which can be utilized by the electrocatalyst to promote the degradation of dyes. This synergy increases the overall degradation efficiency and expands the range of dyes that can be effectively treated [197].
- *Advanced oxidation processes (AOPs):* AOPs, such as electrochemical oxidation, Fenton oxidation, and ozonation, generate highly reactive species to degrade organic pollutants. Integrating electrocatalysis with AOPs allows for the efficient generation and utilization of these reactive species, leading to enhanced dye degradation rates and improved treatment efficiency [198].

By integrating electrocatalysis with other advanced technologies, researchers can develop more efficient and versatile systems for dye degradation, addressing the challenges associated with complex dye molecules.

4.7.4 Emerging Trends and Future Prospects

In the field of electrocatalysis for dye degradation, several emerging trends and future prospects can be identified:

- *Nanomaterials:* The utilization of nanomaterials, such as metal NPs, nanowires, and nanostructured materials, offers unique properties and increased surface-to-volume ratios, leading to enhanced catalytic performance. The incorporation of nanomaterials into electrocatalysts holds great potential for further improving the efficiency of dye degradation processes [199, 170].
- *Artificial intelligence (AI):* AI-based approaches, such as machine learning and data analytics, can be applied to optimize electrocatalyst design, predict catalytic activity, and guide experimental synthesis. AI techniques can accelerate the discovery and development of efficient electrocatalysts, facilitating the advancement of dye degradation technologies [200].

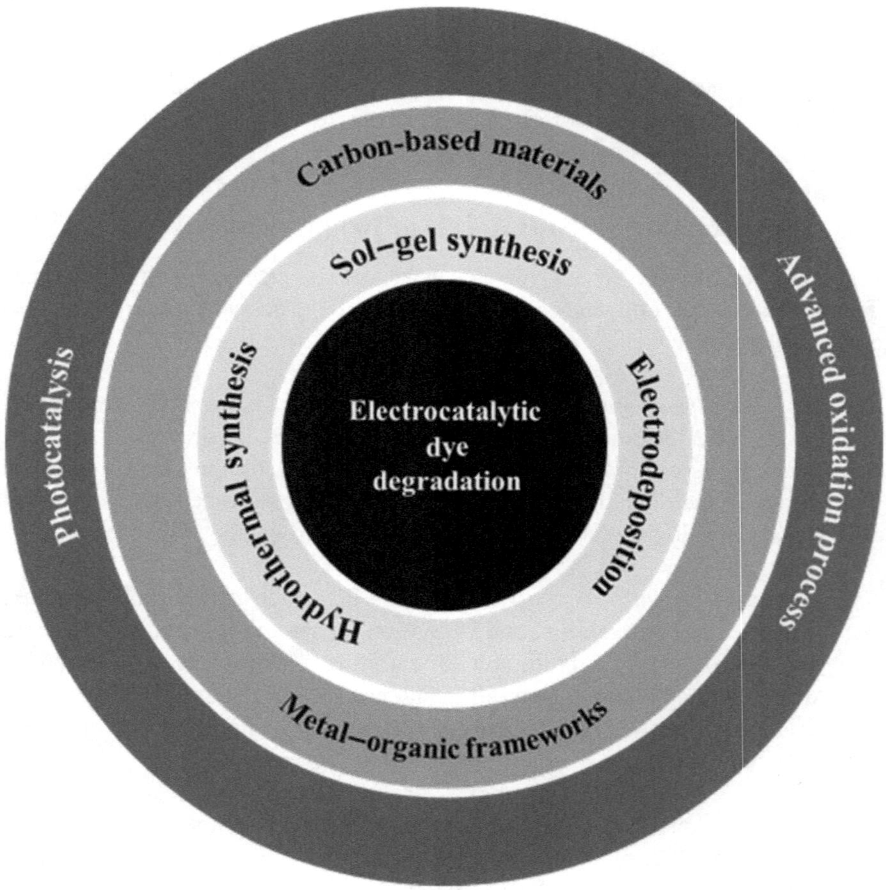

FIGURE 4.3 A schematic diagram for the various components involved in the electrocatalysis for dye degradation.

- *Sustainability and green processes:* The development of sustainable and environmentally friendly electrocatalytic systems is gaining importance. This includes the use of renewable energy sources, the design of recyclable catalysts, and the implementation of green synthesis methods. Future prospects lie in the integration of electrocatalysis with sustainable practices to ensure minimal environmental impact [201].

As research in electrocatalysis progresses, these emerging trends and future prospects hold promise for further advancements in the field, paving the way for more efficient and sustainable dye degradation processes (Figure 4.3).

4.8 CHALLENGES AND LIMITATIONS

4.8.1 Catalyst Stability and Durability

One of the key challenges in electrocatalysis for prolonged dye degradation processes is maintaining the stability and durability of the catalysts. Electrocatalysts are exposed to harsh reaction conditions, such as high temperatures, corrosive electrolytes, and reactive intermediates, which can lead to catalyst degradation and loss of activity over time. Some specific challenges associated with catalyst stability and durability include:

- *Catalyst corrosion:* Electrolytes used in dye degradation processes can be corrosive, leading to the degradation of the catalyst material. This corrosion can result in the loss of active sites and a decrease in catalytic activity [202].
- *Catalyst poisoning:* Dyes may contain impurities or by-products that can adsorb onto the catalyst surface, blocking the active sites and reducing the catalytic activity. These impurities can be difficult to remove and may cause irreversible damage to the catalyst [203].
- *Catalyst deactivation:* Prolonged operation can lead to catalyst deactivation due to surface fouling, aggregation, or structural changes. Over time, catalyst particles may lose their morphology, and surface area, or undergo structural transformations that reduce their catalytic performance [204].

To address these challenges, researchers are exploring various strategies. One approach is to develop catalyst materials with improved corrosion resistance and stability under harsh conditions. For example, using corrosion-resistant metals, metal alloys, or protective coatings on the catalyst surface can enhance stability and durability. Additionally, incorporating catalytic support materials or modifiers can improve the catalyst's resistance to poisoning and deactivation.

4.8.2 Catalyst Fouling and Electrode Surface Modification

Catalyst fouling refers to the accumulation of unwanted species or contaminants on the electrode surface, which can hinder the electrocatalytic activity in dye degradation processes. Several mechanisms contribute to catalyst fouling:

1. *Adsorption of dye molecules:* Dye molecules can adsorb onto the catalyst surface, reducing the available active sites for electrocatalysis. This adsorption can be particularly problematic if the dye molecules have a high affinity for the catalyst surface.
2. *Precipitation or deposition of reaction by-products:* During the dye degradation process, reaction by-products can form and deposit on the catalyst surface, blocking active sites and inhibiting catalytic activity. This can occur if the by-products have low solubility or are not easily removed from the electrode surface.
3. *Surface passivation:* Some compounds present in the dye solution or electrolyte can form a passivating layer on the catalyst surface, preventing efficient electron transfer and limiting catalytic activity. This can occur due to the formation of insulating films or unwanted reaction products.

To mitigate fouling effects, electrode surface modification techniques can be employed. These modifications aim to enhance the stability and activity of the catalyst by:

1. *Introducing protective coatings:* Applying thin films or coatings on the electrode surface can protect the catalyst from fouling by creating a barrier between the catalyst and the dye solution or reaction by-products.
2. *Designing tailored surface properties:* Surface modifications can be used to alter the surface chemistry, charge, or roughness of the electrode, making it less prone to fouling. For example, introducing hydrophobic or hydrophilic groups on the surface can influence the adsorption behavior of dye molecules.
3. *Implementing catalyst supports:* Catalysts can be immobilized or supported on materials that have a high surface area, promoting better dispersion and reducing the likelihood of fouling. These supports can also act as diffusion barriers, preventing unwanted species from reaching the catalyst surface.

4.8.3 Energy Efficiency and Cost Considerations

The energy efficiency and cost implications of electrocatalysis for dye degradation are important considerations for practical implementation. Some key factors to address include:

1. *Energy consumption:* Electrochemical processes typically require a supply of electrical energy, and the energy efficiency of the electrocatalytic system is crucial. High energy consumption can lead to increased operational costs and environmental impact. Improving energy efficiency involves optimizing the design of the system, such as reducing resistive losses, minimizing overpotentials, and selecting efficient electrode materials.
2. *Catalyst cost:* The cost of electrocatalysts can significantly impact the overall feasibility and economics of the dye degradation process. Precious

metal catalysts, such as platinum, are effective but expensive. Developing alternative catalyst materials that are abundant, low cost, and still exhibit high catalytic activity is an active area of research. Additionally, catalyst recovery and recycling strategies can help reduce costs by extending the catalyst's lifespan.

3. *Electrolyte and auxiliary material costs:* The choice of electrolyte and other auxiliary materials, such as supporting electrolytes or additives, can impact the overall cost of the electrocatalytic system. Optimizing the composition and concentration of these materials is important to achieve efficient dye degradation while keeping costs in check.

To improve energy efficiency and cost-effectiveness, researchers are exploring various strategies, including the development of new catalyst materials, the optimization of electrode/electrolyte interfaces, and the integration of renewable energy sources to power the electrochemical system. Additionally, process optimization and scale-up considerations (discussed in Section 4.9.4) can help reduce energy consumption and overall costs [205, 201].

4.8.4 Scale-Up Challenges

Transitioning electrocatalytic systems from lab-scale to industrial applications presents several challenges and considerations:

1. *Reactor design and scalability:* The design and engineering of larger-scale reactors for electrocatalytic systems require careful consideration of mass transfer, flow distribution, and electrode configuration. Scaling up can introduce new challenges related to the efficient distribution of reactants, effective removal of products, and minimization of ohmic losses.
2. *Stability and durability:* Ensuring the stability and durability of the electrocatalytic system over prolonged operation at an industrial scale is critical. Large-scale systems may be subjected to more demanding conditions and longer operating times, which can exacerbate catalyst degradation and lead to decreased performance.
3. *Cost considerations:* The cost of scaling up electrocatalytic systems should be carefully evaluated. The larger quantities of materials required, infrastructure investments, and maintenance costs must be taken into account to assess the economic viability of the scaled-up process.
4. *Safety and regulatory compliance:* Industrial-scale electrocatalytic systems must comply with safety regulations and environmental standards. These regulations govern aspects such as the handling and disposal of electrolytes, waste management, and potential risks associated with the system's operation.

To address these challenges, collaborative efforts between researchers, engineers, and industry experts are essential. Pilot-scale studies can provide valuable insights into the scalability and performance of electrocatalytic systems, enabling the identification of potential bottlenecks and optimization opportunities before large-scale implementation.

4.8.5 Regulatory and Environmental Considerations

The implementation of electrocatalysis for dye degradation must take into account regulatory requirements and environmental considerations. Some key aspects to consider include:

1. *Regulatory compliance:* Electrochemical processes, including dye degradation, may be subject to specific regulations and standards depending on the jurisdiction. These regulations govern factors such as wastewater discharge limits, permissible concentrations of certain chemicals, and the handling of hazardous materials. Compliance with these regulations is essential to ensure the process meets legal requirements.
2. *Environmental impact:* Electrochemical processes should be assessed for their environmental impact, including energy consumption, water usage, and the generation of by-products or waste. Minimizing the use of hazardous materials, implementing efficient catalyst recovery strategies, and reducing energy consumption through process optimization can help mitigate the environmental footprint of the electrocatalytic system.
3. *Life cycle assessment:* Conducting a life cycle assessment (LCA) of the electrocatalytic process can provide a comprehensive evaluation of its environmental impact throughout its entire life cycle, from raw material extraction to end-of-life considerations. LCA can help identify areas for improvement and guide decision-making toward more sustainable and environmentally friendly approaches.

By considering and addressing regulatory and environmental aspects, electrocatalysis for dye degradation can be implemented in a manner that meets both regulatory requirements and sustainability goals. Collaboration between researchers, industry stakeholders, and regulatory bodies is crucial to ensure responsible and compliant deployment of electrocatalytic systems.

4.9 CASE STUDIES AND APPLICATIONS

4.9.1 Electrochemical Degradation of Textile Dyes

Electrocatalytic treatment is an effective approach for the treatment of textile-polluted water. It is becoming a more practical method, as this process does not require any additional chemicals and can operate at room temperature and pressure [206–208].

In a recent study, Kuleyin et al. [209] investigated the effect of the electro-Fenton process for degradation of textile wastewater using graphite plate as anode and cathode in batch and continuous operations. The electro-Fenton process was found an efficient approach that has several properties like 89% of color, 93% of COD, and

58% of TOC removal taking place at pH 3 and the current intensity 1.65 A, Fe^{2+} concentration of 2 mM and flow rate 25 mL/min obtained from degraded wastewater.

As textile wastewater contains a majority of azo dyes, it has been extensively studied by several researchers. Recently in 2021, Belal et al. [134] have seriously examined Yellow 28 textile dye's degradation with IrO_2/Ti meshed electrode and Na_2SO_4 or NaCl as a supporting electrolyte through the electrochemical decolorization method. Efficient variables like pH, current density, beginning dye concentrations, and supporting electrolyte concentrations were observed, and found that NaCl electrolyte is more efficient than Na_2SO_4.

In the year 2020, textile wastewater containing Acid Mixture and Disperse Red 167 dyes was examined. The purification was carried out through a continuous anodic dissolution of aluminum alloy sacrificial anode for artificially aerated Cu–Al alloy galvanic (macro-corrosion) cells. At last, the concentration of the acid Mixture and Disperse Red 167 reduced to 32% and 99% respectively [208].

4.9.2 Treatment of Industrial Dyeing Wastewater

Electrocatalysis technology offers efficient degradation of wastewater obtained from industrial dyeing processes. It is an emerging technology for refractory pollutants existing at low concentrations in textile wastewater [210 211]. In this process electrochemical reaction occurs at the electrode surface to speed up the breakdown and removal of organic contaminants found in the wastewater. Basically, it is two types, electrochemical advanced oxidation processes (EAOPs) [212–219] and electrochemical advanced reduction processes (EARPs) [220, 221].

In electrochemical advanced oxidation processes (EAOPs), oxidation of water takes place at the surface of anode to form hydroxyl radicals. High over-potential electrode materials like doped-SnO_2, PbO_2, TIO_2, and BDD are required to design efficient electrochemical devices. For further enhanced efficiency of the device, the DET (direct electron transfer) pathway is more crucial as it transfers the electrons from the electrode surface to the anode without using any mediator [222–226].

For degradation of oxidized contaminants present in the wastewater, an electrochemical advanced reduction process is introduced. By the combination of activation methods like UV light, electron beam, and microwave and reducing agents like sulfite, ferrous the oxidized contaminants can degrade easily [227, 228].

4.9.3 Integrated Electrocatalytic Technology in Dye Wastewater Treatment

Integrated electrocatalysis promotes the breakdown of toxic organic compounds into less harmful substances [21]. In this approach, catalytic technology combined with oxidization electrocatalytic in a setup like photoelectric catalysis for degradation.

Several researchers proposed various combinations for the treatment of wastewater. In general, the removal rate depends upon several factors like concentration, voltage, decolorization rate, and time. Various photocatalysts like titanium dioxide, tungsten trioxide, and bismuth tungstate are used to degrade the textile wastewater, while titanium dioxide is a widely used photocatalyst as it shows magnificent photovoltaic conversion efficiency [229, 230].

Shen et al. [227] conducted a degradation effect for treating dye wastewater using the nano-TiO_2 catalyst and Co–Bi–PbO_2/Ti anode composition. They concluded that the optimal voltage for the treatment process was around 3 V and the electrolyte concentration was determined to be 0.01 mol/L Na_2SO_4 which leads to an increase in the decolorization rate by 0.15 times with the improvement in COD removal.

Bessegato et al. [228] conducted a study using boron-doped TiO_2 nanotube photoelectrodes as the photoanode under UV–visible spectrophotometer irradiation for the photocatalytic treatment of dye wastewater. The results indicated that the optimal conditions for the photocatalytic degradation of acid red 151 dyes were found to be a pH of 2.0 and a potential of 2.0 V which was carried in just 90 minutes of time.

Three-dimensional electrode reactors had great potential in the degradation of wastewater. When titanium dioxide was doped with three-dimensional electrodes and found that the degradation efficiency of methyl orange reached 98.76% at 35 minutes around 1.0 V [229].

4.9.4 Removal of Synthetic Dyes from Aqueous Solutions

Currently, azo derivates are extensively used as synthetic dyes in the textile industry. There are several treatments employed for the removal of synthetic dyes from industrial wastewater [230]. The technique involves adsorption, coagulation, photocatalytic decolorization and oxidization, membrane filtration, biological treatment, and enzymatic decomposition. Based upon the type, composition, concentration, and amount present of organic containments are the necessary properties to choose an efficient technology for the removal of synthetic dye.

In the adsorption process, sulfonated coals, activated carbon, silica, and acid-activated clay are used as adsorbents. The molecule present in the dye is adsorbed on the surface of the adsorbent and then the water is removed by filtration method [231, 232]. Whereas in the coagulation method aluminum sulfate or ferric chloride forms insoluble flocs in the pollutant water and they can separate through sedimentation [233].

Photocatalyst helps to separate the color and facilitate oxidation reaction. Photocatalyst absorbs a photon and generates charged species to react with the molecules of wastewater and degrade the reacting species into decoloration. In some cases, photocatalysts produce some free radicals, which can oxidize the containments and make them less toxic substances [234].

The membrane filtration method involves the use of a semipermeable membrane to remove the dyes from wastewater [235]. But in the case of biological treatment, enzymes or microorganisms degrade the dye through sludge treatment or enzyme treatment and this process is less costly than other techniques [236].

Enzymatic decomposition is the famous technique for the degradation of azo derivatives. Isoenzymes, horseradish peroxidase, and veratryl alcohol are the significant enzymes for the decomposition of synthetic dye [237].

4.10 CONCLUSIONS

This chapter has provided important findings and advancements in the field of electrocatalysis for sustainable wastewater treatment. The main findings include the successful design and implementation of catalysts for efficient dye degradation, advancements in process optimization techniques, and the development of sustainable electrocatalytic systems.

4.10.1 Future Directions

There are several potential future research directions that can further enhance the field of electrocatalysis. These include the design of novel catalysts with improved activity and selectivity, the exploration of new process optimization strategies, and the development of sustainable electrocatalytic systems that minimize energy consumption and waste generation. Additionally, investigating the potential application of electrocatalysis in the degradation of other pollutants and the integration of renewable energy sources for more sustainable wastewater treatment are important areas for future exploration.

4.10.2 Importance of Electrocatalysis for Sustainable Wastewater Treatment

Electrocatalysis emerges as a significant and efficient approach for dye degradation in wastewater treatment. Its importance lies in its ability to promote sustainable practices by utilizing catalysts that can selectively and effectively degrade dyes, minimizing the environmental impact. By optimizing electrocatalytic systems and processes, it is possible to achieve efficient dye removal while reducing energy consumption and waste generation. Electrochemical techniques have the potential to revolutionize wastewater treatment, offering a greener and more sustainable solution to address the challenges of dye pollution in our environment.

ACKNOWLEDGMENTS

The authors express their gratitude to GITAM Deemed to be University, Visakhapatnam, and the DST-FIST Program 2014 (SR/FST/ETI-373/2016).

REFERENCES

1. Muhd Julkapli, N., Bagheri, S., & Bee Abd Hamid, S. (2014). Recent advances in heterogeneous photocatalytic decolorization of synthetic dyes. *The Scientific World Journal, 2014*, 1–25. https://doi.org/10.1155/2014/692307
2. Zuorro, A., & Lavecchia, R. (2014). Evaluation of UV/H_2O_2 advanced oxidation process (AOP) for the degradation of diazo dye Reactive Green 19 in aqueous solution. *Desalination and Water Treatment*, *52*(7–9), 1571–1577. https://doi.org/10.1080/19443994.2013.787553

3. Litter, M. I., & Quici, N. (2010). Photochemical advanced oxidation processes for water and wastewater treatment. *Recent Patents on Engineering*, *4*(3), 217–241. https://doi.org/10.2174/187221210794578574
4. Stasinakis, A. S. (2008). Use of selected advanced oxidation processes (AOPs) for wastewater treatment- A mini review. *Global NEST Journal*, *10*, 376.
5. Lorimer, J. P., Mason, T. J., Plattes, M., Phull, S. S., & Walton, D. J. (2001). Degradation of dye effluent. *Pure and Applied Chemistry*, *73*(12), 1957–1968. https://doi.org/10.1351/pac200173121957
6. Al-Tohamy, R., Ali, S. S., Li, F., Okasha, K. M., Mahmoud, Y. A.-G., Elsamahy, T., Jiao, H., Fu, Y., & Sun, J. (2022). A critical review on the treatment of dye-containing wastewater: ecotoxicological and health concerns of textile dyes and possible remediation approaches for environmental safety. *Ecotoxicology and Environmental Safety*, *231*, 113160. https://doi.org/10.1016/j.ecoenv.2021.113160
7. Saxena, S., & Raja, A. S. M. (2014). Natural dyes: sources, chemistry, application and sustainability issues. In S. Muthu (eds.) *Roadmap to Sustainable Textiles and Clothing. Textile Science and Clothing Technology* (pp. 37–80). Springer, Singapore. https://doi.org/10.1007/978-981-287-065-0_2
8. Dadrasnia, A., Shahsavari, N., & Emenike, C. U. (2013). Remediation of contaminated sites. In V. Kutcherov and A. Kolesnikov (eds.), *Hydrocarbon*. InTech. https://doi.org/10.5772/51591
9. Chua, L. H. R. (2016). Micro-structural characterisation of non-easel painted artworks. Thesis. http://hdl.handle.net/10453/101877
10. Chattopadhyay, D. P. (2011). Chemistry of dyeing. In *Handbook of Textile and Industrial Dyeing* (pp. 150–183). Elsevier. https://doi.org/10.1533/9780857093974.1.150
11. Tretiak, S., & Mukamel, S. (2002). Density matrix analysis and simulation of electronic excitations in conjugated and aggregated molecules. *Chemical Reviews*, *102*(9), 3171–3212. https://doi.org/10.1021/cr0101252
12. Menger, F. M. (1991). Groups of organic molecules that operate collectively. *Angewandte Chemie International Edition in English*, *30*(9), 1086–1099. https://doi.org/10.1002/anie.199110861
13. Pavithra, K. G., Kumar, P. S., Jaikumar, V., & Rajan, P. S. (2019). Removal of colorants from wastewater: a review on sources and treatment strategies. *Journal of Industrial and Engineering Chemistry*, *75*, 1–19. https://doi.org/10.1016/j.jiec.2019.02.011
14. Tchounwou, P. B., Yedjou, C. G., Patlolla, A. K., & Sutton, D. J. (2012). *Heavy Metal Toxicity and the Environment* (pp. 133–164). DOI: 10.1007/978-3-7643-8340-4_6
15. Oturan, M. A. (2000). An ecologically effective water treatment technique using electrochemically generated hydroxyl radicals for in situ destruction of organic pollutants: application to herbicide. *Journal of Applied Electrochemistry*, *30*(4), 475–482. https://doi.org/10.1023/A:1003994428571
16. Rakotomalala, Q., Khoun, L., Leblond, C., & Sigrist, J.-F. (2021). An advanced semi-analytical model for the study of naval shock problems. *Journal of Sound and Vibration*, *511*, 116317. https://doi.org/10.1016/j.jsv.2021.116317
17. Le, T. X. H., Bechelany, M., Lacour, S., Oturan, N., Oturan, M. A., & Cretin, M. (2015). High removal efficiency of dye pollutants by electron-Fenton process using a graphene based cathode. *Carbon*, *94*, 1003–1011. https://doi.org/10.1016/j.carbon.2015.07.086
18. An, J., Feng, Y., Zhao, Q., Wang, X., Liu, J., & Li, N. (2022). Electrosynthesis of H_2O_2 through a two-electron oxygen reduction reaction by carbon based catalysts: from

mechanism, catalyst design to electrode fabrication. *Environmental Science and Ecotechnology*, *11*, 100170. https://doi.org/10.1016/j.ese.2022.100170

19. Clematis, D., & Panizza, M. (2021). Application of boron-doped diamond electrodes for electrochemical oxidation of real wastewaters. *Current Opinion in Electrochemistry*, *30*, 100844. https://doi.org/10.1016/j.coelec.2021.100844
20. Sun, H., Zhang, Y., Yang, J., Xu, Q., & Li, J. (2018). Electrocatalysis in dye degradation for wastewater treatment: current status, challenges, and perspectives. *Chemical Engineering Journal*, *332*, 616–631.
21. Wu, Z., Ma, M., & Zheng, X. (2020). Electrocatalytic degradation of dyes: mechanisms, influencing factors, and recent advances. *Environmental Science and Pollution Research*, *27*(11), 12067–12083.
22. Sharma, P., Singh, R., & Kumar, V. (2019). Electrocatalytic degradation of organic dyes in wastewater: a review. *Journal of Water Process Engineering*, *31*, 100867.
23. Yang, J., Tian, J., Xie, T., & Zhao, D. (2021). Recent advances in electrocatalysis for wastewater treatment: mechanisms, catalysts, and perspectives. *Chemical Engineering Journal*, *405*, 126822.
24. Anwar, S., Khan, F., Zhang, Y., & Djire, A. (2021). Recent development in electrocatalysts for hydrogen production through water electrolysis. *International Journal of Hydrogen Energy*, *46*(63), 32284–32317. https://doi.org/10.1016/j.ijhydene.2021.06.191
25. Zhao, S. (2016). Metal oxides as electrocatalysts at oxygen electrodes in electrochemical systems. Doctoral Dissertations. 1272. htp://digitalcommons.uconn.edu/dissertations/1272.
26. Jiang, Q., Ren, Y., Yang, Y., Wang, L., Dai, L., & He, Z. (2022). Recent advances in carbon-based electrocatalysts for vanadium redox flow battery: mechanisms, properties, and perspectives. *Composites Part B: Engineering*, *242*, 110094. https://doi.org/10.1016/j.compositesb.2022.110094
27. Vasileff, A., Zheng, Y., & Qiao, S. Z. (2017). Carbon solving carbon's problems: recent progress of nanostructured carbon-based catalysts for the electrochemical reduction of CO_2. *Advanced Energy Materials*, *7*(21), 1700759. https://doi.org/10.1002/aenm.201700759
28. Xue, Y., Sun, S., Wang, Q., Dong, Z., & Liu, Z. (2018). Transition metal oxide-based oxygen reduction reaction electrocatalysts for energy conversion systems with aqueous electrolytes. *Journal of Materials Chemistry A*, *6*(23), 10595–10626. https://doi.org/10.1039/C7TA10569J
29. Liu, Y., Chen, Z., Li, Z., Zhao, N., Xie, Y., Du, Y., Xuan, J., Xiong, D., Zhou, J., Cai, L., & Yang, Y. (2022). CoNi nanoalloy-Co-N_4 composite active sites embedded in hierarchical porous carbon as bi-functional catalysts for flexible Zn–air battery. *Nano Energy*, *99*, 107325. https://doi.org/10.1016/j.nanoen.2022.107325
30. Hua, L., Ma, H., & Zhang, L. (2013). Degradation process analysis of the azo dyes by catalytic wet air oxidation with catalyst CuO/γ-Al_2O_3. *Chemosphere*, *90*(2), 143–149. https://doi.org/10.1016/j.chemosphere.2012.06.018
31. Gosavi, V. D., & Sharma, S. (2013). A general review on various treatment methods for textile wastewater. *Journal of Environmental Science, Computer Science and Engineering & Technology*, *3*(1), 29–39.
32. Dimoglo, A., Utlu, B., Öztürk, D., Gökmen-Erdogan, K. (2023). Influence of the electrocatalytic anode nature on dye destruction. *Chemistry Select*, 8, e202303185. https://doi.org/10.1002/slct.202303185
33. Seema, S., Ritesh, P., Vimal, C.S, L., Shang-L., & Nidheesh, P.V. (2023). A critical review on the degradation mechanism of textile effluent during electrocatalytic

oxidation: Removal optimization and degradation pathways. *Journal of Environmental Chemical Engineering*, *11*(6) 111277. https://doi.org/10.1016/j.jece.2023.111277
34. Abdulgalim, B.I., Nabi, S.S., Asiyat, G.M., Nidheesh, P. V., & Mehmet A.O. (2023). Electrochemical oxidation of azo dyes in water: a review. *Environmental Chemistry Letters*, 21, 2863–2911. https://doi.org/10.1007/s10311-023-01610-5
35. van der Zee, F. P., & Villaverde, S. (2005). Combined anaerobic–aerobic treatment of azo dyes – a short review of bioreactor studies. *Water Research*, *39*, 1425–1440. DOI: 10.1016/j.watres.2005.03.007
36. García-Montaño, J., Domènech, X., García-Hortal, J. A., Torrades, F., & Peral, J. (2008). The testing of several biological and chemical coupled treatments for Cibacron Red FN-R azo dye removal. *Journal of Hazardous Materials*, *154*(1–3), 484–490. https://doi.org/10.1016/j.jhazmat.2007.10.050
37. Chu, W. (2000). Quantitative prediction of direct and indirect dye ozonation kinetics. *Water Research*, *34*(12), 3153–3160. https://doi.org/10.1016/S0043-1354(00)00043-9
38. Prado, A. G. S., Miranda, B. S., & Jacintho, G. V. M. (2003). Interaction of indigo carmine dye with silica modified with humic acids at solid/liquid interface. *Surface Science*, *542*(3), 276–282. https://doi.org/10.1016/S0039-6028(03)00990-7
39. Vaiano, V., Sacco, O., Sannino, D., Stoller, M., Ciambelli, P., & Chianese, A. (2016). Photocatalytic removal of phenol by ferromagnetic n-$TiO_2/SiO_2/Fe_3O_4$ nanoparticles in presence of visible light irradiation. *Chemical Engineering Transaction*, *47*, 235–240. https://doi.org/10.3303/CET1647040
40. Chen, Q.-S., Solla-Gullón, J., Sun, S.-G., & Feliu, J. M. (2010). The potential of zero total charge of Pt nanoparticles and polycrystalline electrodes with different surface structure: the role of anion adsorption in fundamental electrocatalysis. *Electrochimica Acta*, *55*(27), 7982–7994. https://doi.org/10.1016/j.electacta.2010.03.050
41. Hayes, M., & Kuhn, A. T. (1980). Determination of platinum catalyst surface area with potentiodynamic techniques – effect of experimental parameters. *Applications of Surface Science*, *6*(1), 1–14. https://doi.org/10.1016/0378-5963(80)90050-1
42. Thirsk, H. R. (1972). A guide to the study of electrode kinetics, Academic Press, New York.10.1604/9780126877502
43. Li, X., Cui, Y., Feng, Y., Xie, Z., & Gu, J.-D. (2005). Reaction pathways and mechanisms of the electrochemical degradation of phenol on different electrodes. *Water Research*, *39*(10), 1972–1981. https://doi.org/10.1016/j.watres.2005.02.021
44. Wabner, D., & Grambow, C. (1985). Reactive intermediates during oxidation of water lead dioxide and platinum electrodes. *Journal of Electroanalytical Chemistry and Interfacial Electrochemistry*, *195*(1), 95–108. https://doi.org/10.1016/0022-0728(85)80008-5
45. Comninellis, C., & Pulgarin, C. (1991). Anodic oxidation of phenol for waste water treatment. *Journal of Applied Electrochemistry*, *21*(8), 703–708. https://doi.org/10.1007/BF01034049
46. Feng, Y., Yang, L., Liu, J., & Logan, B. E. (2016). Electrochemical technologies for wastewater treatment and resource reclamation. *Environmental Science: Water Research & Technology*, *2*(5), 800–831. https://doi.org/10.1039/C5EW00289C
47. Ammar, S., Asma, M., Oturan, N., Abdelhedi, R., & Oturan, M. A. (2012). Electrochemical degradation of anthraquinone dye alizarin red: role of the electrode material. *Current Organic Chemistry*, *16*(17), 1978–1985. https://doi.org/10.2174/13852721280325161

48. Markovic, M., Jovic, M., Stankovic, D., Mutic, J., Roglic, G., & Manojlovic, D. (2014). Toxicity screening after electrochemical degradation of reactive textile dyes. *Polish Journal of Environmental Studies*, *23*. https://doi.org/10.15244/pjoes/28298
49. Jain, R., Sharma, N., & Radhapyari, K. (2009). Removal of hazardous azo dye metanil yellow from industrial wastewater using electrochemical technique. *European Water*, *27/27*, 43–52.
50. Hammer, B., & Norskov, J. K. (1995). Why gold is the noblest of all the metals. *Nature*, *376*(6537), 238–240. https://doi.org/10.1038/376238a0
51. Jain, P. K., Huang, X., El-Sayed, I. H., & El-Sayed, M. A. (2008). Noble metals on the nanoscale: optical and photothermal properties and some applications in imaging, sensing, biology, and medicine. *Accounts of Chemical Research*, *41*(12), 1578–1586. https://doi.org/10.1021/ar7002804
52. Kannan, P., & John, S. A. (2011). Fabrication of conducting polymer-gold nanoparticles film on electrodes using monolayer protected gold nanoparticles and its electrocatalytic application. *Electrochimica Acta*, *56*(20), 7029–7037. https://doi.org/10.1016/j.electacta.2011.06.004
53. Žutić, V., Svetličić, V., Clavilier, J., & Chevalet, J. (1987). Supramolecular phenomena in organic redox films at electrodes. *Journal of Electroanalytical Chemistry and Interfacial Electrochemistry*, *219*(1–2), 183–195. https://doi.org/10.1016/0022-0728(87)85039-8
54. Kim, J., Yeom, C., & Kim, Y. (2016). Electrochemical degradation of organic dyes with a porous gold electrode. *Korean Journal of Chemical Engineering*, *33*(6), 1855–1859. https://doi.org/10.1007/s11814-016-0033-6
55. (a)Frei, M. S., Mondelli, C., García-Muelas, R., Kley, K. S., Puértolas, B., López, N., Safonova, O. v., Stewart, J. A., Curulla Ferré, D., & Pérez-Ramírez, J. (2019). Atomic-scale engineering of indium oxide promotion by palladium for methanol production via CO_2 hydrogenation. *Nature Communications*, *10*(1), 3377; (b). Shiva Kumar, S., & Himabindu, V. (2020). Boron-doped carbon nanoparticles supported palladium as an efficient hydrogen evolution electrode in PEM water electrolysis. *Renewable Energy*, *146*, 2281–2290. https://doi.org/10.1016/j.renene.2019.08.068; (c) Chen, M., Maeda, N., Baiker, A., & Huang, J. (2018). Hydrogenation of acetophenone on Pd/silica–alumina catalysts with tunable acidity: mechanistic insight by in situ ATR-IR spectroscopy. *ACS Catalysis*, *8*(7), 6594–6600. https://doi.org/10.1021/acscatal.8b00169; (d) Qin, X., Li, H., Xie, S., Li, K., Jiang, T., Ma, X.-Y., Jiang, K., Zhang, Q., Terasaki, O., Wu, Z., & Cai, W.-B. (2020). Mechanistic analysis-guided Pd-based catalysts for efficient hydrogen production from formic acid dehydrogenation. *ACS Catalysis*, *10*(6), 3921–3932. https://doi.org/10.1021/acscatal.0c00225; (e. Portney, N. G., & Ozkan, M. (2006). Nano-oncology: drug delivery, imaging, and sensing. *Analytical and Bioanalytical Chemistry*, *384*(3), 620–630. https://doi.org/10.1007/s00216-005-0247-7; (f) Rajan, C., 2011. Nanotechnology in groundwater remediation. *International Journal of Environmental Science and Development*, *2*(3), 182; (g Shi, Y., Huang, X.-K., Wang, Y., Zhou, Y., Yang, D.-R., Wang, F.-B., Gao, W., & Xia, X.-H. (2019). Electronic metal–support interaction to modulate MoS_2-supported Pd nanoparticles for the degradation of organic dyes. *ACS Applied Nano Materials*, *2*(6), 3385–3393. https://doi.org/10.1021/acsanm.9b00297
56. Popli, S. A., Patel, P., Date, M., Ruparelia, J., & Patel, U. D. (2021). Rapid electrocatalytic reduction of azo dyes and phenolic compounds in the presence of metallic palladium. *Separation and Purification Technology*, *254*, 117658. https://doi.org/10.1016/j.seppur.2020.117658

57. Trasatti, S., & Buzzanca, G. (1971). Ruthenium dioxide: a new interesting electrode material. Solid state structure and electrochemical behaviour. *Journal of Electroanalytical Chemistry and Interfacial Electrochemistry*, *29*(2), A1–A5. https://doi.org/10.1016/S0022-0728(71)80111-0
58. Takasu, Y., & Murakami, Y. (2000). Design of oxide electrodes with large surface area. *Electrochimica Acta*, *45*(25–26), 4135–4141. https://doi.org/10.1016/S0013-4686(00)00534-X
59a. Jeon, W., Lee, W., Yoo, Y. W., An, C. H., Han, J. H., Kim, S. K., & Hwang, C. S. (2014). Chemistry of active oxygen in RuO_x and its influence on the atomic layer deposition of TiO_2 films. *Journal Material Chemistry C*, *2*(46), 9993–10001. https://doi.org/10.1039/C4TC01381F
59b. Alonso-Vante, N., Malakhov, I. V., Nikitenko, S. G., Savinova, E. R., & Kochubey, D. I. (2002). The structure analysis of the active centers of Ru-containing electrocatalysts for the oxygen reduction. An in situ EXAFS study. *Electrochimica Acta*, *47*(22–23), 3807–3814. https://doi.org/10.1016/S0013-4686(02)00351-1
60. Rakesh, S., & Ananda, S. (2012). Electrochemical degradation of acridine orange dye at Ru-doped platinum anode in aqueous solution. *International Journal of Chemistry and Applications*, *4*(3), 227–239.
61. Shilpa, R, Charan Kumar H. C., Ananda, S., & Rai, R. S. (2018). Preparation and characterization of Ru/graphite modified electrode: a kinetic investigation of electrochemical degradation of acridine orange dye in aqueous solution. *Journal of Emerging Technologies and Innovative Research*, *5*(7), 1807533.
62. Xiong, S., Tang, Y., Ng, H. S., Zhao, X., Jiang, Z., Chen, Z., Ng, K. W., & Loo, S. C. J. (2013). Specific surface area of titanium dioxide (TiO_2) particles influences cyto- and photo-toxicity. *Toxicology*, *304*, 132–140. https://doi.org/10.1016/j.tox.2012.12.015
63. Wei, H., Luo, J.-W., Li, S.-S., & Wang, L.-W. (2016). Revealing the origin of fast electron transfer in TiO_2-based dye-sensitized solar cells. *Journal of the American Chemical Society*, *138*(26), 8165–8174. https://doi.org/10.1021/jacs.6b03524
64. Lee, J., Kim, J., & Choi, W. (2011). TiO_2 photocatalysis for the redox conversion of aquatic pollutants. In *Aquatic Redox Chemistry* (pp. 199–222). American Chemical Society. https://doi.org/10.1021/bk-2011-1071.ch010
65. Gomathi, E., Balraj, B., & Kumaraguru, K. (2018). Electrochemical degradation of scarlet red dye from aqueous environment by titanium-based dimensionally stable anodes with SS electrodes. *Applied Biological Chemistry*, *61*(3), 289–293. https://doi.org/10.1007/s13765-018-0357-5
66. Chang, N., Liu, J., Ji, Y., Liu, J., & Chen, Y. (2023). Kinetic study of Rhodamine B degradation of electro-catalysis by TiO_2/activated semi-coke composite as tiny electrode. *Journal of Sol–Gel Science and Technology*, *106*(3), 684–698. https://doi.org/10.1007/s10971-023-06087-w
67. Padmanabhan, N. T., & John, H. (2020). Titanium dioxide based self-cleaning smart surfaces: a short review. *Journal of Environmental Chemical Engineering*, *8*(5), 104211. https://doi.org/10.1016/j.jece.2020.104211
68. Li, L., Yan, J., Wang, T., Zhao, Z.-J., Zhang, J., Gong, J., & Guan, N. (2015). Sub-10 nm rutile titanium dioxide nanoparticles for efficient visible-light-driven photocatalytic hydrogen production. *Nature Communications*, *6*(1), 5881. https://doi.org/10.1038/ncomms6881
69. Lan, Y., Lu, Y., & Ren, Z. (2013). Mini review on photocatalysis of titanium dioxide nanoparticles and their solar applications. *Nano Energy*, *2*(5), 1031–1045. https://doi.org/10.1016/j.nanoen.2013.04.002

70. Chen, D., Cheng, Y., Zhou, N., Chen, P., Wang, Y., Li, K., Huo, S., Cheng, P., Peng, P., Zhang, R., Wang, L., Liu, H., Liu, Y., & Ruan, R. (2020). Photocatalytic degradation of organic pollutants using TiO_2-based photocatalysts: a review. *Journal of Cleaner Production*, *268*, 121725. https://doi.org/10.1016/j.jclepro.2020.121725
71. Kotz, R., Stucki, S., & Carcer, B. (1991). Electrochemical waste water treatment using high overvoltage anodes. Part I: physical and electrochemical properties of SnO_2 anodes. *Journal of Applied Electrochemistry*, *21*(1), 14–20. https://doi.org/10.1007/BF01103823
72. Zhang, Y., Zou, J., He, Z., Zhao, Y., Kang, X., Zhao, Y., & Miao, Z. (2021). Facile synthesis of SnO_2 nanostructures for enhanced electrochemical hydrogen evolution reaction. *Journal of Alloys and Compounds*, *865*, 158597. https://doi.org/10.1016/j.jallcom.2021.158597
73. Zhang, W., Qin, Q., Dai, L., Qin, R., Zhao, X., Chen, X., Ou, D., Chen, J., Chuong, T. T., Wu, B., & Zheng, N. (2018). Electrochemical reduction of carbon dioxide to methanol on hierarchical Pd/SnO_2 nanosheets with abundant Pd–O–Sn interfaces. *Angewandte Chemie International Edition*, *57*(30), 9475–9479. https://doi.org/10.1002/anie.201804142
74. Liu, S., Xiao, J., Lu, X. F., Wang, J., Wang, X., & Lou, X. W. (David). (2019). Efficient electrochemical reduction of CO_2 to HCOOH over Sub-2 nm SnO_2 quantum wires with exposed grain boundaries. *Angewandte Chemie International Edition*, *58*(25), 8499–8503. https://doi.org/10.1002/anie.201903613
75. Yang, Y., Fei, H., Ruan, G., Li, L., Wang, G., Kim, N. D., & Tour, J. M. (2015). Carbon-free electrocatalyst for oxygen reduction and oxygen evolution reactions. *ACS Applied Materials & Interfaces*, *7*(37), 20607–20611. https://doi.org/10.1021/acsami.5b04887
76. Liu, Z., Guo, B., Hong, L., & Lim, T. H. (2006). Microwave heated polyol synthesis of carbon-supported PtSn nanoparticles for methanol electrooxidation. *Electrochemistry Communications*, *8*(1), 83–90. https://doi.org/10.1016/j.elecom.2005.10.019
77. McNab, T. K., Fox, R. A., & Boyle, A. J. F. (1968). Some magnetic properties of magnetite (Fe_3O_4) microcrystals. *Journal of Applied Physics*, *39*(12), 5703–5711. https://doi.org/10.1063/1.1656035
78. Flanders, P. J., & Remeika, J. P. (1965). Magnetic properties of hematite single crystals. *Philosophical Magazine: A Journal of Theoretical Experimental and Applied Physics*, *11*(114), 1271–1288. https://doi.org/10.1080/14786436508224935
79. Strangway, D. W., Honea, R. M., McMahon, B. E., & Larson, E. E. (1968). The magnetic properties of naturally occurring goethite. *Geophysical Journal International*, *15*(4), 345–359. https://doi.org/10.1111/j.1365-246X.1968.tb00191.x
80. Morrish, A. H., & Yu, S. P. (1955). Dependence of the coercive force on the density of some iron oxide powders. *Journal of Applied Physics*, *26*(8), 1049–1055. https://doi.org/10.1063/1.1722134
81. Lopes, A., Martins, S., Morão, A., Magrinho, M., & Gonçalves, I. (2004). Degradation of a textile dye C. I. Direct Red 80 by electrochemical processes. *Portugaliae Electrochimica Acta*, *22*(3), 279–294. https://doi.org/10.4152/pea.200403279
82. Muthukumar, M., Karuppiah, M. T., & Raju, G. B. (2007). Electrochemical removal of CI Acid Orange 10 from aqueous solutions. *Separation and Purification Technology*, *55*(2), 198–205. https://doi.org/10.1016/j.seppur.2006.11.014

83. Stanković, D. M., Ognjanović, M., Espinosa, A., del Puerto Morales, M., Bessais, L., Zehani, K., Antić, B., & Dojcinović, B. (2019). Iron oxide nanoflower-based screen print electrode for enhancement removal of organic dye using electrochemical approach. *Electrocatalysis*, *10*(6), 663–671. https://doi.org/10.1007/s12678-019-00554-1
84. Tang, Y., Zheng, S., Cao, S., Xue, H., & Pang, H. (2020). Advances in the application of manganese dioxide and its composites as electrocatalysts for the oxygen evolution reaction. *Journal of Materials Chemistry A*, *8*(36), 18492–18514. https://doi.org/10.1039/D0TA05985D
85. Noda, Y., Ohno, K., & Nakamura, S. (2016). Momentum-dependent band spin splitting in semiconducting MnO_2: a density functional calculation. *Physical Chemistry Chemical Physics*, *18*(19), 13294–13303. https://doi.org/10.1039/C5CP07806G
86. Sun, B. C., Zhao, W. K., Han, C. B., Zheng, J. Y., Yan, H., Yang, Z. C., Sun, L., Wang, X., & Song, X. (2023). Oxygen vacancies modified MnS/MnO_2 heterostructure anode catalyst for efficiently electrocatalytic removal of dye wastewater. *Journal of Alloys and Compounds*, *942*, 169037. https://doi.org/10.1016/j.jallcom.2023.169037
87. Sotgiu, G., Tortora, L., & Petrucci, E. (2015). Influence of surface roughening of titanium substrate in the electrochemical activity of manganese oxide thin film electrode in anodic oxidation of dye-containing solutions. *Journal of Applied Electrochemistry*, *45*(7), 787–797. https://doi.org/10.1007/s10800-015-0827-y
88. Doumbi, R. T., Noumi, G. B., & Domga, T. (2021). Electrochemical degradation of synthetic textile wastewater by C/MnO_2 electrode assessed by surface response methodology. *Avicenna Journal of Environmental Health Engineering*, *8*(2), 116–125. https://doi.org/10.34172/ajehe.2021.15
89. Abdiryim, T., Xiao-Gang, Z., & Jamal, R. (2005). Comparative studies of solid-state synthesized polyaniline doped with inorganic acids. *Materials Chemistry and Physics*, *90*(2–3), 367–372. https://doi.org/10.1016/j.matchemphys.2004.10.036
90. Stejskal, J., & Gilbert, R. G. (2002). Polyaniline. Preparation of a conducting polymer (IUPAC Technical Report). *Pure and Applied Chemistry*, *74*(5), 857–867. https://doi.org/10.1351/pac200274050857
91. Stejskal, J. (2020). Interaction of conducting polymers, polyaniline and polypyrrole, with organic dyes: polymer morphology control, dye adsorption and photocatalytic decomposition. *Chemical Papers*, *74*(1), 1–54. https://doi.org/10.1007/s11696-019-00982-9
92. Stejskal, J., & Prokeš, J. (2020). Conductivity and morphology of polyaniline and polypyrrole prepared in the presence of organic dyes. *Synthetic Metals*, *264*, 116373. https://doi.org/10.1016/j.synthmet.2020.116373
93. Shi, M., Zhang, Y., Bai, M., & Li, B. (2017). Facile fabrication of polyaniline with coral-like nanostructure as electrode material for supercapacitors. *Synthetic Metals*, *233*, 74–78. https://doi.org/10.1016/j.synthmet.2017.09.007
94. Shi, M., Bai, M., & Li, B. (2018). Acid Red 27-crosslinked polyaniline with nanofiber structure as electrode material for supercapacitors. *Materials Letters*, *212*, 259–262. https://doi.org/10.1016/j.matlet.2017.10.107
95. Minisy, I. M., Salahuddin, N. A., & Ayad, M. M. (2019). Chitosan/polyaniline hybrid for the removal of cationic and anionic dyes from aqueous solutions. *Journal of Applied Polymer Science*, *136*(6), 47056. https://doi.org/10.1002/app.47056
96. Gao, Y., Zhu, W., Li, Y., Zhang, Q., Chen, H., Zhang, J., & Huang, T. (2022). Anthraquinone (AQS)/polyaniline (PANI) modified carbon felt (CF) cathode for selective H_2O_2 generation and efficient pollutant removal in electro-Fenton.

Journal of Environmental Management, 304, 114315. https://doi.org/10.1016/j.jenvman.2021.114315

97. Haque, Md. M., Smith, W. T., & Wong, D. K. Y. (2015). Conducting polypyrrole films as a potential tool for electrochemical treatment of azo dyes in textile wastewaters. *Journal of Hazardous Materials, 283*, 164–170. https://doi.org/10.1016/j.jhazmat.2014.07.038
98. Wang, L.-X., Li, X.-G., & Yang, Y.-L. (2001). Preparation, properties and applications of polypyrroles. *Reactive and Functional Polymers, 47*(2), 125–139. https://doi.org/10.1016/S1381-5148(00)00079-1
99. Zhang, Z., Sun, J., Dou, M., Ji, J., & Wang, F. (2017). Nitrogen and phosphorus codoped mesoporous carbon derived from polypyrrole as superior metal-free electrocatalyst toward the oxygen reduction reaction. *ACS Applied Materials & Interfaces, 9*(19), 16236–16242. https://doi.org/10.1021/acsami.7b03375
100. Curran, D., Grimshaw, J., & Perera, S. D. (1991). Poly(pyrrole) as a support for electrocatalytic materials. *Chemical Society Reviews, 20*(3), 391. https://doi.org/10.1039/cs9912000391
101. Zhang, G., Wang, S., Zhao, S., Fu, L., Chen, G., & Yang, F. (2011). Oxidative degradation of azo dye by hydrogen peroxide electrogenerated in situ on anthraquinone monosulphonate/polypyrrole composite cathode with heterogeneous $CuO/\gamma\text{-}Al_2O_3$ catalyst. *Applied Catalysis B: Environmental, 106*(3–4), 370–378. https://doi.org/10.1016/j.apcatb.2011.05.042
102. Zia, J., Fatima, F., & Riaz, U. (2021). A comprehensive review on the photocatalytic activity of polythiophene-based nanocomposites against degradation of organic pollutants. *Catalysis Science & Technology, 11*(20), 6630–6648. https://doi.org/10.1039/D1CY01129D
103. Jeon, S. S., Yang, S. J., Lee, K.-J., & Im, S. S. (2010). A facile and rapid synthesis of unsubstituted polythiophene with high electrical conductivity using binary organic solvents. *Polymer, 51*(18), 4069–4076. https://doi.org/10.1016/j.polymer.2010.07.013
104. Xing, D., Zhou, P., Liu, Y., Wang, Z., Wang, P., Zheng, Z., Dai, Y., Whangbo, M.-H., & Huang, B. (2021). Atomically dispersed cobalt-based species anchored on polythiophene as an efficient electrocatalyst for oxygen evolution reaction. *Applied Surface Science, 545*, 148943. https://doi.org/10.1016/j.apsusc.2021.148943
105. Bora, C., Pegu, R., Saikia, B. J., & Dolui, S. K. (2014). Synthesis of polythiophene/graphene oxide composites by interfacial polymerization and evaluation of their electrical and electrochemical properties. *Polymer International, 63*(12), 2061–2067. https://doi.org/10.1002/pi.4739
106. Roncali, J., Blanchard, P., & Frere, P. (2005). 3,4-Ethylenedioxythiophene (EDOT) as a versatile building block for advanced functional π-conjugated systems. *Journal of Materials Chemistry, 15*(16), 1589–1610. https://doi.org/10.1039/B415481A
107. Fan, J., Shao, W., Xu, G., Cui, X. T., & Luo, X. (2014). Preparation and electrochemical catalytic application of nanocrystalline cellulose doped poly(3,4-ethylenedioxythiophene) conducting polymer nanocomposites. *RSC Advances, 4*(46), 24328–24333. https://doi.org/10.1039/C4RA02796E
108. Lattach, Y., Deniset-Besseau, A., Guigner, J.-M., & Remita, S. (2013). Radiation chemistry as an alternative way for the synthesis of PEDOT conducting polymers under "soft" conditions. *Radiation Physics and Chemistry, 82*, 44–53. https://doi.org/10.1016/j.radphyschem.2012.09.009
109. Coletta, C., Cui, Z., Archirel, P., Pernot, P., Marignier, J.-L., & Remita, S. (2015). Electron-induced growth mechanism of conducting polymers: a coupled experimental

and computational investigation. *Journal of Physical Chemistry B*, *119*(16), 5282–5298. https://doi.org/10.1021/acs.jpcb.5b02632
110. Tong, L., Skorenko, K. H., Faucett, A. C., Boyer, S. M., Liu, J., Mativetsky, J. M., Bernier, W. E., & Jones, W. E. (2015). Vapor-phase polymerization of poly(3,4-ethylenedioxythiophene) (PEDOT) on commercial carbon coated aluminum foil as enhanced electrodes for supercapacitors. *Journal of Power Sources*, *297*, 195–201. https://doi.org/10.1016/j.jpowsour.2015.06.128
111. Yoon, H., Chang, M., & Jang, J. (2007). Formation of 1D poly(3,4-ethylenedioxythiophene) nanomaterials in reverse microemulsions and their application to chemical sensors. *Advanced Functional Materials*, *17*(3), 431–436. https://doi.org/10.1002/adfm.200600106
112. Choi, S., Boo, J.-H., Sohn, H., & Kim, S. (2014). Quality dependence of vapor phase-polymerized poly(3,4-ethylenedioxythiophene) nanofilm on substrate pre-treatment methods. *Journal of Nanoscience and Nanotechnology*, *14*(12), 9005–9010. https://doi.org/10.1166/jnn.2014.10077
113. Zhang, L., Jamal, R., Zhao, Q., Wang, M., & Abdiryim, T. (2015). Preparation of PEDOT/GO, PEDOT/MnO_2, and PEDOT/GO/MnO_2 nanocomposites and their application in catalytic degradation of methylene blue. *Nanoscale Research Letters*, *10*(1), 148. https://doi.org/10.1186/s11671-015-0859-6
114. Asadian, E., Shahrokhian, S., & Iraji Zad, A. (2020). ZIF-8/PEDOT @ flexible carbon cloth electrode as highly efficient electrocatalyst for oxygen reduction reaction. *International Journal of Hydrogen Energy*, *45*(3), 1890–1900. https://doi.org/10.1016/j.ijhydene.2019.11.124
115. Abdullah, U., Ali, M., & Pervaiz, E. (2021). An inclusive review on recent advancements of cadmium sulfide nanostructures and its hybrids for photocatalytic and electrocatalytic applications. *Molecular Catalysis*, *508*, 111575. https://doi.org/10.1016/j.mcat.2021.111575
116. Yu, S., Liu, Q., Yang, W., Han, K., Wang, Z., & Zhu, H. (2013). Graphene–CeO_2 hybrid support for Pt nanoparticles as potential electrocatalyst for direct methanol fuel cells. *Electrochimica Acta*, *94*, 245–251. https://doi.org/10.1016/j.electacta.2013.01.149
117. Mansor, N., Miller, T. S., Dedigama, I., Jorge, A. B., Jia, J., Brázdová, V., Mattevi, C., Gibbs, C., Hodgson, D., Shearing, P. R., Howard, C. A., Cora, F., Shaffer, M., Brett, D. J. L., & McMillan, P. F. (2016). Graphitic carbon nitride as a catalyst support in fuel cells and electrolyzers. *Electrochimica Acta*, *222*, 44–57. https://doi.org/10.1016/j.electacta.2016.11.008
118. Ganesan, P., Staykov, A., Shu, H., Uejima, M., & Nakashima, N. (2020). Designing an Fe^{III}-doped nickel sulfide/carbon nanotube hybrid catalyst for alkaline electrolyte membrane water electrolyzers and Zn–air battery performances. *ACS Applied Energy Materials*, *3*(11), 10961–10975. https://doi.org/10.1021/acsaem.0c01931
119. Liu, Z., Xu, X., Fang, J., Zhu, X., & Li, B. (2012). Synergistic degradation of Eosin Y by photocatalysis and electrocatalysis in UV irradiated solution containing hybrid BiOCl/TiO_2 particles. *Water, Air, & Soil Pollution*, *223*(5), 2783–2798. https://doi.org/10.1007/s11270-011-1066-4
120. Pahra, S., Sangabathula, O., Sharma, C. S., & Devi, P. (2023). A noble metal-free candle soot derived carbon electrocatalyst for simultaneous H_2 generation and wastewater treatment. *Journal of Physics and Chemistry of Solids*, *173*, 111106. https://doi.org/10.1016/j.jpcs.2022.111106
121. Pirkarami, A., Rasouli, S., & Ghasemi, E. (2022). CdS@NiCo-LDH hybrid photoelectrocatalyst with enhanced photocatalytic activity: a convenient and stable

hybrid for wastewater treatment. *Journal of Alloys and Compounds*, *911*, 164736. https://doi.org/10.1016/j.jallcom.2022.164736

122. Listorti, A., O'Regan, B., & Durrant, J. R. (2011). Electron transfer dynamics in dye-sensitized solar cells. *Chemistry of Materials*, *23*(15), 3381–3399. https://doi.org/10.1021/cm200651e
123. Rauf, M. A., & Ashraf, S. S. (2009). Radiation induced degradation of dyes – an overview. *Journal of Hazardous Materials*, *166*(1), 6–16. https://doi.org/10.1016/j.jhazmat.2008.11.043
124. Prajapat, K., Dhonde, M., Sahu, K., Bhojane, P., Murty, V., & Shirage, P. M. (2023). The evolution of organic materials for efficient dye-sensitized solar cells. *Journal of Photochemistry and Photobiology C: Photochemistry Reviews*, *55*, 100586. https://doi.org/10.1016/j.jphotochemrev.2023.100586
125. Katoh, R., & Furube, A. (2014). Electron injection efficiency in dye-sensitized solar cells. *Journal of Photochemistry and Photobiology C: Photochemistry Reviews*, *20*, 1–16. https://doi.org/10.1016/j.jphotochemrev.2014.02.001
126. Jiang, Y., Zhao, H., Liang, J., Yue, L., Li, T., Luo, Y., Liu, Q., Lu, S., Asiri, A. M., Gong, Z., & Sun, X. (2021). Anodic oxidation for the degradation of organic pollutants: anode materials, operating conditions and mechanisms. A mini review. *Electrochemistry Communications*, *123*, 106912. https://doi.org/10.1016/j.elecom.2020.106912
127. Spadaro, J. T., Isabelle, L., & Renganathan, V. (1994). Hydroxyl radical mediated degradation of azo dyes: evidence for benzene generation. *Environmental Science & Technology*, *28*(7), 1389–1393. https://doi.org/10.1021/es00056a031
128. Ledakowicz, S., & Pazdzior, K. (2021). Recent achievements in dyes removal focused on advanced oxidation processes integrated with biological methods. *Molecules*, *26*(4), 870. https://doi.org/10.3390/molecules26040870
129. Nosaka, Y., & Nosaka, A. (2016). Understanding hydroxyl radical (•OH) generation processes in photocatalysis. *ACS Energy Letters*, *1*(2), 356–359. https://doi.org/10.1021/acsenergylett.6b00174
130. Heard, D. M., & Lennox, A. J. J. (2020). Electrode materials in modern organic electrochemistry. *Angewandte Chemie International Edition*, *59*(43), 18866–18884. https://doi.org/10.1002/anie.202005745
131. Etacheri, V., di Valentin, C., Schneider, J., Bahnemann, D., & Pillai, S. C. (2015). Visible-light activation of TiO_2 photocatalysts: advances in theory and experiments. *Journal of Photochemistry and Photobiology C: Photochemistry Reviews*, *25*, 1–29. https://doi.org/10.1016/j.jphotochemrev.2015.08.003
132. Teissie, J. (2017). Involvement of reactive oxygen species in membrane electropermeabilization. In *Handbook of Electroporation* (pp. 473–487). Springer International Publishing. https://doi.org/10.1007/978-3-319-32886-7_40
133. Selvaraj, V., Swarna Karthika, T., Mansiya, C., & Alagar, M. (2021). An over review on recently developed techniques, mechanisms and intermediate involved in the advanced azo dye degradation for industrial applications. *Journal of Molecular Structure*, *1224*, 129195. https://doi.org/10.1016/j.molstruc.2020.129195
134. Belal, R. M., Zayed, M. A., El-Sherif, R. M., & Abdel Ghany, N. A. (2021). Advanced electrochemical degradation of basic yellow 28 textile dye using IrO_2/Ti meshed electrode in different supporting electrolytes. *Journal of Electroanalytical Chemistry*, *882*, 114979. https://doi.org/10.1016/j.jelechem.2021.114979
135. Xiong, T., Wang, J., Wang, Y., & Wei, Y. (2018). Electrochemical degradation of dyes: mechanisms, influential factors, and research trends. *Environmental Science and Pollution Research*, *25*(20), 19542–19561. DOI: 10.1007/s11356-018-2020-2

136. Cionti, C., Pargoletti, E., Falletta, E., Bianchi, C. L., Meroni, D., & Cappelletti, G. (2022). Combining pH-triggered adsorption and photocatalysis for the remediation of complex water matrices. *Journal of Environmental Chemical Engineering*, *10*(5), 108468. https://doi.org/10.1016/j.jece.2022.108468
137. Greijer Agrell, H., Lindgren, J., & Hagfeldt, A. (2003). Degradation mechanisms in a dye-sensitized solar cell studied by UV–VIS and IR spectroscopy. *Solar Energy*, *75*(2), 169–180. https://doi.org/10.1016/S0038-092X(03)00248-2
138. Yang, R.-Y., Chen, H.-Y., & Lai, F.-D. (2012). Performance degradation of dye-sensitized solar cells induced by electrolytes. *Advances in Materials Science and Engineering*, *2012*, 1–4. https://doi.org/10.1155/2012/902146
139. Su, X., Zhang, M., Gao, W., & Yan, Y. (2017). A study of electrochemical degradation of reactive dyes on different anodes. *Journal of Chemistry*, *2017*, 6391819. DOI: 10.1155/2017/6391819
140. Zhao, S., Ribbing, C.-G., & Wackelgard, E. (2005). New method to optimize a solar absorber graded film profile. *Solar Energy*, *78*(1), 125–130. https://doi.org/10.1016/j.solener.2004.06.010
141. Sirés, I., Brillas, E., & Oturan, M. A. (2014). Electro-Fenton process and related electrochemical technologies based on Fenton's reaction chemistry. *Chemical Reviews*, *114*(24), 11527-11588. DOI: 10.1021/cr4006698
142. Li, Q., Ma, J., Zhang, Y., Zhang, G., & Sun, S. (2018). Electrochemical degradation of acid orange 7 using boron-doped diamond electrode: role of active species and degradation pathways. *Chemical Engineering Journal*, *334*, 1711–1720. DOI: 10.1016/j.cej.2017.12.089
143. Kabir, M. H., & Lockwood, F. C. (2016). Electrochemical decolorization and degradation of acid dyes in alkaline media. *Environmental Science & Technology*, *50*(21), 12023–12030. DOI: 10.1021/acs.est.6b03253
144. Cheng, J., Liu, S., Wang, Y., & Qiu, J. (2018). Enhanced electrocatalytic activity of a 3D macroporous nitrogen-doped graphene/MnO_2 composite electrode for the electrochemical degradation of dyes. *Chemical Engineering Journal*, *334*, 2008–2018. DOI: 10.1016/j.cej.2017.11.151
145. Krishnan, S., Jaiganesh, P. S., Karunakaran, A., Kumarasamy, K., & Lin, M.-C. (2021). The effect of pH on the photocatalytic degradation of cationic and anionic dyes using polyazomethine/ZnO and polyazomethine/TiO_2 nanocomposites. *International Journal of Applied Science and Engineering*, *18*(5), 1–8. https://doi.org/10.6703/IJASE.202109_18(5).008
146. Pan, B., Liu, B., Wang, S., Lv, Y., Du, H., & Zhang, Y. (2023). Understanding the hydroxyl adsorption behavior at Pt electrode surface in high-temperature alkaline solutions. *Chinese Journal of Chemical Engineering*, *54*, 173–179. https://doi.org/10.1016/j.cjche.2022.04.012
147. Salleh, M. A. M., Mahmoud, D. K., Karim, W. A. W. A., & Idris, A. (2011). Cationic and anionic dye adsorption by agricultural solid wastes: a comprehensive review. *Desalination*, *280*(1–3) 1–13. https://doi.org/10.1016/j.desal.2011.07.019
148. Verma, S., Tirumala Rao, B., Singh, R., & Kaul, R. (2021). Photocatalytic degradation kinetics of cationic and anionic dyes using Au–ZnO nanorods: role of pH for selective and simultaneous degradation of binary dye mixtures. *Ceramics International*, *47*(24), 34751–34764. https://doi.org/10.1016/j.ceramint.2021.09.014
149. Aquino, J. M., Rodrigo, M. A., Rocha-Filho, R. C., Saez, C., & Canizares, P. (2012). Influence of the supporting electrolyte on the electrolyses of dyes with conductive-diamond anodes. *Chemical Engineering Journal*, *184*, 221–227. https://doi.org/10.1016/j.cej.2012.01.044

150. Keyikoglu, R., Can, O. T., Aygun, A., & Tek, A. (2019). Comparison of the effects of various supporting electrolytes on the treatment of a dye solution by electrocoagulation process. *Colloid and Interface Science Communications*, *33*, 100210. https://doi.org/10.1016/j.colcom.2019.100210
151. Kuang, L., Zhao, Y., Zhang, W., & Ge, S. (2016). Roles of reactive oxygen species and holes in the photodegradation of cationic and anionic dyes by TiO_2 under UV irradiation. *Journal of Environmental Engineering*, *142*(2). https://doi.org/10.1061/(ASCE)EE.1943-7870.0001032
152. Zainal, Z., Lee, C. Y., Hussein, M. Z., Kassim, A., & Yusof, N. A. (2005). Effect of supporting electrolytes in electrochemically-assisted photodegradation of an azo dye. *Journal of Photochemistry and Photobiology A: Chemistry*, *172*(3), 316–321. https://doi.org/10.1016/j.jphotochem.2004.12.021
153. Masud, & Kim, H. K. (2023). Redox shuttle-based electrolytes for dye-sensitized solar cells: comprehensive guidance, recent progress, and future perspective. *ACS Omega*, *8*(7), 6139–6163. https://doi.org/10.1021/acsomega.2c06843
154. Aguedach, A., Brosillon, S., Morvan, J., & Lhadi, E. K. (2008). Influence of ionic strength in the adsorption and during photocatalysis of reactive black 5 azo dye on TiO_2 coated on non-woven paper with SiO_2 as a binder. *Journal of Hazardous Materials*, *150*(2), 250–256. https://doi.org/10.1016/j.jhazmat.2007.04.086
155. Akpan, U. G., & Hameed, B. H. (2009). Parameters affecting the photocatalytic degradation of dyes using TiO_2-based photocatalysts: a review. *Journal of Hazardous Materials*, *170*(2–3), 520–529. https://doi.org/10.1016/j.jhazmat.2009.05.039
156. Uranga-Flores, A., de la Rosa-Juarez, C., Gutierrez-Granados, S., de Moura, D. C., Martínez-Huitle, C. A., & Peralta Hernández, J. M. (2015). Electrochemical promotion of strong oxidants to degrade Acid Red 211: effect of supporting electrolytes. *Journal of Electroanalytical Chemistry*, *738*, 84–91. https://doi.org/10.1016/j.jelechem.2014.11.030
157. Chow, H., Ingelsson, M., Roberts, E. P. L., & Pham, A. L.-T. (2021). How does periodic polarity reversal affect the faradaic efficiency and electrode fouling during iron electrocoagulation? *Water Research*, *203*, 117497. https://doi.org/10.1016/j.watres.2021.117497
158. Kwak, W.-J., Kim, H., Petit, Y. K., Leypold, C., Nguyen, T. T., Mahne, N., Redfern, P., Curtiss, L. A., Jung, H.-G., Borisov, S. M., Freunberger, S. A., & Sun, Y.-K. (2019). Deactivation of redox mediators in lithium-oxygen batteries by singlet oxygen. *Nature Communications*, *10*(1), 1380. https://doi.org/10.1038/s41467-019-09399-0
159. Rountree, E. S., McCarthy, B. D., Eisenhart, T. T., & Dempsey, J. L. (2014). Evaluation of homogeneous electrocatalysts by cyclic voltammetry. *Inorganic Chemistry*, *53*(19), 9983–10002. https://doi.org/10.1021/ic500658x
160. Wang, S., Xu, Z., Wu, X., Zhao, H., Zhao, J., Liu, J., Yan, C., & Fan, X. (2020). Analyses and optimization of electrolyte concentration on the electrochemical performance of iron-chromium flow battery. *Applied Energy*, *271*, 115252. https://doi.org/10.1016/j.apenergy.2020.115252
161. Devadi, M. A. H., Krishna, M., Murthy, H. N. N., & Sathyanarayana, B. S. (2014). Statistical optimization for photocatalytic degradation of methylene blue by Ag–TiO_2 nanoparticles. *Procedia Materials Science*, *5*, 612–621. https://doi.org/10.1016/j.mspro.2014.07.307
162. Mohan, S., & Rajasekaran, N. (2011). Influence of electrolyte pH on composition, corrosion properties and surface morphology of electrodeposited Cu–Ni alloy. *Surface Engineering*, *27*(7), 519–523. https://doi.org/10.1179/026708410X12786785573472

163. Kumar, A., & Pandey, G. (2017). A review on the factors affecting the photocatalytic degradation of hazardous materials. *Material Science & Engineering International Journal*, *1*(3), 106–114. https://doi.org/10.15406/mseij.2017.01.00018
164. Mohtar, S. S., Aziz, F., Ismail, A. F., Sambudi, N. S., Abdullah, H., Rosli, A. N., & Ohtani, B. (2021). Impact of doping and additive applications on photocatalyst textural properties in removing organic pollutants: a review. *Catalysts*, *11*(10), 1160. https://doi.org/10.3390/catal11101160
165. Park, H., Park, Y., Kim, W., & Choi, W. (2013). Surface modification of TiO_2 photocatalyst for environmental applications. *Journal of Photochemistry and Photobiology C: Photochemistry Reviews*, *15*, 1–20. https://doi.org/10.1016/j.jphotochemrev.2012.10.001
166. Elumalai, N. K., Vijila, C., Jose, R., Uddin, A., & Ramakrishna, S. (2015). Metal oxide semiconducting interfacial layers for photovoltaic and photocatalytic applications. *Materials for Renewable and Sustainable Energy*, *4*(3), 11. https://doi.org/10.1007/s40243-015-0054-9
167. Li, S.-H., Zhao, Y., Chu, J., Li, W.-W., Yu, H.-Q., & Liu, G. (2013). Electrochemical degradation of methyl orange on Pt–Bi/C nanostructured electrode by a square-wave potential method. *Electrochimica Acta*, *92*, 93–101. https://doi.org/10.1016/j.electacta.2013.01.012
168. Zhao, G., Cui, X., Liu, M., Li, P., Zhang, Y., Cao, T., Li, H., Lei, Y., Liu, L., & Li, D. (2009). Electrochemical degradation of refractory pollutant using a novel microstructured TiO_2 nanotubes/Sb-doped SnO_2 electrode. *Environmental Science & Technology*, *43*(5), 1480–1486. https://doi.org/10.1021/es802155p
169. Kariyajjanavar, P., Jogttappa, N., & Nayaka, Y. A. (2011). Studies on degradation of reactive textile dyes solution by electrochemical method. *Journal of Hazardous Materials*, *190*(1–3), 952–961. https://doi.org/10.1016/j.jhazmat.2011.04.032
170. Hamad, H., Bassyouni, D., El-Ashtoukhy, E.-S., Amin, N., & Abd El-Latif, M. (2018). Electrocatalytic degradation and minimization of specific energy consumption of synthetic azo dye from wastewater by anodic oxidation process with an emphasis on enhancing economic efficiency and reaction mechanism. *Ecotoxicology and Environmental Safety*, *148*, 501–512. https://doi.org/10.1016/j.ecoenv.2017.10.061
171. Zhang, C., Zhang, Z., He, Z., & Fu, D. (2017). New insights into the relationship between anode material, supporting electrolyte and applied current density in anodic oxidation processes. *Electrochimica Acta*, *229*, 55–64. https://doi.org/10.1016/j.electacta.2017.01.134
172. Ruiz, E. J., Hernández-Ramírez, A., Peralta-Hernández, J. M., Arias, C., & Brillas, E. (2011). Application of solar photoelectro-Fenton technology to azo dyes mineralization: effect of current density, Fe^{2+} and dye concentrations. *Chemical Engineering Journal*, *171*(2), 385–392. https://doi.org/10.1016/j.cej.2011.03.004
173. Khan, M. Z., Song, R.-H., Hussain, A., Lee, S.-B., Lim, T.-H., & Hong, J.-E. (2020). Effect of applied current density on the degradation behavior of anode-supported flat-tubular solid oxide fuel cells. *Journal of the European Ceramic Society*, *40*(4), 1407–1417. https://doi.org/10.1016/j.jeurceramsoc.2019.11.017
174. Martínez-Huitle, C. A., & Ferro, S. (2006). Electrochemical oxidation of organic pollutants for the wastewater treatment: direct and indirect processes. *Chemical Society Reviews*, *35*(12), 1324–1340. https://doi.org/10.1039/B517632H
175. An, H., Cui, H., Zhang, W., Zhai, J., Qian, Y., Xie, X., & Li, Q. (2012). Fabrication and electrochemical treatment application of a microstructured TiO_2-NTs/Sb–SnO_2/PbO_2 anode in the degradation of C.I. Reactive Blue 194 (RB 194). *Chemical Engineering Journal*, *209*, 86–93. https://doi.org/10.1016/j.cej.2012.07.089

176. Fernandes, A. (2004). Electrochemical degradation of C. I. Acid Orange 7. *Dyes and Pigments*, *61*(3), 287–296. https://doi.org/10.1016/j.dyepig.2003.11.008
177. Chen, X., & Chen, G. (2006). Anodic oxidation of Orange II on Ti/BDD electrode: variable effects. *Separation and Purification Technology*, *48*(1), 45–49. https://doi.org/10.1016/j.seppur.2005.07.024
178. Zaher, A., el Rouby, W. M. A., & Barakat, N. A. M. (2020). Influences of tungsten incorporation, morphology and calcination temperature on the electrocatalytic activity of Ni/C nanostructures toward urea elimination from wastewaters. *International Journal of Hydrogen Energy*, *45*(15), 8082–8093. https://doi.org/10.1016/j.ijhydene.2020.01.090
179. Polymeros, G., Baldizzone, C., Geiger, S., Grote, J. P., Knossalla, J., Mezzavilla, S., Keeley, G. P., Cherevko, S., Zeradjanin, A. R., Schüth, F., & Mayrhofer, K. J. J. (2016). High temperature stability study of carbon supported high surface area catalysts – expanding the boundaries of ex-situ diagnostics. *Electrochimica Acta*, *211*, 744–753. https://doi.org/10.1016/j.electacta.2016.06.105
180. Bartholomew, C. H., Agrawal, P. K., & Katzer, J. R. (1982). Sulfur poisoning of metals. *Advances in Catalysis*, *31*, 135–242. https://doi.org/10.1016/S0360-0564(08)60454-X
181. Awad, H. S., & Galwa, N. A. (2005). Electrochemical degradation of Acid Blue and Basic Brown dyes on Pb/PbO_2 electrode in the presence of different conductive electrolyte and effect of various operating factors. *Chemosphere*, *61*(9), 1327–1335. https://doi.org/10.1016/j.chemosphere.2005.03.054
182. Rocha, J. H. B., Solano, A. M. S., Fernandes, N. S., da Silva, D. R., Peralta-Hernandez, J. M., & Martinez-Huitle, C. A. (2012). Electrochemical degradation of Remazol Red BR and Novacron Blue C-D dyes using diamond electrode. *Electrocatalysis*, *3*(1), 1–12. https://doi.org/10.1007/s12678-011-0070-1
183. Sun, S.-P., Li, C.-J., Sun, J.-H., Shi, S.-H., Fan, M.-H., & Zhou, Q. (2009). Decolorization of an azo dye Orange G in aqueous solution by Fenton oxidation process: effect of system parameters and kinetic study. *Journal of Hazardous Materials*, *161*(2–3), 1052–1057. https://doi.org/10.1016/j.jhazmat.2008.04.080
184. Ullah, R., Naeemullah, & Tuzen, M. (2023). Photocatalytic removal of organic dyes by titanium doped alumina nanocomposites: using multivariate factorial and kinetics models. *Journal of Molecular Structure*, *1285*, 135509. https://doi.org/10.1016/j.molstruc.2023.135509
185. Panizza, M., & Cerisola, G. (2008). Removal of colour and COD from wastewater containing acid blue 22 by electrochemical oxidation. *Journal of Hazardous Materials*, *153*(1–2), 83–88. https://doi.org/10.1016/j.jhazmat.2007.08.023
186. Bensalah, N., Alfaro, M. A. Q., & Martínez-Huitle, C. A. (2009). Electrochemical treatment of synthetic wastewaters containing Alphazurine A dye. *Chemical Engineering Journal*, *149*(1–3), 348–352. https://doi.org/10.1016/j.cej.2008.11.031
187. Martínez-Huitle, C. A., Ferro, S., & de Battisti, A. (2004). Electrochemical incineration of oxalic acid. *Electrochimica Acta*, *49*(22–23), 4027–4034. https://doi.org/10.1016/j.electacta.2004.01.083
188. Marselli, B., Garcia-Gomez, J., Michaud, P.-A., Rodrigo, M. A., & Comninellis, Ch. (2003). Electrogeneration of hydroxyl radicals on boron-doped diamond electrodes. *Journal of the Electrochemical Society*, *150*(3), D79. https://doi.org/10.1149/1.1553790
189. Dinesh, A., Kanmani Raja, K., Manikandan, A., Almessiere, M. A., Slimani, Y., Baykal, A., Saeed Alorfi, H., Hussein, M. A., & Khan, A. (2022). Sol–gel combustion synthesis and photocatalytic dye degradation studies of rare earth element

Ce substituted Mn–Zn ferrite nanoparticles. *Journal of Materials Research and Technology*, *18*, 5280–5289. https://doi.org/10.1016/j.jmrt.2022.04.121

190. Dharamalingam, K., Arjun Kumar, B., Ramalingam, G., Sasi Florence, S., Raju, K., Senthil Kumar, P., Govindaraju, S., & Thangavel, E. (2022). The role of sodium dodecyl sulfate mediated hydrothermal synthesis of MoS_2 nanosheets for photocatalytic dye degradation and dye-sensitized solar cell application. *Chemosphere*, *294*, 133725. https://doi.org/10.1016/j.chemosphere.2022.133725
191. Rafique, M., Tahir, R., Khalid, N. R., Tahir, M. B., Irshad, M., Gillani, S. S. A., Usman, A., Shahzad, K., Mahmood Ali, A., & Muhammad, S. (2021). Hydrothermal synthesis of an efficient and visible light responsive pure and strontium doped zinc oxide nano-hexagonal photocatalysts for photodegradation of Rhodamine B dye. *Applied Nanoscience*, *11*(3), 1045–1056. https://doi.org/10.1007/s13204-021-01669-y
192. Abu Ghalwa, N. M., & Zaggout, F. R. (2006). Electrodegradation of methylene blue dye in water and wastewater using lead oxide/titanium modified electrode. *Journal of Environmental Science and Health, Part A*, *41*(10), 2271–2282. https://doi.org/10.1080/10934520600872888
193. Tabti, S., Benchettara, A., Smaili, F., Benchettara, A., & Berrabah, S. E. (2022). Electrodeposition of lead dioxide on Fe electrode: application to the degradation of indigo carmine dye. *Journal of Applied Electrochemistry*, *52*(8), 1207–1217. https://doi.org/10.1007/s10800-022-01709-7
194. Basavaraj, N., Sekar, A., & Yadav, R. (2021). Review on green carbon dot-based materials for the photocatalytic degradation of dyes: fundamentals and future perspective. *Materials Advances*, *2*(23), 7559–7582. https://doi.org/10.1039/D1MA00773D
195. Pereira, R. A., Pereira, M. F. R., Alves, M. M., & Pereira, L. (2014). Carbon based materials as novel redox mediators for dye wastewater biodegradation. *Applied Catalysis B: Environmental*, *144*, 713–720. https://doi.org/10.1016/j.apcatb.2013.07.009
196. Zhang, M., Wang, L., Zeng, T., Shang, Q., Zhou, H., Pan, Z., & Cheng, Q. (2018). Two pure MOF-photocatalysts readily prepared for the degradation of methylene blue dye under visible light. *Dalton Transactions*, *47*(12), 4251–4258. https://doi.org/10.1039/C8DT00156A
197. Suhadolnik, L., Pohar, A., Novak, U., Likozar, B., Mihelic, A., & Ceh, M. (2019). Continuous photocatalytic, electrocatalytic and photo-electrocatalytic degradation of a reactive textile dye for wastewater-treatment processes: batch, microreactor and scaled-up operation. *Journal of Industrial and Engineering Chemistry*, *72*, 178–188. https://doi.org/10.1016/j.jiec.2018.12.017
198. Bazzazan, S., Moeinabadi-Bidgoli, K., Lalami, Z. A., Bazzazan, S., Mehrarya, M., Yeganeh, F. E., Hejabi, F., Akbarzadeh, I., Noorbazargan, H., Jahanbakhshi, M., Hossein-khannazer, N., & Mostafavi, E. (2023). Engineered UIO-66 metal–organic framework for delivery of curcumin against breast cancer cells: an in vitro evaluation. *Journal of Drug Delivery Science and Technology*, 79. https://doi.org/10.1016/j.jddst.2022.104009
199. Mukimin, A., Zen, N., Purwanto, A., Wicaksono, K. A., Vistanty, H., & Alfauzi, A. S. (2017). Application of a full-scale electrocatalytic reactor as real batik printing wastewater treatment by indirect oxidation process. *Journal of Environmental Chemical Engineering*, *5*(5), 5222–5232. https://doi.org/10.1016/j.jece.2017.09.053
200. Qian, W., Xu, S., Zhang, X., Li, C., Yang, W., Bowen, C. R., & Yang, Y. (2021). Differences and similarities of photocatalysis and electrocatalysis in two-dimensional

nanomaterials: strategies, traps, applications and challenges. *Nano-Micro Letters*, *13*(1), 156. https://doi.org/10.1007/s40820-021-00681-9

201. Chang, J.-H., Wang, Y.-L., Dong, C.-D., & Shen, S.-Y. (2020). Electrocatalytic degradation of azo dye by vanadium-doped TiO_2 nanocatalyst. *Catalysts*, *10*(5), 482. https://doi.org/10.3390/catal10050482
202. Yu, N., Lu, X., Song, F., Yao, Y., & Han, E. (2021). Electrocatalytic degradation of sulfamethazine on IrO_2–RuO_2 composite electrodes: influencing factors, kinetics and modeling. *Journal of Environmental Chemical Engineering*, *9*(4), 105301. https://doi.org/10.1016/j.jece.2021.105301
203. Singh, S., Srivastava, V. C., & Mall, I. D. (2013). Mechanism of dye degradation during electrochemical treatment. *Journal of Physical Chemistry C*, *117*(29), 15229–15240. https://doi.org/10.1021/jp405289f
204. Li, F., Huang, L., Zaman, S., Guo, W., Liu, H., Guo, X., & Xia, B. Y. (2022). Corrosion chemistry of electrocatalysts. *Advanced Materials*, *34*(52). https://doi.org/10.1002/adma.202200840
205. Nunes, C., Souza, P., Freitas, A., Silva, M., Rosa, F., & Muniz, E. (2017). Poisoning effects of water and dyes on the [Bmim][BF4] catalysis of poly(ethylene terephthalate) (PET) depolymerization under supercritical ethanol. *Catalysts*, *7*(12), 43. https://doi.org/10.3390/catal7020043.
206. Pieczyńska, A., Ossowski, T., Bogdanowicz, R., & Siedlecka, E. (2019). Electrochemical degradation of textile dyes in a flow reactor: effect of operating conditions and dyes chemical structure. *International Journal of Environmental Science and Technology*, *16*(2), 929–942. https://doi.org/10.1007/s13762-018-1704-0
207. Samarghandi, M. R., Dargahi, A., Shabanloo, A., Nasab, H. Z., Vaziri, Y., & Ansari, A. (2020). Electrochemical degradation of methylene blue dye using a graphite doped PbO_2 anode: optimization of operational parameters, degradation pathway and improving the biodegradability of textile wastewater. *Arabian Journal of Chemistry*, *13*(8), 6847–6864. https://doi.org/10.1016/j.arabjc.2020.06.038
208. Łuba, M., Mikołajczyk, T., Pierożyński, B., Smoczyński, L., Wojtacha, P., & Kuczyński, M. (2020). Electrochemical degradation of industrial dyes in wastewater through the dissolution of aluminum sacrificial anode of Cu/Al macro-corrosion galvanic cell. *Molecules*, *25*(18), 4108. https://doi.org/10.3390/molecules25184108
209. Kuleyin, A., Gök, A., & Akbal, F. (2021). Treatment of textile industry wastewater by electro-Fenton process using graphite electrodes in batch and continuous mode. *Journal of Environmental Chemical Engineering*, *9*(1), 104782. https://doi.org/10.1016/j.jece.2020.104782
210. Al-Tohamy, R., Ali, S. S., Li, F., Okasha, K. M., Mahmoud, Y. A.-G., Elsamahy, T., Jiao, H., Fu, Y., & Sun, J. (2022). A critical review on the treatment of dye-containing wastewater: ecotoxicological and health concerns of textile dyes and possible remediation approaches for environmental safety. *Ecotoxicology and Environmental Safety*, *231*, 113160. https://doi.org/10.1016/j.ecoenv.2021.113160
211. Saratale, R. G., Saratale, G. D., Chang, J. S., & Govindwar, S. P. (2011). Bacterial decolorization and degradation of azo dyes: a review. *Journal of the Taiwan Institute of Chemical Engineers*, *42*(1), 138–157. https://doi.org/10.1016/j.jtice.2010.06.006
212. Moreira, F. C., Boaventura, R. A. R., Brillas, E., & Vilar, V. J. P. (2017). Electrochemical advanced oxidation processes: a review on their application to synthetic and real wastewaters. *Applied Catalysis B: Environmental*, *202*, 217–261. https://doi.org/10.1016/j.apcatb.2016.08.037
213. Barrera-Díaz, C., Cañizares, P., Fernández, F. J., Natividad, R., & Rodrigo, M. A. (2017). Electrochemical advanced oxidation processes: an overview of the current

applications to actual industrial effluents. *Journal of the Mexican Chemical Society, 58*(3). https://doi.org/10.29356/jmcs.v58i3.133
214. Brosler, P., Girão, A. v., Silva, R. F., Tedim, J., & Oliveira, F. J. (2023). Electrochemical advanced oxidation processes using diamond technology: a critical review. *Environments, 10*(2), 15. https://doi.org/10.3390/environments10020015
215. Vellanki, B. P., Batchelor, B., & Abdel-Wahab, A. (2013). Advanced reduction processes: a new class of treatment processes. *Environmental Engineering Science, 30*(5), 264–271. https://doi.org/10.1089/ees.2012.0273
216. Batchelor, B. (2019). Advanced reduction and oxidation–reduction processes for water treatment. In *Encyclopedia of Water* (pp. 1–13). Wiley. https://doi.org/10.1002/9781119300762.wsts0020
217. García-Espinoza, J. D., Robles, I., Durán-Moreno, A., & Godínez, L. A. (2021). Photo-assisted electrochemical advanced oxidation processes for the disinfection of aqueous solutions: a review. *Chemosphere, 274*, 129957. https://doi.org/10.1016/j.chemosphere.2021.129957
218. Wu, J., Zhu, K., Xu, H., & Yan, W. (2019). Electrochemical oxidation of Rhodamine B by PbO_2/Sb–SnO_2/TiO_2 nanotube arrays electrode. *Chinese Journal of Catalysis, 40*(6), 917–927. https://doi.org/10.1016/S1872-2067(19)63342-5
219. Oturan, M. A., & Brillas, E. (2007). Electrochemical advanced oxidation processes (EAOPs) for environmental applications. *Portugaliae Electrochimica Acta, 25*(1), 1–18. https://doi.org/10.4152/pea.200701001
220. Alulema-Pullupaxi, P., Fernández, L., Debut, A., Santacruz, C. P., Villacis, W., Fierro, C., & Espinoza-Montero, P. J. (2021). Photoelectrocatalytic degradation of glyphosate on titanium dioxide synthesized by sol–gel/spin-coating on boron doped diamond (TiO_2/BDD) as a photoanode. *Chemosphere, 278*, 130488. https://doi.org/10.1016/j.chemosphere.2021.130488
221. Ma, D., Han, X., Li, X., & Luo, D. (2023). Photocatalytic degradation of diclofenac in tap water on TiO_2 nanotubes assisted with ozone generated from boron-doped diamond electrode. *Catalysts, 13*(5), 877. https://doi.org/10.3390/catal13050877
222. Guerra-Rodríguez, S., Cediel, N., Rodríguez, E., & Rodríguez-Chueca, J. (2021). Photocatalytic activation of sulfite using Fe(II) and Fe(III) for *Enterococcus* sp. inactivation in urban wastewater. *Chemical Engineering Journal, 408*, 127326. https://doi.org/10.1016/j.cej.2020.127326
223. Wu, S., Shen, L., Lin, Y., Yin, K., & Yang, C. (2021). Sulfite-based advanced oxidation and reduction processes for water treatment. *Chemical Engineering Journal, 414*, 128872. https://doi.org/10.1016/j.cej.2021.128872
224. Garcia-Segura, S., & Brillas, E. (2017). Applied photoelectrocatalysis on the degradation of organic pollutants in wastewaters. *Journal of Photochemistry and Photobiology C: Photochemistry Reviews, 31*, 1–35. https://doi.org/10.1016/j.jphotochemrev.2017.01.005
225. Armaković, S. J., Savanović, M. M., & Armaković, S. (2022). Titanium dioxide as the most used photocatalyst for water purification: an overview. *Catalysts, 13*(1), 26. https://doi.org/10.3390/catal13010026
226. Raza, W., Bahnemann, D., & Muneer, M. (2018). A green approach for degradation of organic pollutants using rare earth metal doped bismuth oxide. *Catalysis Today, 300*, 89–98. https://doi.org/10.1016/j.cattod.2017.07.029
227. Shen, Z., Wu, D., Yang, J., Yuan, T., Wang, W., & Jia, J. (2006). Methods to improve electrochemical treatment effect of dye wastewater. *Journal of Hazardous Materials, 131*(1–3), 90–97. https://doi.org/10.1016/j.jhazmat.2005.09.010

228. Bessegato, G. G., de Almeida, L. C., Ferreira, S. L. C., & Zanoni, M. V. B. (2019). Experimental design as a tool for parameter optimization of photoelectrocatalytic degradation of a textile dye. *Journal of Environmental Chemical Engineering*, *7*(4), 103264. https://doi.org/10.1016/j.jece.2019.103264
229. Pan, G., Jing, X., Ding, X., Shen, Y., Xu, S., & Miao, W. (2019). Synergistic effects of photocatalytic and electrocatalytic oxidation based on a three-dimensional electrode reactor toward degradation of dyes in wastewater. *Journal of Alloys and Compounds*, *809*, 151749. https://doi.org/10.1016/j.jallcom.2019.151749
230. Forgacs, E., Cserháti, T., & Oros, G. (2004). Removal of synthetic dyes from wastewaters: a review. *Environment International*, *30*(7), 953–971. https://doi.org/10.1016/j.envint.2004.02.001
231. Adeyemo, A. A., Adeoye, I. O., & Bello, O. S. (2017). Adsorption of dyes using different types of clay: a review. *Applied Water Science*, *7*(2), 543–568. https://doi.org/10.1007/s13201-015-0322-y
232. Agarwala, R., & Mulky, L. (2023). Adsorption of dyes from wastewater: a comprehensive review. *ChemBioEng Reviews*, *10*(3), 326–335. https://doi.org/10.1002/cben.202200011
233. Iwuozor, K. O. (2019). Prospects and challenges of using coagulation-flocculation method in the treatment of effluents. *Advanced Journal of Chemistry-Section A*, 105–127. https://doi.org/10.29088/SAMI/AJCA.2019.2.105127
234. Das, A., & Adak, M. K. (2022). Photo-catalyst for wastewater treatment: a review of modified Fenton, and their reaction kinetics. *Applied Surface Science Advances*, *11*, 100282. https://doi.org/10.1016/j.apsadv.2022.100282
235. Obotey Ezugbe, E., & Rathilal, S. (2020). Membrane technologies in wastewater treatment: a review. *Membranes*, *10*(5), 89. https://doi.org/10.3390/membranes10050089
236. Jamee, R., & Siddique, R. (2019). Biodegradation of synthetic dyes of textile effluent by microorganisms: an environmentally and economically sustainable approach. *European Journal of Microbiology and Immunology*, *9*(4), 114–118. https://doi.org/10.1556/1886.2019.00018
237. Ollikka, P., Alhonmäki, K., Leppänen, V.-M., Glumoff, T., Raijola, T., & Suominen, I. (1993). Decolorization of azo, triphenyl methane, heterocyclic, and polymeric dyes by lignin peroxidase isoenzymes from *Phanerochaete chrysosporium*. *Applied and Environmental Microbiology*, *59*(12), 4010–4016. https://doi.org/10.1128/aem.59.12.4010-4016.1993

5 Ion-Exchange Materials for Dye Removal

Lalit Singh and Brijesh Shah

5.1 INTRODUCTION: ION EXCHANGE

The concept of ion exchange can be traced back to the late 18th century when scientists observed that certain substances could exchange ions in solution. This early observation laid the foundation for later developments.

In the 19th century, researchers began to study the exchange of ions between solids and solutions. The term "ion exchange" was coined by chemist Hugo Erdmann in 1880 to describe this phenomenon. The first synthetic ion-exchange resin was developed in the early 20th century by English Chemists Thomas W. Campbell and George N. Campbell in 1905. They created a resin by polymerizing phenol and formaldehyde, which exhibited ion-exchange properties. In 1935, American chemists Adams and Holmes synthesized the first commercial ion-exchange resin, known as Amberlite IR-120. This marked a significant milestone in the practical application of ion-exchange technology.

Throughout the mid-20th century, research into ion-exchange materials expanded, leading to the development of a wide range of ion-exchange resins with varying properties and applications. Resins tailored for specific ions and industries emerged.

The introduction of strong (SAC) and weak acid cation (WAC) exchange resins, as well as strong (SBA) and weak base anion (WBA) exchange resins, allowed for selective ion exchange for water softening, deionization, and purification. Ion-exchange technology found applications in industries such as water treatment, pharmaceuticals, food and beverage, nuclear, and more. Throughout the mid-20th century, research into ion-exchange materials expanded, leading to the development of a wide range of ion-exchange resins with varying properties and applications. Resins tailored for specific ions and industries emerged.

The introduction of SAC and WAC exchange resins, as well as SBA and WBA exchange resins, allowed for selective ion exchange for water softening, deionization, and purification. Ion-exchange technology found applications in industries such as water treatment, pharmaceuticals, food and beverage, nuclear, and more.

Today, ion-exchange materials continue to be crucial in various fields, including water treatment, chemical processing, biotechnology, and more. Advances in nanotechnology are enabling the creation of nanostructured ion-exchange materials with enhanced properties. Efforts are being made to integrate ion-exchange technology

DOI: 10.1201/9781003441083-5

with other separation techniques for improved efficiency and selectivity. Sustainability concerns are driving the development of eco-friendly ion-exchange materials and processes.

Water quality worldwide is under threat due to the unprecedented rate of global population, and industrial and climate changes, leading to a freshwater crisis. Among the contributors to this crisis are multiple users and violators of freshwater, including the cosmetic, paint and varnish, leather, pulp and paper, food, and pharmaceutical industries. These industries use a range of dyes, such as methyl orange (MO), Disperse Violet 26, methylene blue (MB), Congo red (CR), Rhodamine B (RhB), crystal violet, and methyl red which are considered the most significant sources of industrial pollutants. It is estimated that approximately 70 lakh tons of dyes are being produced worldwide every year with never-ending demands. The release of these industrial waste dyes into water poses a threat to both human health and the environment. Literature studies reveal that various techniques such as coagulation, biological methods, precipitation, adsorption, and chemical oxidation are used to treat industrial and domestic effluents. However, each of these techniques cannot provide wholesome results, including each method contains specific advantages and disadvantages. For example, the coagulation method for dye and impurity removal has been extensively used in industries, which also prohibits toxic and hazardous intermediates generation. However, sludge formation and its disposal are the major drawbacks. Operational costs and efficiency are the major parameters for the implementation of any treatment method. Hence, ion exchange and adsorption techniques are considered to be the prime solutions having high potential and efficiency for dyewater treatment [1]. Specifically, the ion-exchange method has shown tremendous results in effluent treatment and dye removal. The reusability and specificity of ion exchangers make them the premium treatment option for various plants and industries. *Ion exchange, also known as ion transport, is the process of transporting mobile ions from an external electrolytic solution to ions that are electrostatically bonded to functional groups in a solid matrix (the ion exchanger)* [2]. The ions are stoichiometrically exchanged with equivalent amounts of other ions of the same charge from the ion exchanger without any permanent structural change or physical modification to itself [2,3]. When looking into ion-exchange materials, researchers take into account a number of crucial characteristics, such as the following:

- *Particle size and form:* The rate of ion-exchange reactions depends upon the particle size and its configuration. Altering the size or form of particles significantly changes the time required and efficiency of the ion-exchange process [4,5].
- *Solubility:* The exchanger must exhibit no solubility in the solution medium where ion exchange takes place.
- *Porosity and swelling:* Porosity is defined as the ratio of volume to its mass. The variety in pore size or ratio brings selectivity and specificity to this technique. The penetration of ions into the matrix relies strongly on porosity, which further depends upon polymerization procedures [4, 6]. *The amount of swelling* is directly proportional to the number of hydrophilic functional

groups attached to the polymer matrix and is inversely proportional to the degree of divinyl benzene (DVB) cross-linking present in the resin. Factors like the rate of hydration and volume expansion of pore/resin to adsorb bigger molecules are maneuvered by swelling capacity.

- *Acid–base strength:* The numerous ionogenic groups integrated into the resin determine an exchanger's acid or base strength. These strengths may affect the rate of adsorption by the exchange matrix and also bring selectivity for specific ions.
- *Cross linkage:* The degree (measured in percentage) of cross-linking affects the external physical structure of the matrix pore/resin size. The degree of cross-linkage is controlled by the percent of DVB involved in the copolymerization and the fraction of DVB in the polymer matrix determines the limit to which exchange resin is free to swell and shrink. Resins with low cross-linking can take a considerable amount of water and swell into a soft and gelatinous structure [4, 7].

5.1.1 Classification of Ion-Exchange Materials

The classification of ion-exchange materials can be based on various factors. In particular, the source and chemical composition of the ion exchangers provide valuable insights into the diversity and functionality of these materials. Detailed classification can be seen in Figure 5.1.

5.1.1.1 Classification Based on the Source of Ion Exchange

Natural organic ion exchangers: Natural organic materials like wood, peat, fiber, plant cells, animal cells, etc., possess ion-exchange properties or they can be modified to develop such properties by simple chemical treatments. For instance,

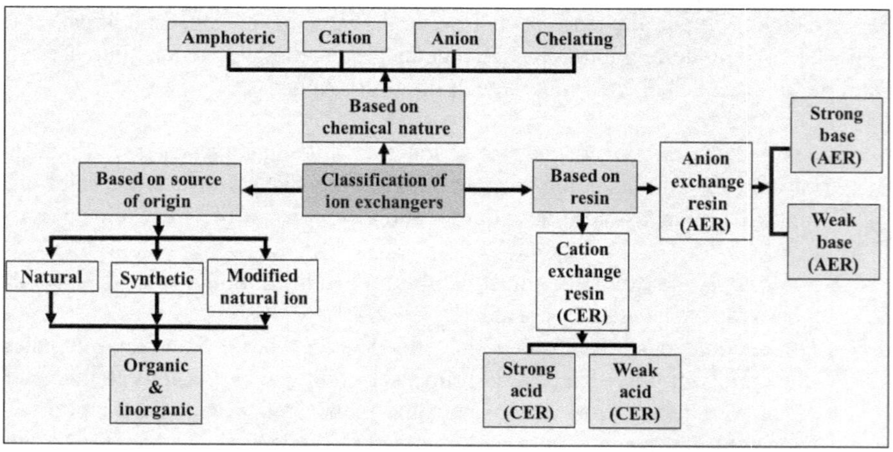

FIGURE 5.1 Classification of ion exchangers based on different sources.

phenolic groups (–OH), which are weakly acidic and swap their hydrogen ions for other cations under neutral or alkaline conditions, and carboxyl groups (–COOH) of amphoteric proteins can both induce the development of such traits in plant and animal cells. The soil containing humin and humic acid has developed these properties because of the presence of decayed plants and animals. Many polysaccharides, proteins, and cellulose (filter paper) materials have the quality of ion exchangers [8].

Natural inorganic ion exchangers: Many natural minerals, such as vermiculite, clay, and zeolites, exhibit ion-exchange properties. Clay being present in abundance naturally is used because of its flexible workability, low permeability, and ion-exchange properties as buffer materials for radioactive waste disposal. Clay, such as illite, kaolinite, and bentonite. Ion-exchange characteristics are present in zeolites such as analcite, chabazite, sodalite, and clinoptilolite [8,9].

Synthetic organic and inorganic ion exchangers: Bakelite was first prepared in 1909 by Baekeland. The well-known resin "Bakelite," which is a hard, insoluble condensation material that can be made by heating phenols and formaldehyde in the presence of base or acid with water elimination, was first produced in 1935 by two chemists Adams and Holmes at the National Chemical Laboratory in Teddington, the United Kingdom. The scientists showed that this structure exchanged hydrogen ions in an alkaline medium and also prepared cationic exchangers by modifying the structure with the sulphonic acid group ($-SO_3H$) [8]. Synthetic ion exchangers, such as polystyrene-based resins, are widely used in commercial applications due to their numerous advantages. Compared to condensed resins, they exhibit greater physical and chemical stability. Additionally, these structures can be modified in specific ways to create a wide range of different products, increasing their versatility and workability. Other materials commonly used for this purpose include cross-linked polymers of phenol and formaldehyde, which share many of the same beneficial properties as polystyrene-based resins [8].

Synthetic inorganic ion exchangers: Synthetic inorganic ion exchangers are solid materials that can selectively exchange ions with their surroundings. These materials are typically composed of metal oxides or zeolites and have a high surface area, which allows for a high degree of ion exchange. Synthetic inorganic ion exchangers are widely used in a variety of applications, including water purification, waste treatment, and industrial processes. Some common examples of synthetic inorganic ion exchangers are zeolites, hydrous oxides, and metal ferrocyanides.

Modified natural ion exchangers: The introduction of groups like phosphate, carbonic, or other acidic functional groups is used to modify the natural organic ion exchangers to improve the exchange capacity and selectivity. Such functional groups could be used to alter cation exchangers made of cellulose, for instance. Natural exchangers and materials' sorption characteristics can be enhanced, for example, clinoptilolite (natural zeolite) in the presence of dilute solution acids/some salt [8, 10,11].

5.1.1.2 Classification Based on the Chemical Nature of Ion Exchange

Cation exchangers: These materials exchange positively charged ions (cations) with the external solution medium. Cation exchangers are of two types, namely, weak acid and strong acid as they differentiate in exchange groups. SAC exchangers generally contain $-SO_3$ functional group and WAC exchangers contain –COO functional groups [2].

Anion exchangers: These materials exchange negatively charged ions (anions) with the external solution medium. The anion exchange materials can be classified into the weak base and strong base categories according to the type of exchange group. Weak base ion exchangers generally act as acid adsorbers. For example, efficient removal of strong acids such as sulfuric acids and hydrochloric acids. However, they are preferred to remove carbon dioxide or silica [2,12].

Amphoteric exchangers: These ion exchangers contain both cation and anion sites making them different from the other monofunctional exchangers. Under viable conditions, they can simultaneously exchange both cations and anions from an external medium. These exchangers depending on their chemical structure, ions' size, and charge have binding preferences for certain ions and groups. For example, Retard ion 11A8 has been used for the separation of cadmium [2,13].

Ion-exchange resins: Ion-exchange resins are cross-linked porous polymer materials containing functional (inorganic) groups. These are small (0.25–0.5 mm radius) microbeads with an insoluble matrix. The beads are porous, proving the exchange of ions fluency and efficiency. The porosity also determines the rate of exchange and provides selectivity to the process respectively. There are multiple types of ion-exchange resin. Polystyrene sulfonate is the major substituent in the production of commercial resins. They are generally referred to as ion-exchange polymers. Figure 5.2 presents a classification of ion-exchange resins [2,14].

SAC resins: SAC resins work similarly to strong acids. SAC resins typically come in two different forms: sodium ($R\text{-}SO_3Na$) or hydrogen ($R\text{-}SO_3H$).

The usual cation exchange process in strong acids:

$$2(R\text{-}SO_3Na) + CaCl_2 \Leftrightarrow (R\text{-}SO_3)_2Ca + 2NaCl$$

(Here, R represents the ion-exchange matrix.)

SAC resins have a cross-linking percentage ranging from 8% to 10%. When its pH changes, its ion-exchange capability is unaffected. Strong acids, such as HCl, can be used to renew the depleted SAC resins. Sodium chloride solution (NaCl) regenerates in the form of sodium salt. It is frequently used to dealkalize and demineralize water [2, 15].

WAC resins: These resins have a carboxylic group (–COOH) as the exchanger. These resins are easily regenerable by stoichiometric concentrations of acid because they have a high bonding capacity for hydrogen ions. With an increase in the solution's pH, WAC resins' ion-exchange capacity rises. WAC has applications in de-alkalization, deionization, softening of water, etc. [2, 16].

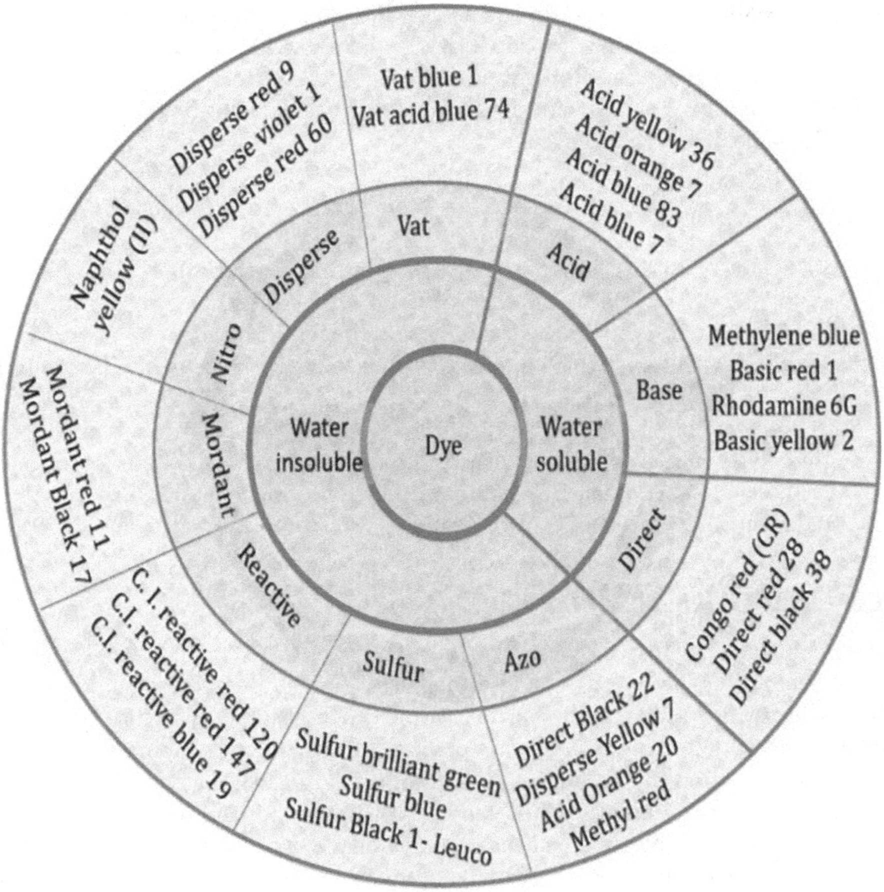

FIGURE 5.2 Dye classification circle (classification of dye with examples).

$$R\text{ - }COOH + NaHCO_3 \Leftrightarrow R\text{ - }COONa + H_2O + CO_2$$

(Here, R represents the ion-exchange matrix)

SBA resins: SBA resins work similarly to strong bases. SBA resins are generally found in hydroxide form: ($R\text{-}NH_3OH$)

The typical SBA exchange reaction:

$$R\text{-}NH_3OH + HNO \Leftrightarrow R\text{-}NH_3NO_3 + H_2O$$

(Here, R represents the ion-exchange matrix.)

SBA resins are used for the de-alkalization and demineralization of water. Concentrated sodium hydroxide (NaOH) solution can be used to renew the SBA resins that have been entirely used.

WBA resins: WBA resins work similarly to weak bases having amine functionality. The typical WBA exchange reaction:

$$R\text{-}NH_2 + HNO_3 \Leftrightarrow R\text{-}NH_3NO_3$$

(Here, R represents the ion-exchange matrix.)

The ability of WBA resins to exchange ions is directly dependent on the pH solution and it is observed that it increases with a decrease in the pH of the solution.

For treating solutions with a pH of greater than 6, WBA resins are typically not used. They are easily regenerable using modest amounts of weak basic salts, such as sodium carbonate or ammonia, which neutralize the resin's use of acid and regenerate the sites [2, 16].

5.2 INTRODUCTION TO THE DYES

The Ecological and Toxicological Association of Dyes (ETAD) and organic pigment manufacturers define dye as "intensely colored or fluorescent organic substances only, which impart color to a substrate by selective absorption of light. They are soluble and go through an application process which, at least temporarily, destroys any crystal structure by absorption, solution, and mechanical retention or by ionic or covalent chemical bonds." Dyes can be broadly categorized on the basis of the nature of extraction (natural and synthetic) and on the water solubility. Further, dyes consist of aromatic molecular structures originating from hydrocarbon framework, which includes structures like xylene, benzene, naphthalene, toluene, and anthracene [17]. Plants, animals, different insects, and minerals are some of the natural sources of dyes, whereas man-made and industrially manufactured synthetic dyes are manufactured using combinations and variations of natural and organic molecules. However, the exponential demand for dyes in day-to-day life inevitably involves their discharge along with toxic organic/inorganic chemicals in the form of industrial effluents. The discharge into the natural water sources not only dampens the water quality but also degrades the quality of aquatic life [1, 18].The major problem regarding dye-based pollution comes from the over-dependency and the variety of applications it is involved in, leading to multiple health hazards and environmental damage. Classification of dyes can be done based on different criteria. In this response, we will be discussing the classification of dyes depending upon solubility, applications, and eco-toxicological effects along with a few examples of each dye. We can see in Table 5.1, the classification of dyes based on their solubility, application, and different eco-toxicological effects.

A technical classification of dyes can be proposed based on the dyeing process and subsequently considering their solubility and chemical properties [33], which can

TABLE 5.1
Classification of dyes based on their solubility, applications, and eco-toxicological effects

Type of Dye	Examples	Structure Example	Water Solubility	Dye Application	Toxic Effects	References
Acid dye	Tartrazine, Acid red 87, Acid orange 7, Acid blue 7	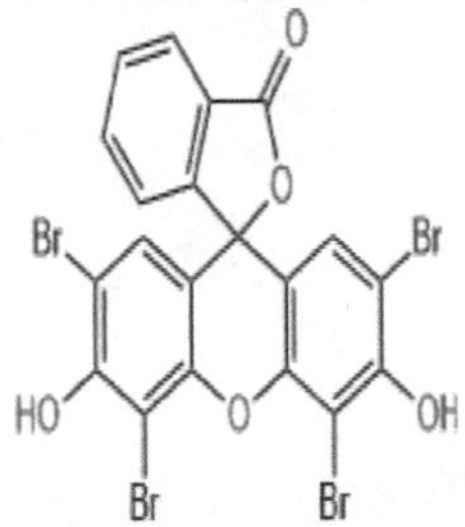 Acid red 87	Soluble	Pharmaceutical, leather and textile industries; nylon wool, silk, and modified acrylics	Diarrhea, vomiting, nausea, carcino-genic and mutagenic effects	[1, 19–22]
Vat dye	Anthraquinone derivatives, vat blue 1, vat acid blue 74	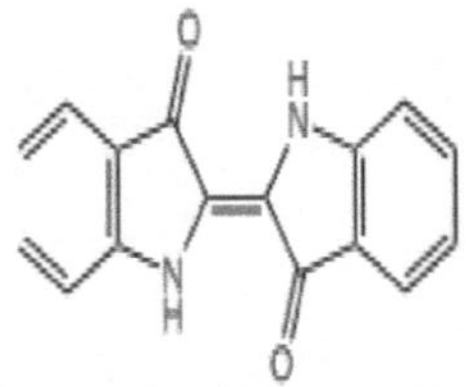 Vat blue 1	Insoluble	Coloring cellulosic fibers: cotton, fibers natural fibers.	Allergic conjunctivitis, rhinitis, and other allergic reaction	[1, 19, 20, 23–25]

(*continued*)

TABLE 5.1 (Continued)
Classification of dyes based on their solubility, applications, and eco-toxicological effects

Type of Dye	Examples	Structure Example	Water Solubility	Dye Application	Toxic Effects	References
Basic dye	Basic blue 9,Basic red 1,Basic red 118	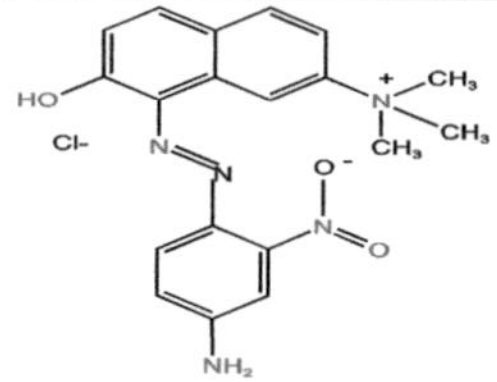 Basic red 118		Paper, polyacrylonitrile-modified nylons, and modified polyesters	Devastating effects on flora and fauna. Detrimental effects on water bodies.	[1, 19, 23]
Direct dye	CR, direct red 28, brilliant yellow, direct black 38	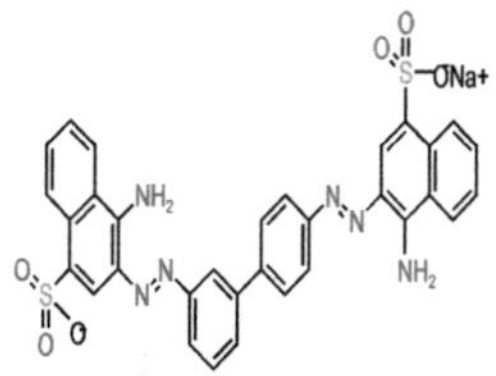 Direct red 28	Soluble	Biological materials, coloring paper products	Carcinogenic; mutagenic, and dermatitis. Dangerous to aquatic life.	[1, 19, 26, 27]
Dispersed dye	Disperse Red 9, disperse Violet 1, disperse red 60	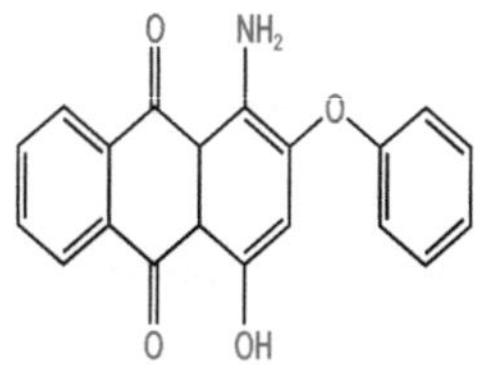 Dispersed red 60		Polyester, nylon, cellulose acetate, and acrylic fibers	Mutagenic; carcinogenic; causes soil and water pollution	[1, 19, 28]

Reactive dye	C.I. reactive red 120, C.I. reactive Black 5, C.I. reactive blue 19	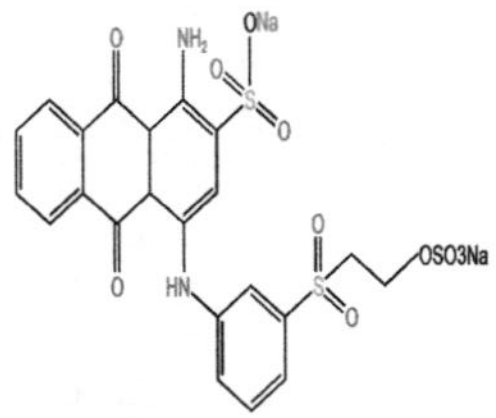 C.I Reactive Blue 19	Dyeing cellulosic, silk, and wool fibers	Allergic reaction in eyes, skin, mucous membrane, and the upper respiratory tract	[1, 19]
Mordant dye	Mordant red 11, Mordant Black 17	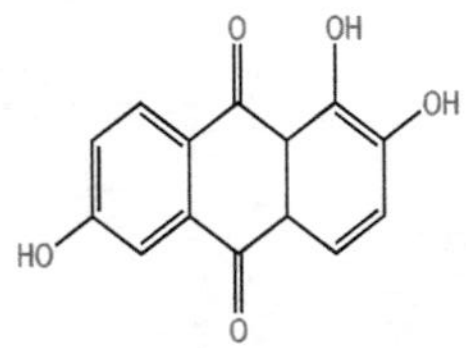 Mordent red 4	Textile fibers such as wool, silk, and leather	Allergic reactions, especially skin	[1, 19, 29, 30]
Azo dye	Direct Black 22, Disperse Yellow7, Acid Orange 20, Methyl red, MO, Trypan blue	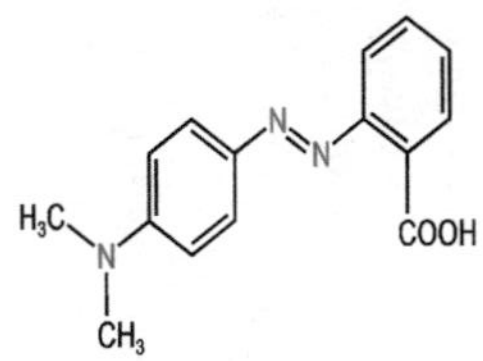 Methyl red	Textile industry for dyeing, process and food coloring	Carcinogenic to humans and animals. Hazardous when inhaled or swallowed: affects the eye, skin, digestive tract. Disturbs aquatic life.	[1, 19, 20, 31, 32]

have an impact on the application of dyes. The variety in dye applications depends upon different methods of dye bonding with the material. Figure 5.2 highlights dye's classification into direct, acid, basic, etc., and a few examples are mentioned for each type. Broadly, dyes can be categorized into two classes, the first being *water-soluble dyes*, and the other *water-insoluble dyes*. However, there are a few dyes whose salts dissolve in water (sulfur and vat dyes) and those that can be dissolved in organic solvents, e.g., fatty dyes [34]. The unprecedented increase in population worldwide has seen dynamic growth in industries and production capacities, leading to major environmental changes. These substantial changes are degrading our health and resources unparallelly [36, 35]. The improper treatment and discharge of industrial effluent containing hazardous chemical sand dye exposure pose substantial risks to aquatic, terrestrial, and human life. The coloring agent (dye) is the primary pollutant that can be visually recognized in industrial wastewater [36, 37, 38]. The dyes containing aromatic groups are hazardous and carcinogenic. They are not only detrimental to life above the earth but below the surface as well. Aquatic life alters multiple folds when chemical composition changes underwater. Even low dye concentration in water can drastically alter the salinity and diminish the perforation of light consequently retarding the rate of photosynthesis [36]. Dye-bearing effluents are a major source of water pollution and as the demand for dyes has increased multiple folds to meet the unprecedented requirements, they become a major polluter. There are more dye effluent volumes because dyes are needed in many different sectors, including textile, printing, plastics, paper, carbide, food, and cosmetics [39–41]. As the discharge withholds many varieties of substances and pigments, each dye pollutant attains a different toxicity threshold, posing a challenge in the treatment procedures and creating different hazards. However, the majority of the contaminants and chemicals in dye effluent discharge streams are not biodegradable and contain cancer-causing qualities [39, 42]. Dyes are highly dispersed aesthetic pollutants that are difficult to treat and handle. The reason is the stability of the molecules in dye molecules, which resists degradation by light, chemical, biological, and other treatments or exposure [43]. A major dye pollution contributor in textile wastewaters, about 50%, is by washing procedure after dyeing and the dyeing procedure itself [39, 43]. According to Mondal [44], dyes are constituents of textile wastewater that cause the biggest and most complicated problems in treatment procedures. The work done by Ghaly et al. [45] suggests domestic household dye effluents concentration range of 10–250 mg/L. It has been calculated that 10–15% of dye pollutants are released during the dyeing process out of the total dye consumption worldwide which exceeds ten thousand tons per year [39, 46, 47]. Direct dyes are feasibly removed by biological treatment [48, 49], adsorption [50–53], and ion exchange [54, 55] as well as membrane processes, coagulation–flocculation [56, 57], ozonation, and oxidation [39, 46 58]. Figure 5.3 shows a diagram of sources and pathways of dye pollution.

Effluent discharge from textile and leather industries having toxic dye pollutants causes significant health concerns for living species, leading to environmental agencies' growing strictness [40]. Additionally, the dark color prevents sunlight from

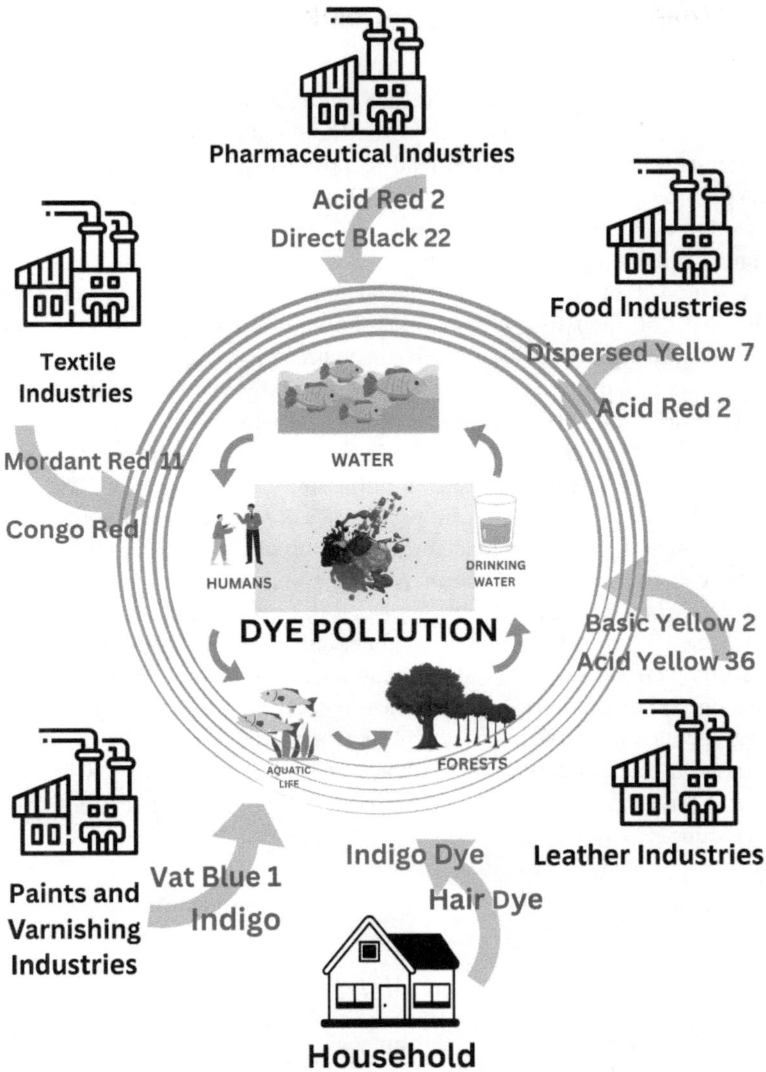

FIGURE 5.3 Sources and pathways of dye pollution.

penetrating water sources, which causes several problems for the ecosystem, including the eutrophication of aquatic ecosystems and bioaccumulation which causes health issues for aquatic life. These problems are all caused by the fact that their wastewater contains toxic pollutants and dyes that are dangerous to the biological world [46]. Hence, the decolorization treatment before its discharge becomes an important aspect of wastewater treatment [39].

5.2.1 Different Techniques Used for the Removal of Dye and Their Limitations

In dye industries, pigments, and dyes, are undoubtedly the essential components, and are highly evident substances, and even the minimal quantities discharged into the environment and water sources lead to possible environmental pollution [59]. Additionally, the dyeing sector uses a significant amount of water, which results in significant pollution emissions.

Around 1 million tons of synthetic dyes, which can be classified as direct, acid, reactive, basic, vat, mordant, disperse, metal complex, and sulfur dyes, are produced annually across all industrial sectors, including those that produce food, paints and varnishes, textiles, paper printing, pharmaceuticals, leather, and cosmetics. As a result, they pose one of the biggest threats to biodiversity and natural resources [60]. With more than 10,000 types of dyes used worldwide in the textile industries, 2% of the dyes are discharged as wastewater effluent from manufacturing operations, while textile and associated industries comprise 10% of dye discharge [61]. The effluents from textile dyeing processes contain dyestuff, which makes up 8–20% of the overall pollution load and is made up primarily of auxiliary chemicals and water. The consequence of the increasing demand for textile products and the products requiring dye application enhances the production and the use of synthetic dyes causing the dye wastewater to become a serious pollution problem [60, 62]. The conventional methods alone cannot effectively decolorize and treat the dyestuff-containing effluents, as the dye molecules are stable to light, heat, and oxidizing agents and resistant to aerobic digestion [60, 61]. Some of the methods are discussed in Table 5.2, with their advantages and disadvantages. Chemical, biological, and physical approaches make up the three main types of industrial color removal technology [60, 63].

TABLE 5.2
Conventional methods for dye – decolorization

Name	Principle	Advantages	Disadvantages	References
		Chemical Methods		
Ozonation	Oxidation using ozone gas	Application in a gaseous state, no alteration of volume	Short half-life (20 minutes), high cost	[64–66]
Fenton method	Radical oxidation of colored compounds while others precipitate out. Oxidation using H_2O_2–Fe(II)	Effective decolorization of both soluble and insoluble dyes	Sludge generation (management and handling)	[65, 67, 68]

TABLE 5.2 (Continued)
Conventional methods for dye – decolorization

Name	Principle	Advantages	Disadvantages	References
Coagulation–flocculation		Economically feasible, excellent color removal	Sludge production	[65, 66, 69]
Electro-coagulation	Producing coagulants using sacrificial anode (Al or Fe) at appropriate current density, which sweeps away the colloidal particles (impurity) to larger flocks by aggregation.	Efficient in dye removal. High destabilization power as compared to the coagulation–flocculation method	High cost, less electrode reliability	[65, 70]
		Physical Methods		
Ion exchange	The stoichiometric and equivalent exchange of ions by ion-exchange resins.	Easy regeneration Low absorbent loss Recovery of solvent after use. Removal of soluble dye.	Pre-treatment is required.	[64, 65, 71]
Membrane filtration	Physical separation	Equally effective over all types of dye.	Production of concentrated sludge, high cost. low energy consumption, simplicity, and environmental friendliness	[65, 72]
Adsorption	Dye removal based on a solid support matrix.	Excellent removal of wide variety of dyes	Regeneration difficulties, costly disposal of adsorbent	[65, 66]
		Biological Methods		
	Treatment based on microbiological degradation	Environmentally friendly	Slow process, need of adequate nutrients, narrow operating	[65, 73]

5.2.2 Role of Ion-Exchange Materials

Some of the common uses of ion-exchange materials are listed below:

1. *Water softening:* The elevated levels of calcium and magnesium ions in hard water result in scaling and reduce the effectiveness of soap. The sodium ions in cation exchange resins are utilized to swap out the calcium and magnesium ions, softening the water.
2. *Food and beverage processing:* Ion-exchange resins are used to remove undesirable ions, colors, or flavors from food and beverage manufacturing, enhancing the quality of the finished product.
3. *Separation and purification processes:* Ion-exchange resins are used in laboratories and the chemical industry to separate and purify particular compounds according to their charge characteristics.
4. *Color removal:* They assist in lowering the pigmentation of wastewater by successfully removing dyes, which is crucial for adhering to environmental standards and making sure that the treated water may be released appropriately or reused.

It is vital to remember that ion-exchange resins' ability to remove dyes may differ depending on the specific dye varieties, quantities, and presence of other pollutants in the wastewater. To obtain the best results in treating dye wastewater, it may occasionally be necessary to combine various treatment techniques such as adsorption, coagulation, and biological treatment.

The adsorption procedure has a number of advantages over other traditional dye removal methods. Low cost, outstanding selectivity, and exceptional capacity for regeneration and reusability are some beneficial aspects of the adsorption method [36, 73]. The liquid–solid intermolecular forces of attraction cause the solute to concentrate at the solid surface matrix when a solution containing an absorbable solute (adsorbate) comes into contact with a solid (adsorbent) material possessing a highly porous surface structure [74]. The charged dye molecules in each solution medium engage strongly with the functional groups (the active sites) on the ion-exchange matrixes to remove dye using the ion-exchange methodology. The separation of dyes from the ion-exchanger material is caused by the development of strong links between the dye molecules [75].

According to research conducted as part of the Romanian Nucleus Project "The utilization of macro-porous resin by developing active and passive nanostructures for wastewater treatment." To effectively remove dyes from wastewater, it has been discovered that a strongly basic anion exchanger with a macro-porous structure, comprising tertiary amine-functionalized polystyrene cross-linked with DVB matrix, is necessary. This finding suggests that the synthesized resin could be a practical solution for wastewater treatment plants seeking to remove dyes from their effluent [40]. A case study based on Purolite A500 and Purolite PFA 500 MB are presented in Table 5.3 with data before and after IER treatment.

A very interesting work by Huang et al. [75] on poly(ethylene terephthalate) (PET) recycling by glycolysis shows how efficient and effective ion exchangers

TABLE 5.3
Ion-exchange resins – Purolite A 500 and Purolite PFA 500 MB

Physicochemical Indicators	Wastewater (Black Acid Dye)	Ion Exchange Resin (Purolite A 500)	Ion-Exchange Resin (Purolite PFA 500 MB)
Color	Dark brown	Light greenish brown	Light yellowish brown
pH	3.11	2.7	2.4
Total solid, mg/L	3118	2711	2344
Total nitrogen, mg/L	38.4	23.9	19.4
Sulfates, mg/L	1.553	109	5.1
Turbidity, FTU	95.6	8.67	10.7

Source: Huang et al. [75].

Physiochemical indicators of wastewater containing before and after IER treatment.

are. Glycolysis is considered one of the most promising methods for PET recycling. Bis(hydroxyethyl) terephthalate (BHET) is obtained as a major by-product of PET glycolysis which is a high-value raw material for the production of polyurethane, hydrophobic textile dyes, etc. [76]. BHET often has undesirable colors, leading to inefficient industrialization and increased costs for its recycling. Additionally, for the first time, Huang et al. evaluated the decolorizing efficacy of eight ion-exchange resins using their rates of color removal and BHET retention (Figure 5.4).

Outperforming all other resins in terms of decolorization effectiveness and product retention was resin D201. The retention efficiency of BHET and the colorant elimination rate were over 99% and 95%, respectively, under ideal circumstances. With five repeated cycles, D201 showed exceptional reusability, while the decolored BHET and its r-PET displayed acceptable chromaticity. Adsorption interactions between the colorant and resin were extensively examined by various characterizations, revealing that electrostatic force, π–π interactions, and hydrogen bonding were the dominant adsorption mechanisms [75]. BHET decolorization has excellent future prospects, e.g., D201 resin's above-mentioned strong performances, and this environmentally friendly decolorization technique can produce waste PET glycolysis products for use in a wider range of applications [75].

Numerous natural and manufactured clays are widely used as adsorbents for the removal of dye from aqueous solutions due to their wide availability, low cost, high porosity, high potential for ion exchange, and nontoxicity [77, 78]. For instance, coal-bearing kaolinite treated with sulfuric acid attained a maximum MB dye adsorption capacity of 101.5 mg/g. Another study examined how RhB gets adsorbed on sodium montmorillonite clay, revealing an adsorption capacity of 42.19 mg/g. Electrostatic attraction occurred during the adsorption process between the positively charged cationic dye and the negatively charged adsorbent surfaces [1, 77, 78].

Furthermore, in the field of dye removal from contaminated water, significant progress has been made employing biosorbents such as *Spirulina platensis*, *Penaeus indicus* shrimp, cellulose, *Ganoderma lucidum*, and wheat flour [79]. Dotto et al.

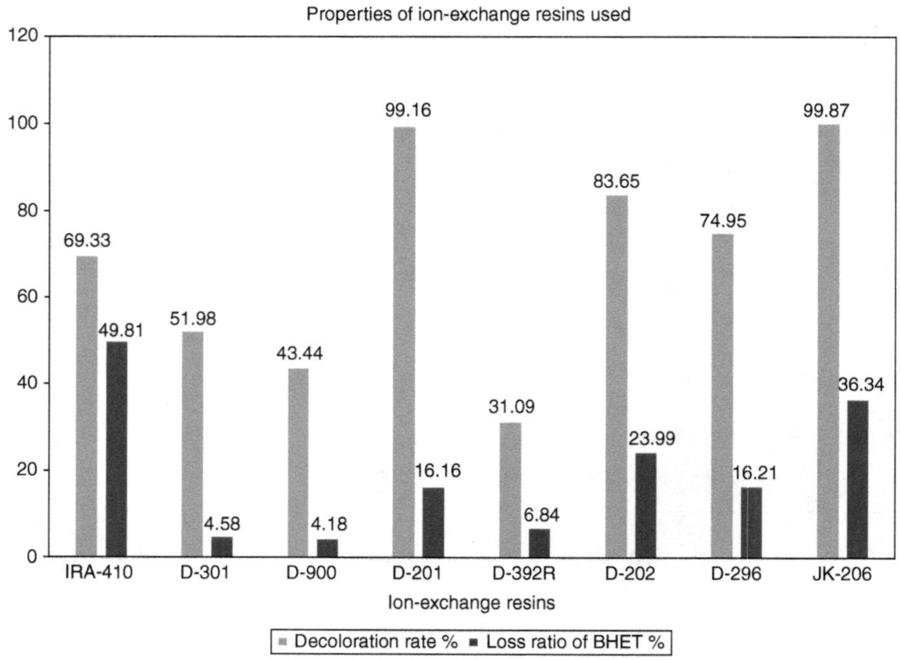

FIGURE 5.4 Comparative analysis of ion-exchange resins used with respect to decoloration rate and the loss ratio of BHET [75].

[79] claim that Acid Blue 9 and FD&C Red No. 40 were successfully adsorbed on the synthetic biosorbent produced by *Spirulina platensis*. For FD&C Red No. 40 and Acid Blue 9 dye, the experimental study revealed a biosorption capacity of 400.3 and 1653.0 mg/g, respectively, at an initial solution pH of 2 and a contact period of 100 minutes [1].

Anionic dyes are frequently employed in a variety of industries, such as the textile, paper, leather, and printing sectors, and if wastewater is not adequately handled, their presence can lead to environmental pollution. To remove the dye, anion exchange resins function as follows:

- *Anionic dye attraction:* Anion exchange resins have functional groups with a positive charge that can attract and bind to anionic dye molecules (often quaternary ammonium groups or tertiary amine groups).
- *Ion-exchange process:* The negatively charged dye molecules are drawn to the positively charged functional groups on the surface of the anion exchange resin when the dye-containing wastewater comes into contact with it. This electrical pull results in an exchange with another anion.
- *Saturation:* As the dye molecules continue to be adsorbed, the capacity of the anion exchange resin for dye removal gradually diminishes until it becomes saturated with dye molecules.
- *Regeneration:* To restore the resin's capacity for further dye removal, the resin is regenerated. Regeneration involves passing a regenerating agent (usually a

strong salt solution, such as sodium chloride or sodium hydroxide) through the resin. The regenerating agent displaces the adsorbed dye molecules from the resin, and they are replaced by chloride ions or hydroxide ions.

Anion exchange resins provide an efficient and selective method for removing anionic dyes from wastewater. However, their effectiveness may depend on factors such as the type of anionic dye present, the concentration of the dye in the wastewater, and the presence of other contaminants that could potentially compete for adsorption sites on the resin.

Cation exchange resins are highly effective for dye removal when dealing with cationic dyes, which are dyes that carry a positive charge. Cationic dyes are widely used in various industries, including textile, paper, and ink manufacturing. Like anionic dyes, their presence in wastewater can cause environmental pollution if not properly treated. Cation exchange resins offer an efficient method for removing cationic dyes from wastewater. Here's how cation exchange resins work for dye removal:

- *Attraction to cationic dyes:* Cation exchange resins have functional groups with a negative charge (often sulfonic acid groups) that can attract and bind to cationic dye molecules.
- *Ion-exchange process:* When the cationic dye-containing wastewater comes into contact with the cation exchange resin, the positively charged dye molecules are attracted to the negatively charged functional groups on the resin's surface. This electrostatic attraction causes the dye molecules to be exchanged with other cations (usually sodium or hydrogen ions) present in the resin.
- *Saturation:* As the dye molecules continue to be adsorbed, the capacity of the cation exchange resin for dye removal gradually diminishes until it becomes saturated with dye molecules.
- *Regeneration:* To restore the resin's capacity for further dye removal, the resin is regenerated. Regeneration involves passing a regenerating agent (usually a strong acid, such as hydrochloric acid) through the resin. The regenerating agent displaces the adsorbed dye molecules from the resin, and they are replaced by sodium or hydrogen ions.

Similarly, in the case of anion exchange resins, the design and optimization of the cation exchange resin system for dye removal should take into account the specific characteristics of the wastewater and the desired level of dye removal efficiency. Proper management of the spent regeneration and the dyes recovered from the regeneration process are also essential for ensuring environmental compliance and sustainable wastewater treatment practices.

5.3 ION-EXCHANGE MECHANISM AND CASE STUDIES

Chemisorption or physisorption: Based on the nature of the bond formation, adsorption processes can be classified into two branches, namely physisorption and chemisorption. Intramolecular forces like van der Waals, electrostatics, or other interactions are involved in physisorption. Without altering the inherent chemical identities of the molecules or ions, intramolecular forces operate between them. In contrast, chemisorption entails the creation and destruction of ionic or covalent intermolecular chemical interactions. Physisorption is reversible by altering the operating temperature or the concentration of the adsorbate as the binding attractive forces are weaker than those of intermolecular chemical bonds. As opposed to the physisorption process, stronger bonds are generated during chemisorption because the attraction forces are chemical in nature [80]. The ion-exchange mechanism, like any other heterogeneous process, involves the back-and-forth transfer of ions via the interphase boundary. (Figure 5.5 illustrates the ion-exchange mechanism.) Ion exchange refers to the dispersion of counterions during the interphase. Ion exchangers can transport counterions, which are exchange ions. Within the framework, counterions are free to move, but to maintain the electroneutrality principle, their movement has to be balanced out by matching counter moves of other ions of identical change. The diffusion of any counterion inside the exchange material is accompanied by replacing an equivalent amount of other counterions. This happens as a consequence of the electroneutrality balancing throughout the phases. The major phases here are inside and outside the ion-exchange material which is the interphase boundary. An electric potential is created when a counterion crosses the interphase boundary, and this potential must be neutralized by the movement of another counterion in the opposite direction [8].

According to the work by Ebrahimian Pirbazari et al. [81], two principal mechanisms play a major role in the removal of the MB (methylene blue) dye on NaOH-treated wheat straw impregnated with Fe_3O_4 (acting as ion-exchange material), which are

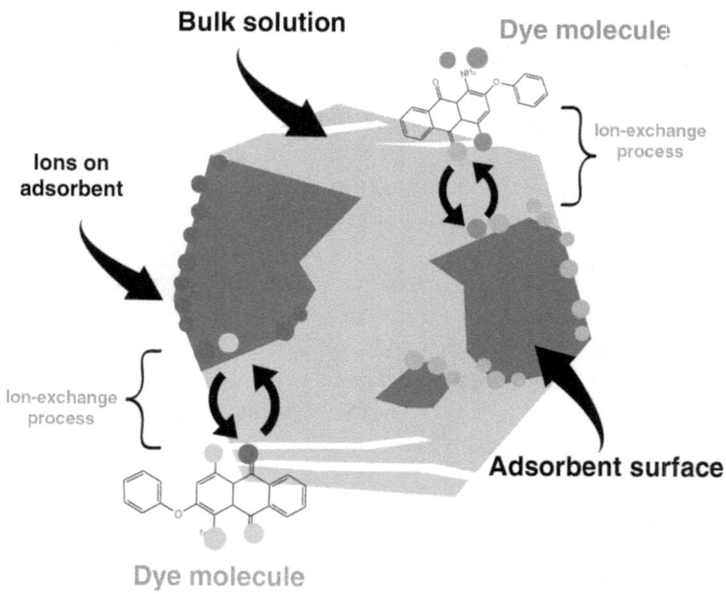

FIGURE 5.5 Ion-exchange mechanism.

surface complex formation and ion exchange between the dye molecule and adsorption material [1]. The adsorption process, which is defined as the association of ions onto various functional groups that are available and active, on the surface of the adsorbent material, and electrostatic interaction between the dye-absorbate material surface, includes the mechanism of surface complex formation. According to Siddiqui et al., the interaction between the –OH groups (on MnO_2/BC) and the acceptor groups present on the MB molecule is what causes H-bonds to form between MB and MnO_2/BC (bamboo charcoal monolith hybrids) [82]. Additionally, the adsorption process typically involves multiple simultaneous mechanisms and interactions. For instance, p–p interactions, intermolecular H-bonding, and electrostatic interactions all play a role in the Coomassie Brilliant Blue R 250 dye's ability to bind to adsorbent surfaces [1, 83].

In recent years, a number of unconventional adsorbents have drawn significant interest as viable, cost-effective replacements for pricey adsorbent materials to remove harmful pollutants [1]. This includes the use of widely accessible agriculture, waste materials including industrial, natural resources, biological wastes, etc. Prior to being used as adsorbents, these waste materials undergo numerous procedures, such as chemical processing, decomposition, and conversion to powder form [1]. In light of this, various waste materials can be used to absorb harmful colors.

Hybrid nanomaterials: Due to their greater surface area and high adsorption-to-mass ratio, nanomaterials have been widely utilized in water treatment applications. As a result, hybrid nanomaterials, which are composed of two or more nanoparticles, have been shown to have a variety of uses, including the removal of colors from contaminated water [1].

1. *Carbon-based hybrid nanocomposites:* Similar to other carbon-based nanocomposites, carbon-based hybrid nanocomposites have facile synthesis, cost-effectiveness, availability, non-toxicity, high porosity, etc.
   After being treated with RhB and MB, ultrafine nickel/carbon (dose: 2 g/L) showed an adsorption capacity of 5.269 and 7.415 mg/g, respectively [1,84]. In another investigation, methyl blue and acid fuchsine dyes were removed using a porous silicon–carbon–nitrogen (Si–C–N) hybrid, which had an adsorption capacity of 1327.7 and 1084.5 mg/g, respectively [1,85].
2. *Graphene and reduced graphene oxide (GO) nanocomposites:* Dyes like; Direct Red 81, Indosol SFGL direct blue, crystal violet, MO, and MB, all have been successfully removed from wastewater using GO as an adsorbent [1, 86–87]. The functionalized GO with hydroxyl and carboxylic groups and the active functional groups in the dye have strong interactions in the adsorption mechanism [1, 89, 90]. Additionally, numerous investigations on GO and reduced graphene oxide (rGO)-based nanocomposites for the adsorption of dye from contaminated water have been published.
   To remove CR and MO dye, Zheng et al. [91] created a 3D hierarchical GO-NiFe layered double hydroxide (LDH) sandwich hybrid. Here, both sides of the GO are completely shielded by the ultrathin NiFe-LDH nanosheets, creating a sandwich-like shape. The hybrid had stronger adsorption phenomena

for CR and MO, as shown by the adsorption capacity values of 489 and 438 mg/g, respectively. This higher adsorption affinity was explained by the existence of ion-exchange processes and electrostatic attraction between the dye molecules and hybrid adsorbents [1].

In another work, to remove MB dye, Heidarizad et al. [92] employed GO/magnesium oxide nanocomposites and succeeded in 833 mg/g of adsorption capacity at a contact time of up to 60 minutes [1].

3. *Polymers and their nanocomposites:* Due to their ease of fabrication, highly effective surface area, high selectivity, interesting doping/de-doping chemistry, electrical transport properties, strong binding affinities, and porous nature, the polymer-based adsorbents like PANI/GO, polyaniline (PANI), polypyrrole, PANI/PPy copolymer, and chitosan have found enormous applications in the field of dye treatment [1,93, 94]. The majority of conducting polymer composites follow the physisorption, hydrogen bonding, p–p interactions, and electrostatic interaction mechanisms for dye adsorption [1,95]. Additionally, the polymer's inclusion of active groups (such as amine and imine) makes the adsorption process easier.

Due to multiple benefits and properties, including its straightforward synthesis, presence of –NH– groups, doping ability, great physicochemical properties, mechanical flexibility, stability, low cost, and the simple availability of its monomer, PANI is one of the most studied conducting polymers [1, 96, 97]. Polypyrrole is an alternative polymer being researched for the removal of colors from wastewater [1,98].

Maximum adsorption capacities for CR on PANI and PPY were 250.01 and 66.6 mg/g, respectively [1,98]. Additionally, the findings of the experiment showed that adsorption effectiveness increased with reaction time and adsorbent dosage. The equilibrium adsorption results best corresponded with the Langmuir isotherm model, while the kinetic data fit well with the pseudo-second-order model.

In a different investigation, the adsorption of CR and sunset yellow on a PPY-multi-walled carbon nanotube (MWCNT) composite resulted in adsorption capacities of 212.1 and 147 mg/g, respectively [1,99]. Electrostatic attraction and p–p electron donor–acceptor interaction were implicated in the adsorption mechanism.

Smita et al. [100] employed PANI to remove a hazardous textile dye (MO) from wastewater with an efficiency of 92% in under 5 hours. The mechanistic investigation showed that the dye's adsorption was caused by an electrostatic contact between the counterions of the dye molecules and the adsorbent [1].

Due to their superior adsorption capacity, polymeric nanohybrid materials have recently gained considerable interest in the field of wastewater treatment. Reactive Black and Reactive Violet-4 dyes, for instance, were treated with starch/PANI, and their respective adsorption capacities were 811.30 and 578.39 mg/g [1, 101].

The single-component equilibrium adsorption was better explained by the Toth isotherm model than dye removal was by the modified Freundlich model.

Additionally, Wang et al. [102] removed MB dye using PANI/TiO_2 with a maximum adsorption capacity of 458.10 mg/g, and the findings of the experiment were closely associated with the Langmuir adsorption isotherm. The responsible adsorption processes were chemical adsorption, membrane diffusion, and intraparticle diffusion, while the responsible adsorption mechanisms were H-bonding, electrostatic interaction, and coordination interaction. Electrostatic contact and hydrogen bonding are the key mechanisms by which MB binds to the surface of PANI, primarily on amino groups [1].

One of the most affordable biopolymers for dye removal that may be obtained from natural resources is chitosan. It has drawn a lot of attention in comparison to other commercial adsorbents because of its distinctive qualities, including cationic charge, high adsorption capacity, macromolecular structure, abundance, and affordability [1, 103,104]. Due to its biocompatibility, biodegradability, antibacterial characteristics, and nontoxicity, chitosan is a desirable source of natural polymers for the adsorption of contaminants from wastewater [1,97]. However, it is typically employed in the form of a composite due to its subpar mechanical qualities, small surface area, pH sensitivity, and low porosity. In light of this, Janaki et al. [105] reported that CR, Coomassie Brilliant Blue, and Remazol brilliant blue R sulfonated anionic dye were successfully removed by a PANI/chitosan composite with removal efficiencies of 95.4%, 98.2%, and 99.8%, respectively. The nonsulfonated cationic dye MB, on the other hand, had a clearance effectiveness of only 10.6% [1].

Polyvinyl alcohol (PVA) was utilized as an adsorbent by Agarwal et al. [106] to remove bromothymol and MB from wastewater. Both the Freundlich and Langmuir models provided good fits for the relevant adsorption isotherms. In 10 minutes, the adsorbent reached its maximum adsorption capacity, which is equivalent to 276.2 and 123.3 mg/g, respectively [1]. The dye sorption was thought to be regulated by electrostatic interaction, p–p interactions, and intermolecular H-bonding, according to the investigation on the adsorption mechanism.

Metal-organic frameworks (MOFs): Due to their controlled topologies and constrained geometries, as well as their finely adjustable pore architectures, MOFs have received a lot of interest as adsorbents. In addition, it is expected that the vast surface areas, versatility, polar/polarizable bonds, and potential for host–guest interactions due to chemical alteration of the organic ligands and/or inorganic subunits will each have a special function [1, 107]. Additionally, it was discovered that MIL-100(Fe) and MIL-100(Cr)-derived MOFs were effective adsorbents for removing MO and MB dye molecules from aqueous solution. For MO and MB, MIL-100(Fe) showed an adsorption capacity of 1045.2 and 736.2 mg/g, while MIL-100(Cr) demonstrated a capacity of 211.8 and 645.3 mg/g [1, 108]. The MB molecules and MOF engage in hydrophobic or p–p interactions as part of the adsorption process. It was also observed that, when the concentration of MB was increased from 30 to 300 mg/L, the adsorption capacity of a magnetic MOF rose from 84 to 245 mg/g, respectively [1, 109].

Due to their distinctive qualities, such as their high reactivity, small size, and vast surface area, metal oxide-based nano-adsorbents have been used extensively in wastewater treatment in recent years. For the adsorptive decolorization of CR dye on a Fe_2O_3–Al_2O_3 nanohybrid, Mahapatra et al. [110] observed a maximum adsorption capacity of 416.66 mg/g at pH 7. The interaction between the oxy-hydroxide group of the nanohybrid material and the amine functional group of the CR dye molecules was the main cause of this enhanced adsorption capacity [1].

The removal of dyes from the contaminated water has been accomplished using a variety of nonmagnetic oxide hybrid nanomaterials as adsorbents. Due to its large specific surface area and positive charge on its surface, MO was able to adsorb 1057.9 mg/g onto nano dimensional Co/Cr-codoped ZnO, according to Li et al. [111]. For the elimination of CR dye in 12 hours, Lei et al. [112] reported a maximum adsorption capacity of 397 mg/g on ZnO–Al_2O_3. This adsorbent was composed of nanosheets with a thickness of approximately 60 nm that held together microspheres with a diameter of 12–16 mm.

Ultimately the choice of adsorbent depends on factors like the type of dye, its chemical properties, the available infrastructure, and economic considerations. Researchers often focus on modifying and optimizing adsorbents to enhance their dye removal efficiency and selectivity. Additionally, sustainable and cost-effective options are of increasing interest to address environmental concerns in dye removal processes.

Critical factors influencing dye adsorption: The solution pH, temperature, initial dye concentration, contact time, and adsorbent dose are critical factors in the adsorptive removal of dyes and have the potential to alter the efficiency of the material (Table 5.4).

Further, *the initial dye concentration* has a major impact on the adsorption phenomena. Multiple observations and studies indicate that an increase in dye concentration shows a positive trend only up to the threshold limit. Hence, we can establish a directly proportional relationship between the dye concentration and the adsorption efficiency. Further, the adsorption frequency and efficiency depend upon the available active sites. The initial acceleration is due to the abundant availability of unsaturated and active sites on the material. As the process begins, available active sites decrease leading to a reduction in adsorption, which later comes to a halt [1,113,114]. According to work done by Liu et al. [118], when utilizing cellulose-g-poly(acrylic acid-co-acrylamide) as an adsorbent material for the starting concentration of acid blue and MB of 200 mg/L, respectively, it was shown to have adsorption capacities of 1602 and 1814 mg/g [118]. According to this fact, a high starting concentration typically translates into a high adsorption capacity.

The temperature also has a prominent effect on the capacities and efficiency of dye adsorption. Furthermore, a temperature variation is helpful in identifying whether the adsorption process is endothermic or exothermic. In an exothermic process, as the temperature increases, the adsorption capacity decreases, whereas an endothermic process shows an increased capacity of adsorption with the temperature rise [1,115].

The solution pH plays an essential role in the dye removal from polluted water over exchange material. The work done by Zhou et al. [113] depicts the pH variation affecting the ionization level and surface charge between the dye and absorbent material [1]. Further, the low and high pH favors the adsorption of anionic and cationic dyes, respectively [114]. This was supported by research by Daneshvar et al. and Phoemphoonthanyakit et al. [119], who found that Acid Blue 25 had an adsorption

TABLE 5.4
Critical factors influencing the dye removal process

Critical Factors	Influence on Adsorption	Salient Features	Remarks	References
Solution pH	pH variation affects the reaction between the adsorbent and the dye molecule by affecting the ionization level and surface charge of adsorbent.	Crucial role in dye adsorption.	On based one salt present, dye effluent may be acidic or basic.	[1,113, 114]
Temperature	Increased adsorption capacity with increased temperature depicts the endothermic nature, whereas a decrease in adsorption capacity and increase in temperature shows the exothermic nature of reactions.	Shows whether the adsorption is endothermic or exothermic. (Nature of adsorption.)	In general, an increase in temperature shows an increase in adsorption capacity	[1,115, 116]
Initial dye concentration	Increased dye concentration increases the adsorption capacity until the unsaturated active sites of the adsorbent become saturated and occupied.	Increased dye concentration; increases the adsorption capacity until the active sites get saturated.		[1,114, 117]
Contact time	Positive growth of adsorption seen, until equilibrium between the active adsorbent sites and dye molecules is established.	Shows the contact time between the adsorbate and adsorbent.	High contact time increases the energy and cost of the treatment.	[1,116]
Adsorbent dose (resin, membrane, etc.)	Generally, an increased adsorbent material provides more active sites for dye removal. Increases the efficiency of the technique.	Depicts the amount of adsorbent used for dye removal.	Treatment cost increases.	[1,114, 116]

capacity of 1093 mg/g at pH 2 and Rhodamine 6G had an adsorption capacity of 600 mg/g at pH 7 [1,119,120]. Generally, higher the **adsorbent dose,** the greater the positive effects on the adsorptive dye removal. This is mainly accounted for, because of the higher number of available active adsorption sites [114]. Further, a higher dose may cause congestion and competition over the limited active sites of the adsorbent material, leading to reduced efficiency results. According to the work done by Khan and Nazir [121], a dose of 0.5 g/L of a Fe_2O_3/chitosan–bamboo saw-dust composite material, obtained an adsorption level of 217.39 mg/g for bromothymol blue. In contrast, Ebrahimian Pirbazari et al. [81] determined an adsorption capacity of 1374.6 mg/g for MB (methyl blue) consisting adsorbent material of NaOH-treated wheat straw material mixed with Fe_3O_4 nanoparticles with 1.0 g/L of its dosage. These results and findings demonstrate the positive effects of using a higher adsorbent material dose for increased results [1].

Contact time can have both negative and positive effects on adsorption efficiencies and potential. Until the equilibrium is reached between the dye molecules and adsorbent material, we expect to see an exponential increase in the adsorption rate. However, after the equilibrium is established, no further adsorption can occur as the threshold capacity of adsorption is reached. Increasing the contact time further will not increase the adsorption rate. This can be well understood by considering some examples. Work by Khan and Nazir [121] depicts an adsorption capacity of 217.39 mg/g for bromothymol blue dye with 30 minutes contact time over a Fe_2O_3/chitosan-bamboo saw-dust composite material [1]. Hanif et al. [122] observed the adsorption capacity while maintaining the concentrations of acid blue-2445 (25 mg/L) and MO dye (100 mg/L) and the adsorbent dose (0.1 g). Results showed that as contact time increased, so did the adsorption of both colors on anion exchange membrane BI. However, after 2 hours, MO and acid blue-2445 had adsorbed to their maximum extent (the threshold limit) on the anion exchange membrane, rendering further adsorption useless [1].

Understanding and optimizing these critical factors are essential for designing efficient dye adsorption processes using ion-exchange materials or other adsorbents. The interactions between these factors can be complex and may vary depending on the specific dye and adsorbent system. Also, the choice of dye removal method depends on factors like the type of dye, its concentration, available infrastructure, environmental regulations, and economic feasibility. Often, a combination of techniques may be required to achieve efficient and comprehensive dye removal from wastewater.

5.4 FUTURE ASPECTS AND NEW TECHNIQUES

In recent years, major developments in adsorbents and ion-exchange materials have been attracting substantial attention as potential economic alternatives to costly materials to remove toxic dye and pollutants [124]. This includes utilizing abundant agricultural, industrial, and natural resources, biowastes, etc. with modification for pollutant removal [1]. Future aspects of ion-exchange materials for dye removal involve several key areas of development. Enhanced material synthesis techniques are anticipated, enabling the creation of materials with improved surface properties and

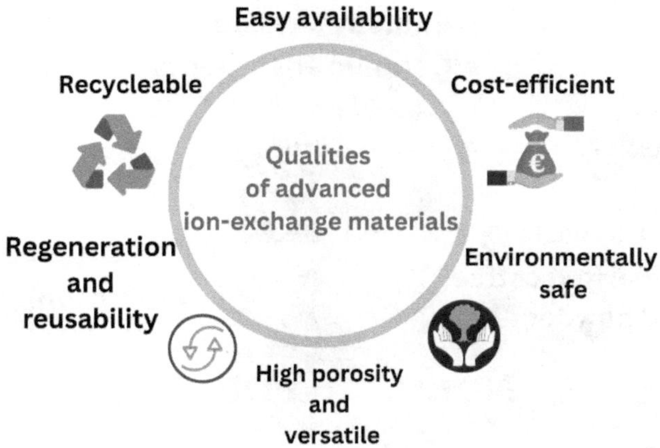

FIGURE 5.6 Ion-exchange material qualities.

ion-exchange capacities. Researchers are exploring modifications at the molecular level to tailor materials for specific dye classes, resulting in higher selectivity and efficiency. Adsorption and ion exchange are the most preferred and flexible techniques for dye removal because of their ease of operation, high efficiency, recyclability, and lower cost. These techniques can be implemented for both the pilot/small-scale and plant-scale wastewater treatment facilities, making them the preferred choice. The adsorption ability and efficiency depend on the choice of adsorbent/exchange material selected for the decolorization of wastewater. Therefore, materials should have easy availability, cost-effectiveness, high porosity, recycling and regenerating ability, and a higher active site ratio (Figure 5.6). However, even after substantial developments, hardships continue to exist in developing low-cost, highly efficient, exchangers and adsorbents with enhanced activity providing long-term stability. Integrating agro-industrial waste which is eco-friendly and several natural and organic materials, with potential biodegradable nanomaterials prohibiting human and environmental hazards can be the best alternative.

Figure 5.7 highlights some examples of emerging materials that can be used for dye removal. Also, the choice of nanomaterials as adsorbents and integrating them with naturally existing materials in wastewater treatment depends upon their broad surface area and high adsorption capacities. Costs associated with manufacturing and maintaining nano-adsorbents, however, provide a significant barrier to their commercial usage in any industrial wastewater treatment [1,124]. Recently, materials having dual characteristics and being environmentally responsible have emerged as the talking point in the scientific community. LDHs are one of those materials showing adsorptive degradation which is been widely reported. LDHs are a class of nanoscale materials that include interlayer anions as well as trivalent and divalent cationic layers. The feature that makes LHDs a potent alternative is their applicability and flexibility. It allows a large variety of cations and anions in their respective layers, which increases its functionality. Commonly used ions used are: M^{2+} (Mg^{2+} , Co^{2+}, Cu^{2+}, Ni^{2+}, Cd^{2+}, or Zn^{2+}) and M^{3+} species (Al^{3+}, Cr^{3+}, Ga^{3+}, or Fe^{3+}). Since the

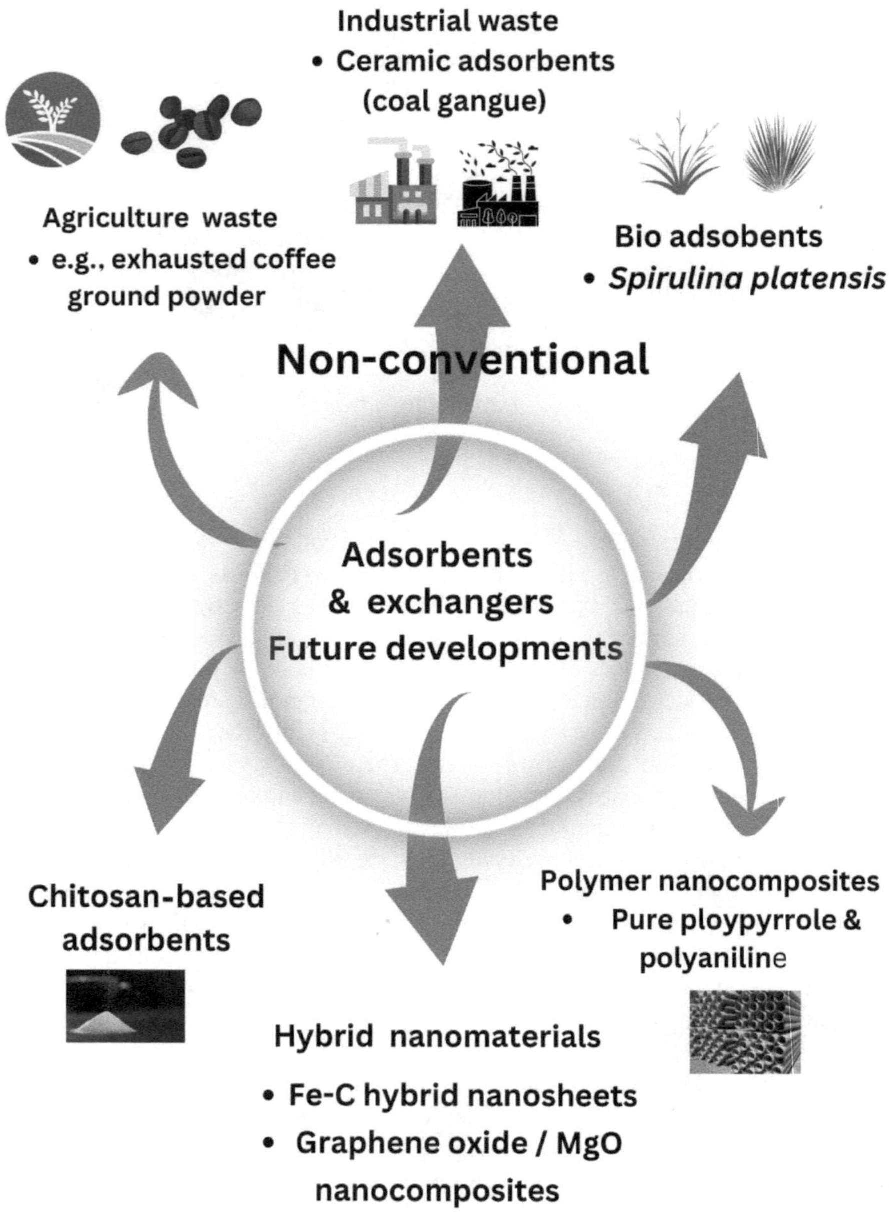

FIGURE 5.7 Future adsorbents and exchange materials.

last two decades, researchers have been examining LDHs' many properties to determine whether they may be used as catalysts [125], hosts for genes and molecules [125,126], functional hybrid nanostructured materials [127,128], and controlled drug release systems [129,130].

Advanced techniques are being integrated with ion-exchange materials to enhance dye removal efficiency. Hybrid materials, combining ion exchange with other mechanisms like adsorption or catalysis, are being investigated for synergistic effects. Furthermore, the integration of nanotechnology and nanomaterials is poised to revolutionize the field, allowing for increased surface area and better interaction with dyes. In terms of applications, the future holds promise for the implementation of ion-exchange materials in decentralized water treatment systems, where their efficiency and ease of operation can provide accessible and clean water solutions to remote areas. Moreover, their integration into industrial processes for dye removal can lead to more sustainable and environmentally responsible practices.

In conclusion, ion-exchange materials for dye removal are an evolving field with exciting prospects. Future developments are expected in material design, synthesis techniques, sustainability, and the integration of advanced technologies. These advancements will contribute to more efficient, selective, and eco-friendly dye removal processes, addressing both environmental concerns and technological demands.

5.5 CONCLUDING REMARKS

The colored dye wastewater discharge in the environment has degraded the quality of freshwater resources and compelled the scientific community to look for more efficient, green, and reliable sources of treatment. This chapter contributes to highlighting the conventional methods and new emerging techniques to tackle the dye wastewater problem. Among all the different techniques, ion exchange and adsorption techniques showed potential and were preferred because of their ease of applicability, re-usability, higher efficiency, and cost-effectiveness. The biggest advantage of these techniques is the flexibility they offer and the countless modifications that can be done, as per the requirement. Hybrid-nanomaterials, polymers and their nanocomposites, industrial and agricultural wastes, and bio-adsorbents are some successful examples that need more attention and application on both small and large scales. Factors like pH, contact time, initial dye concentration, material dosage, and temperature were identified as critical factors that influence the dye removal process and its efficiency.

ACKNOWLEDGMENT

One of the authors Dr. Brijesh Shah would like to thank the Navrachana University, Vadodara, Gujarat, for providing the research fund in terms of the "NUV-Seed Grant (NUV/Seed Grant 2022/22/03)" to carry out research work.

ABBREVIATIONS

AER anion exchange resins
BHET bis(hydroxyethyl) terephthalate
CER cation exchange resins
CR Congo red

DVB divinyl benzene
ETAD the ecological and toxicological association of dyes
IER ion-exchange resins
LDH layered double hydroxide
MB methylene blue
MO methyl orange
PANI polyaniline
PET poly(ethylene terephthalate)
PPY polypyrrole
RhB Rhodamine B
SAC strong acid cation
SBA strong base anion
WAC weak acid cation
WBA weak base anion

REFERENCES

1. Dutta, S., Gupta, B., Srivastava, S. K., and Gupta, A. K. Recent advances on the removal of dyes from wastewater using various adsorbents: a critical review. *Materials Advances*, 2(14), 4497–4531(2021). DOI: 10.1039/d1ma00354b.
2. Sharma, S., Yadav, A., and Ahmad, W. The classification, characterization, and application of ion exchange resins: a general survey. *SSRN Electronic Journal*, 1–22 (2018). DOI: 10.2139/ssrn.3299226.
3. de Dardel, F., and Arden, T. V. Ion exchangers. In: *Ullmann's Encyclopedia of Industrial Chemistry*. Weinheim (2002).
4. Srikanth, M. V., Sunil, S. A., Rao, N. S., Uhumwangho, M. U., and Ramana Murthy, K. V. Ion-exchange resins as controlled drug delivery carriers. *Journal of Scientific Research*, 2(3), 597 (2010). DOI: 10.3329/jsr.v2i3.4991.
5. Helfferich, F. *Ion Exchange*. New York: McGraw-Hill Book Company Inc., pp. 72–94 (1962).
6. Jeong, S., and Park, K. Development of sustained release fast-disintegrating tablets using various polymer-coated ion-exchange resin complexes. *International Journal of Pharmaceutics*, 353(1–2), 195–204 (2008). DOI: 10.1016/j.ijpharm.2007.11.033.
7. Van Abbe, N., and Rees, J. Amberlite Resin XE-88 as a tablet disintegrant. *Journal of the American Pharmaceutical Association (Scientific Ed.)*, 47(7), 487–489 (1958). DOI: 10.1002/jps.3030470707.
8. Kumar, S., and Jain, S. History, Introduction, and kinetics of ion exchange materials. *Journal of Chemistry*, 2013, 1–13 (2013). DOI: 10.1155/2013/95764.
9. Ehrampoush, M. H., Moussavi, G., Ghaneian, M., Rahimi, S., and Ahmadian, M. Removal of methylene blue dye from textile simulated sample using tubular reactor and TiO_2/UV-C photocatalytic process. *Iranian Journal of Environmental Health Science & Engineering*, 8(1), 35–40 (2011).
10. Adams, B. A., and Holmes, E. L. Adsorptive properties of synthetic resins. *Journal of the Society of Chemical Industry (London)*, 54(1), 1–6 (1935). DOI: 10.1002/jctb.5000540101.
11. Chernjatskaja, N. B. Sorption of strontiumon clinoptilolite and heulandite. *Radiochemistry*, 27, 618–621 (1988).

12. Siddiqui, W. A., and Khan, S. A. Inamuddin, synthesis, characterization and ion-exchange properties of a new and novel 'organic–inorganic' hybrid cation-exchanger: poly(methyl methacrylate) Zr(IV)phosphate. *Colloids and Surfaces A: Physicochemical and Engineering Aspects*, 295, 193 (2007). DOI: 10.1016/j.colsurfa.2006.08.053.
13. Singh, K. D., Singh, S., and Srivastava, B. Synthesis characterization and analytical application of Zr(IV) triethylammonium phosphate. *Indian Journal of Chemistry*, 11, 23–28 (2002).
14. Sairam Sundaram, C., and Meenakshi, S. Fluoride sorption using organic–inorganic hybrid type ion exchangers. *Journal of Colloid and Interface Science*, 333(1), 58–62 (2002). DOI: 10.1016/j.jcis.2009.01.022.
15. Varshney, K., Tayal, N., and Gupta, U. Acrylonitrile based cerium (IV) phosphate as a new mercury selective fibrous ion-exchanger. *Colloids and Surfaces A: Physicochemical and Engineering Aspects*, 145(1–3), 71–81 (1998). DOI: 10.1016/s0927-7757(98)00657-8.
16. Varshney, K. G., Gupta, P., and Tayal, N..Synthesis, characterization and applications of a new phase of crystalline and mercury selective acrylamide cerium (IV) phosphate: a novel fibrous ion exchanger. *Indian Journal of Chemistry Section A: Inorganic, Physical, Theoretical & Analytical*, 42(1), 89–93 (2003).
17. Definitions of a dye and a pigment Colour Index. URL: https://colour-index.com/definitions-of-a-dye-and-a-pigment.
18. Yaseen, D. A., and Scholz, M. Textile dye wastewater characteristics and constituents of synthetic effluents: a critical review. *International Journal of Environmental Science and Technology*, 16(2), 1193–1226 (2018). DOI: 10.1007/s13762-018-2130-z.
19. Benkhaya, S., M'rabet, S., and El Harfi, A. A review on classifications, recent synthesis and applications of textile dyes. *Inorganic Chemistry Communications*, 115, 107891 (2020). DOI: 10.1016/j.inoche.2020.107891.
20. Yamjala, K., Nainar, M. S., and Ramisetti, N. R. Methods for the analysis of azo dyes employed in food industry – a review. *Food Chemistry*, 192, 813–824 (2016). DOI: 10.1016/j.foodchem.2015.07.085.
21. Davies, L., Cabrita, G., Ferreira, R., Carias, C., Novais, J., and Martins-Dias, S. Integrated study of the role of *Phragmites australis* in azo-dye treatment in a constructed wetland: from pilot to molecular scale. *Ecological Engineering*, 35(6), 961–970 (2009). DOI: 10.1016/j.ecoleng.2008.08.001.
22. Alasl, M. K., Marandi, R., Khosravi, M., and Seyyedi, K. Treatment of dye solution containing colored index acid yellow 36 by electrocoagulation using iron electrodes. *International Journal of Environmental Science and Technology*, 2(4), 365–371 (2006).
23. Jain, K., Madamwar, D., and Tiwari, O. *Mapping of Research Outcome on Remediation of Dyes, Dye Intermediates and Textile Industrial Waste*, University Press, Sardar Patel University (2019).
24. Burkinshaw, S., and Son, Y. A. The dyeing of supermicrofibre nylon with acid and vat dyes. *Dyes and Pigments*, 87(2), 132–138 (2010). DOI: 10.1016/j.dyepig.2010.03.009.
25. Muthuraman, G., and Teng, T. T. Extraction of methyl red from industrial wastewater using xylene as an extractant. *Progress in Natural Science*, 19(10), 1215–1220 (2009). DOI: 10.1016/j.pnsc.2009.04.002.
26. Jalandoni-Buan, A. C., Decena-Soliven, A. L. A., Cao, E. P., Barraquio, V. L., and Barraquio, W. L. Characterization and identification of Congo red decolorizing

bacteria from monocultures and consortia. *Philippine Journal of Science*, 139(1), 71–78 (2010).

27. Sponza, D. T., and Işık, M. Reactor performances and fate of aromatic amines through decolorization of Direct Black 38 dye under anaerobic/aerobic sequentials. *Process Biochemistry*, 40(1), 35–44 (2005). DOI: 10.1016/j.procbio.2003.11.030.
28. Baughman, G. L., and Weber, E. J. Estimation of water solubility and octanol/water partition coefficient of hydrophobie dyes. *Dyes and Pigments*, 16(4), 261–271 (1991). DOI: 10.1016/0143-7208(91)85016-2.
29. Shalaby, A. A., and Mohamed, A. A. Determination of acid dissociation constants of Alizarin Red S, methyl orange, bromothymol blue and bromophenol blue using a digital camera. *RSC Advances*, 10(19), 11311–11316 (2020). DOI: 10.1039/c9ra10568a.
30. Millington, K. R., Fincher, K. W., and King, A. L. Mordant dyes as sensitisers in dye-sensitised solar cells. *Solar Energy Materials and Solar Cells*, 91(17), 1618–1630 (2007). DOI: 10.1016/j.solmat.2007.05.020.
31. Berradi, M., Hsissou, R., Khudhair, M., Assouag, M., Cherkaoui, O., El Bachiri, A., and El Harfi, A. Textile finishing dyes and their impact on aquatic environs. *Heliyon*, 5(11), 02711 (2019). DOI: 10.1016/j.heliyon.2019.e02711.
32. Yadav, A. K., Jain, C. K., and Malik, D. S. Toxic characterization of textile dyes and effluents in relation to human health hazards. *Journal of Sustainable Environmental Research*, 3(1), 95–102 (2014).
33. Wawrzkiewicz, M. Zastosowanie sorbentów różnego typu w procesie usuwania barwników z roztworów wodnych i ścieków przemysłowych. *Przemysl Chemiczny*, 45–52 (2012).
34. Wawrzkiewicz, M., and Hubicki, Z. Anion exchange resins as effective sorbents for removal of acid, reactive, and direct dyes from textile wastewaters. *Ion Exchange – Studies and Applications*, 1,37–72 (2015). DOI: 10.5772/60952.
35. Rajabi, M., Mahanpoor, K., and Moradi, O. Removal of dye molecules from aqueous solution by carbon nanotubes and carbon nanotube functional groups: critical review. *RSC Advance*, 7(74), 47083–47090 (2017). DOI: 10.1039/c7ra09377b.
36. Hanif, F., Ehsan, S., Zafar, S., Akhtar, M., Khan, M. I., Warsi, M. F., Mubarik, S., Hassan, W., Shakir, I., and Manzoor, S. Adsorptive removal of methyl orange and acid blue-2445 from binary system by anion exchange membrane BI: non-linear and linear form of isotherms. *Desalination and Water Treatment*, 194, 290–301 (2020). DOI: 10.5004/dwt.2020.25864.
37. Awomeso, J. A. Studies on the pollution of water body by textile industry effluents in Lagos, Nigeria. *Journal of Applied Science Environmental Sanitation*, 5,353–359 (2010).
38. Almomani, F., Bhosale, R., Khraisheh, M., Kumar, A., and Almomani, T. Heavy metal ions removal from industrial wastewater using magnetic nanoparticles (MNP), *Applied Surface Science*, 506, 144924 (2020). DOI: 10.1016/j.apsusc.2019.144924.
39. Naim, M. M., Al-harby, N. F., El Batouti, M., and Elewa, M. M. Macro-reticular ion exchange resins for recovery of direct dyes from spent dyeing and soaping liquors. *Molecules*, 27(5), 1593 (2022). DOI: 10.3390/molecules27051593.
40. Deaconu, M., and Senin, R. Adsorption decolorization technique of textile/leather-dye containing effluents. *International Journal of Waste Resources*, 6(2), 1–7 (2016). DOI: 10.4172/2252-5211.1000212.
41. Sen, T. K. Review on dye removal from its aqueous solution into alternative cost effective and non-conventional adsorbents. *Journal of Chemical and Process Engineering* (2013).1, 104. DOI: 10.17303/jce.2014.105.

42. Kumar, A., and Sehgal, M. Hydrogen fuel cell technology for a sustainable future: a review. *SAE Technical Papers on CD-ROM/SAE Technical Paper Series* (2018). DOI: 10.4271/2018-01-1307.
43. Joshi, M. J., Bansal, R., and Purwar, R. Colour removal from textile effluents. *IJFTR*, 29(2), 239–259 (2004).
44. Mondal, S. Methods of dye removal from dye house effluent – an overview. *Environmental Engineering Science*, 25(3), 383–396 (2008). DOI: 10.1089/ees.2007.0049.
45. Ghaly, A. E., Ananthashankar, R., Alhattab, M., and Ramakrishnan, V.V. , Production, characterization and treatment of textile effluents: a critical review. *Journal of Chemical Engineering & Process Technology*, 5(01), 1–18 (2013). DOI: 10.4172/2157-7048.1000182.
46. Gupta, V. K., Kumar, R., Nayak, A., Saleh, T. A., and Barakat, M. Adsorptive removal of dyes from aqueous solution onto carbon nanotubes: a review. *Advances in Colloid and Interface Science*, 193–194, 24–34 (2013). DOI: 10.1016/j.cis.2013.03.003.
47. Gomez, V., Larrechi, M., and Callao, M. Kinetic and adsorption study of acid dye removal using activated carbon. *Chemosphere*, 69(7), 1151–1158 (2007).
48. Donkadokula, N. Y., Kola, A. K., Naz, I., and Saroj, D. (2020). A review on advanced physico-chemical and biological textile dye wastewater treatment techniques. *Reviews in Environmental Science and Bio/Technology*, 19(3), 543–560 (2007). DOI: 10.1007/s11157-020-09543-z.
49. Dutta, S., and Bhattacharjee, J. A comparative study between physicochemical and biological methods for effective removal of textile dye from wastewater. In: *Development in Wastewater Treatment Research and Processes: Innovative Microbe-Based Applications for Removal of Chemicals and Metals in Wastewater Treatment Plants*. Elsevier, Ch. 1, pp. 1–21 (2022). DOI: 10.1016/b978-0-323-85657-7.00003-1.
50. Sinha, S., Behera, S. S., Das, S., Basu, A., Mohapatra, R. K., Murmu, B. M., Dhal, N. K., Tripathy, S. K., and Parhi, P. K. Removal of Congo Red dye from aqueous solution using Amberlite IRA-400 in batch and fixed bed reactors. *Chemical Engineering Communications*, 205(4), 432–444 (2018). DOI: 10.1080/00986445.2017.1399366.
51. Tang, S., Xia, D., Yao, Y., Chen, T., Sun, J., Yin, Y., Shen, W., and Peng, Y. Dye adsorption by self-recoverable, adjustable Amphiphilic Graphene aerogel. *Journal of Colloid and Interface Science*, 554, 682–691 (2019). DOI: 10.1016/j.jcis.2019.07.041.
52. Marrakchi, F., Hameed, B., and Hummadi, E. Mesoporous biohybrid epichlorohydrin crosslinked chitosan/carbon–clay adsorbent for effective cationic and anionic dyes adsorption. *International Journal of Biological Macromolecules*, 163, 1079–1086 (2020). DOI: 10.1016/j.ijbiomac.2020.07.032.
53. Mogale, R., Akpomie, K. G., Conradie, J., and Longer, E. H. Dye adsorption of aluminium- and zirconium-based metal organic frameworks with azobenzene dicarboxylate linkers. *Journal of Environmental Management*, 304, 114166 (2022). DOI: https://doi.org/10.1016/j.jenvman.2021.114166
54. Hassan, M. M., and Carr, C. M. A critical review on recent advancements of the removal of reactive dyes from dyehouse effluent by ion-exchange adsorbents. *Chemosphere*, 209, 201–219 (2018). DOI: 10.1016/j.chemosphere.2018.06.043.
55. Joseph, J., Radhakrishnan, R. C., Johnson, J. K., Joy, S. P., and Thomas, J. Ion-exchange mediated removal of cationic dye-stuffs from water using ammonium phosphomolybdate. *Materials Chemistry and Physics*, 242, 122488 (2020). DOI: 10.1016/j.matchemphys.2019.122488.

56. Kono, H., and Kusumoto, R. Removal of anionic dyes in aqueous solution by flocculation with cellulose ampholytes. *Journal of Water Process Engineering*, 7, 83–93 (2015). DOI: 10.1016/j.jwpe.2015.05.007.
57. Le, O. T. H., Tran, L. N., Doan, V. T., Pham, Q. V., Ngo, A. V., and Nguyen, H. H. Mucilage extracted from dragon fruit peel (*Hylocereus undatus*) as flocculants for treatment of dye wastewater by coagulation and flocculation process. *International Journal of Polymer Science,* 2020, 1–9 (2020). DOI: 10.1155/2020/7468343.
58. Ghuge, S., and Saroha, A. Degradation of azo dye in ozonation by noble metal supported mesoporous catalyst. *International Journal of Environment and Waste Management*, 1(1), (2022). DOI: 10.1504/ijewm.2022.10032506.
59. Ejder-Korucu, M., Gurses, A., Dogar, C., Sharma, S. K., and Acikyildiz, M. Removal of organic dyes from industrial effluents: an overview of physical and biotechnological applications. In: Sharma, S. K. (Ed.), *Green Chemistry for Dyes Removal from Wastewater: Research Trends and Applications*. Scrivener Publishing, Canada, pp. 1–34 (2015).
60. Gurses, A., Güneş, K., and Şahin, E. Removal of dyes and pigments from industrial effluents. In: *Green Chemistry and Water Remediation: Research and Applications*, pp. 135–187 (2021). DOI: 10.1016/b978-0-12-817742-6.00005-0.
61. Hassaan, M. A., and Nemr, A. E. Health and environmental impacts of dyes: mini review. *American Journal of Environmental Science and Engineering*, 1(3), 64 (2017). DOI: 10.11648/j.ajese.20170103.11.
62. Chequer, F. D., De Oliveira, G. R., Ferraz, E. A., Cardoso, J. C., Zanoni, M. B., and de Oliveira, D. P. Textile dyes: dyeing process and environmental impact. *Eco-Friendly Textile Dyeing and Finishing*, 6(6), 151–176 (2013). DOI: 10.5772/53659.
63. Robinson, T., McMullan, G., Marchant, R., and Nigam, P. Remediation of dyes in textile effluent: a critical review on current treatment technologies with a proposed alternative. *Bioresource Technology*, 77(3), 247–255 (2001). DOI: 10.1016/s0960-8524(00)00080-8.
64. Verma, A. K., Dash, R. R., and Bhunia, P. A review on chemical coagulation/flocculation technologies for removal of colour from textile wastewaters. *Journal of Environmental Management*, 93(1), 154–168 (2012). DOI: 10.1016/j.jenvman.2011.09.012.
65. Hao, O. J., Kim, H., and Chiang, P. C. Decolorization of wastewater. *Critical Reviews in Environmental Science and Technology*, 30(4), 449–505 (2000).
66. Adewuyi, Y. G. Sonochemistry: environmental science and engineering applications. *Industrial & Engineering Chemistry Research*, 40(22), 4681–4715 (2001). DOI: 10.1021/ie010096l.
67. Arslan-Alaton, I. A review of the effects of dye-assisting chemicals on advanced oxidation of reactive dyes in wastewater. *Coloration Technology*, 119(6), 345–353 (2003). DOI: 10.1111/j.1478-4408.2003.tb00196.x.
68. Ciabatti, I., Tognotti, F., and Lombardi, L. Treatment and reuse of dyeing effluents by potassium ferrate. *Desalination*, 250(1), 222–228 (2010). DOI: 10.1016/j.desal.2009.06.019.
69. Phalakornkule, C., Polgumhang, S., Tongdaung, W., Karakat, B., and Nuyut, T. Electrocoagulation of blue reactive, red disperse and mixed dyes, and application in treating textile effluent. *Journal of Environmental Management*, 91(4), 918–926 (2010). DOI: 10.1016/j.jenvman.2009.11.008.
70. Slokar, Y., and Majcen Le Marechal, A. Methods of decoloration of textile wastewaters. *Dyes and Pigments*, 37(4), 335–356 (1998). DOI: 10.1016/s0143-7208(97)00075-2.

71. Marcucci, M., Nosenzo, G., Capannelli, G., Ciabatti, I., Corrieri, D., and Ciardelli, G. Treatment and reuse of textile effluents based on new ultrafiltration and other membrane technologies. *Desalination*, 138(1–3), 75–82 (2001).
72. Sandhya, S., and Swaminathan, K. Kinetic analysis of treatment of textile wastewater in hybrid column upflow anaerobic fixed bed reactor. *Chemical Engineering Journal*, 122(1–2), 87–92 (2006). DOI: 10.1016/j.cej.2006.04.006.
73. Tripathi, A., and Rawat Ranjan, M. Heavy metal removal from wastewater using low cost adsorbents. *Journal of Bioremediation & Biodegradation*, 6(6) (2015). DOI: 10.4172/2155-6199.1000315.
74. Kandisa, R. V., Saibaba, N. K. V., Shaik, B., and Gopinath, R. Dye removal by adsorption: a review. *Journal of Bioremediation & Biodegradation*, 7(6), (2016). DOI: 10.4172/2155-6199.1000371.
75. Huang, R., Zhang, Q., Yao, H., Lu, X., Zhou, Q., and Yan, D. Ion-exchange resins for efficient removal of colorants in bis(hydroxyethyl) terephthalate. *ACS Omega*, 6(18), 12351–12360 (2021). DOI: 10.1021/acsomega.1c01477.
76. Yun, X., Xin-yi, Y., Dun-hong, G., Yong-bo, D., and Liang, S. Preparation and characterization of waterborne alkyd-amino baking coatings based on waste polyethylene terephthalate. *Royal Society Open Science*, 7(1), 191447 (2020). DOI: 10.1098/rsos.191447.
77. Gao, W., Zhao, S., Wu, H., Deligeer, W., and Asuha, S. Direct acid activation of kaolinite and its effects on the adsorption of methylene blue. *Applied Clay Science*, 126, 98–106 (2016). DOI: 10.1016/j.clay.2016.03.006.
78. Xue, A., Zhou, S., Zhao, Y., Lu, X., and Han, P. Adsorption of reactive dyes from aqueous solution by silylated palygorskite. *Applied Clay Science*, 48(4), 638–640 (2010). DOI: 10.1016/j.clay.2010.03.011.
79. Dotto, G. L., Esquerdo, V. M., Vieira, M. L. G., and De Almeida Pinto, L. A. Optimization and kinetic analysis of food dyes biosorption by *Spirulina platensis*. *Colloids and Surfaces B: Biointerfaces*, 91, 234–241, (2012). DOI: 10.1016/j.colsurfb.2011.11.008.
80. de Haan, A. B., Eral, H. B., and Schuur, B. Adsorption and ion exchange. In: *Industrial Separation Processes*. Ch. 6, pp. 155–194 (2020).
81. Ebrahimian Pirbazari, A., Saberikhah, E., and Habibzadeh Kozani, S. Fe_3O_4–wheat straw: preparation, characterization and its application for methylene blue adsorption. *Water Resources and Industry*, 7–8, 23–37 (2014). DOI: 10.1016/j.wri.2014.09.001.
82. Siddiqui, S. I., Manzoor, O., Mohsin, M., and Chaudhry, S. A. Nigella sativa seed based nanocomposite-MnO_2/BC: an antibacterial material for photocatalytic degradation, and adsorptive removal of methylene blue from water. *Environmental Research*, 171, 328–340 (2019). DOI: 10.1016/j.envres.2018.11.044.
83. Thamer, B. M., Aldalbahi, A., Moydeen, A. M., Al-Enizi, A. M., El-Hamshary, H., and El-Newehy, M. H. Fabrication of functionalized electrospun carbon nanofibers for enhancing lead-ion adsorption from aqueous solutions. *Scientific Reports*, 9(1), 1–13 (2019). DOI: 10.1038/s41598-019-55679-6.
84. Kim, T. S., Song, H. J., Dar, M. A., Lee, H. J., and Kim, D. W. Fast adsorption kinetics of highly dispersed ultrafine nickel/carbon nanoparticles for organic dye removal. *Applied Surface Science*, 439, 364–370 (2018). DOI: 10.1016/j.apsusc.2018.01.061.
85. Meng, L., Zhang, X., Tang, Y., Su, K., and Kong, J. Hierarchically porous silicon–carbon–nitrogen hybrid materials towards highly efficient and selective adsorption of organic dyes. *Scientific Reports*, 5(1), 7910 (2015).
86. Bezerra de Araujo, C. M., Filipe Oliveira do Nascimento, G., Rodrigues Bezerra da Costa, G., Santos da Silva, K., Salgueiro Baptisttella, A. M., Gomes Ghislandi,

M., and Alves da Motta Sobrinho, M. Adsorptive removal of dye from real textile wastewater using graphene oxide produced via modifications of hummers method. *Chemical Engineering Communication*, 206, 1375–1387, 2018. DOI: 10.1080/00986445.2018.1534232.

87. Yang, S., Chen, S., Chang, Y., Cao, A., Liu, Y., and Wang, H. Removal of methylene blue from aqueous solution by graphene oxide. *Journal of Colloid and Interface Science*, 359(1), 24–29 (2011). DOI: 10.1016/j.jcis.2011.02.064.
88. Sivakumar, M., Yadav, S., Hung, W., and Lai, J. One-pot eco-friendly synthesis of edge-carboxylate graphene via dry ball milling for enhanced removal of acid and basic dyes from single or mixed aqueous solution. *Journal of Cleaner Production*, 263, 121498 (2020). DOI: 10.1016/j.jclepro.2020.121498.
89. De Assis, L. K., Damasceno, B. S., Carvalho, M. N., Oliveira, E. H. C., and Ghislandi, M. G. Adsorption capacity comparison between graphene oxide and graphene nanoplatelets for the removal of coloured textile dyes from wastewater. *Environmental Technology*, 41, 2360–2371 (2019). DOI: 10.1080/09593330.2019.1567603]
90. Kalita, H., Tyagi, H., and Aslam, M. Surface-tailored graphene oxide paper: an efficient filter for dye pollutants. *Environmental Science*, 6(4), 963–975 (2020). DOI: 10.1039/c9ew01129c.
91. Zheng, Y., Cheng, B., You, W., Wang, Y., and Ho, W. 3D hierarchical graphene oxide–NiFe LDH composite with enhanced adsorption affinity to Congo red, methyl orange and Cr(VI) ions. *Journal of Hazardous Materials*, 369, 214–225 (2019). DOI: 10.1016/j.jhazmat.2019.02.013.
92. Heidarizad, M., and Şengor, S. S. Synthesis of graphene oxide/magnesium oxide nanocomposites with high-rate adsorption of methylene blue. *Journal of Molecular Liquids*, 224, 607–617 (2016).
93. Muhammad, A., Shah, A. A., and Bilal, S. Comparative study of the adsorption of Acid Blue 40 on polyaniline, magnetic oxide and their composites: synthesis, characterization and application. *Materials*, 12(18), 2854 (2019). DOI: 10.3390/ma12182854.
94. Kubra, K. T., Salman, M. S., Znad, H., and Hasan, M. N. Efficient encapsulation of toxic dye from wastewater using biodegradable polymeric adsorbent. *Journal of Molecular Liquids*, 329, 115541 (2021). DOI: 10.1016/j.molliq.2021.115541.
95. Bober, P., Minisy, I. M., Acharya, U., Pfleger, J., Babayan, V., Kazantseva, N. E., Hodan, J., & Stejskal, J. Conducting polymer composite aerogel with magnetic properties for organic dye removal. *Synthetic Metals*, 260, 116266 (2020). DOI: 10.1016/j.synthmet.2019.116266.
96. Acharya, S., Sahoo, S., Sonal, S., Lee, J. H., Mishra, B. K., and Nayak, G. C. Adsorbed Cr(VI) based activated carbon/polyaniline nanocomposite: a superior electrode material for asymmetric supercapacitor device. *Composites Part B – Engineering*, 193, 107913 (2020). DOI: 10.1016/j.compositesb.2020.107913.
97. Nasar, A., and Mashkoor, F. Application of polyaniline-based adsorbents for dye removal from water and wastewater – a review. *Environmental Science and Pollution Research*, 26(6), 5333–5356 (2019). DOI: 10.1007/s11356-018-3990-y.
98. Chafai, H., Laabd, M., Elbariji, S., Bazzaoui, M., and Albourine, A. Study of Congo red adsorption on the polyaniline and polypyrrole. *Journal of Dispersion Science and Technology*, 38(6), 832–836 (2016). DOI: 10.1080/01932691.2016.1207185.
99. Aliabadi, R. S., and Mahmoodi, N. O. Synthesis and characterization of polypyrrole, polyaniline nanoparticles and their nanocomposite for removal of azo dyes; sunset yellow and Congo red. *Journal of Cleaner Production*, 179, 235–245 (2018). DOI: 10.1016/j.jclepro.2018.01.035.

100. Smita, J., Dipika, J., and Shraddha, K. Polyaniline for removal of methyl orange dye from waste water. *International Journal of Science Engineering and Management*, 1, 1–6 (2016).
101. Janaki, V., Vijayaraghavan, K., Oh, B., Lee, K., Muthuchelian, K., Ramasamy, A. K., and Kamala-Kannan, S. Starch/polyaniline nanocomposite for enhanced removal of reactive dyes from synthetic effluent. *Carbohydrate Polymers*, 90(4), 1437–1444 (2012). DOI: 10.1016/j.carbpol.2012.07.012.
102. Wang, N., Chen, J., Wang, J., Feng, J., and Yan, W. Removal of methylene blue by polyaniline/TiO_2 hydrate: adsorption kinetic, isotherm and mechanism studies. *Powder Technology*, 347, 93–102 (2019). DOI: 10.1016/j.powtec.2019.02.049.
103. Vakili, M., Rafatullah, M., Salamatinia, B., Abdullah, A. Z., Ibrahim, M. H., Tan, K. B., Gholami, Z., and Amouzgar, P. Application of chitosan and its derivatives as adsorbents for dye removal from water and wastewater: a review. *Carbohydrate Polymers*, 113, 115–130 (2014). DOI: 10.1016/j.carbpol.2014.07.007.
104. Muzzarelli, R. A., Boudrant, J., Meyer, D., Manno, N., DeMarchis, M., and Paoletti, M. G. Current views on fungal chitin/chitosan, human chitinases, food preservation, glucans, pectins and inulin: a tribute to Henri Braconnot, precursor of the carbohydrate polymers science, on the chitin bicentennial. *Carbohydrate Polymers*, 87(2), 995–1012 (2012). DOI: 10.1016/j.carbpol.2011.09.063.
105. Janaki, V., Oh, B., Shanthi, K., Lee, K., Ramasamy, A. K., and Kamala-Kannan, S. Polyaniline/chitosan composite: an eco-friendly polymer for enhanced removal of dyes from aqueous solution. *Synthetic Metals*, 162(11–12), 974–980 (2012). DOI: 10.1016/j.synthmet.2012.04.015.
106. Agarwal, S., Sadegh, H., Monajjemi, M., Hamdy, A. S., Ali, G. a. M., Memar, A., Shahryari-Ghoshekandi, R., Tyagi, I., and Gupta, V. K. Efficient removal of toxic bromothymol blue and methylene blue from wastewater by polyvinyl alcohol. *Journal of Molecular Liquids*, 218, 191–197 (2016). DOI: 10.1016/j.molliq.2016.02.060.
107. Haque, E., Lo, V., Minett, A. I., Harris, A. T., and Church, T. L. Dichotomous adsorption behaviour of dyes on an amino-functionalized metal-organic framework, amino-MIL-101(Al). *Journal of Materials Chemistry: A, Materials for Energy and Sustainability*, 2(1), 193–203 (2014). DOI: 10.1039/c3ta13589f.
108. Tong, M., Liu, D., Yang, Q., Devautour-Vinot, S., Maurin, G., and Zhong, C. Influence of framework metal ions on the dye capture behavior of MIL-100 (Fe, Cr) MOF type solids. *Journal of Materials Chemistry. A, Materials for Energy and Sustainability*, 1(30), 8534 (2013). DOI: 10.1039/c3ta11807j.
109. Zhao, X., Liu, S., Tang, Z., Niu, H., Cai, Y., Meng, W., Wu, F., and Giesy, J. P. Synthesis of magnetic metal-organic framework (MOF) for efficient removal of organic dyes from water. *Scientific Reports*, 5(1) 1–10 (2015). DOI: 10.1038/srep11849.
110. Mahapatra, A., Mishra, B. G., and Hota, G. Adsorptive removal of Congo red dye from wastewater by mixed iron oxide–alumina nanocomposites. *Ceramics International*, 39(5), 5443–5451 (2013). DOI: 10.1016/j.ceramint.2012.12.052.
111. Li, Z., Sun, Y., Jian-Wei, X., Xing, Y., and Meng, A. One-step synthesis of Co/Cr-codoped ZnO nanoparticle with superb adsorption properties for various anionic organic pollutants and its regeneration. *Journal of Hazardous Materials*, 352, 204–214 (2018). DOI: 10.1016/j.jhazmat.2018.03.049.
112. Lei, C., Pi, M., Xu, D., Jiang, C., and Cheng, B. Fabrication of hierarchical porous ZnO–Al_2O_3 microspheres with enhanced adsorption performance. *Applied Surface Science*, 426, 360–368 (2017). DOI: 10.1016/j.apsusc.2017.07.095.

113. Zhou, Y., Lu, J., Zhou, Y., and Liu, Y. Recent advances for dyes removal using novel adsorbents: a review. *Environmental Pollution*, 252, 352–365 (2019). DOI: 10.1016/j.envpol.2019.05.072.
114. Salleh, M. A. M., Mahmoud, D. K., Karim, W. A. W. A., and Idris, A. Cationic and anionic dye adsorption by agricultural solid wastes: a comprehensive review. *Desalination*, 280(1–3), 1–13 (2011). DOI: 10.1016/j.desal.2011.07.019.
115. Ofomaja, A., and Ho, Y., Equilibrium sorption of anionic dye from aqueous solution by palm kernel fibre as sorbent. *Dyes Pigments*, 74, 60–66 (2007).
116. Katheresan, V., Kansedo, J., and Lau, S. Y. Efficiency of various recent wastewater dye removal methods: a review. *Journal of Environmental Chemical Engineering*, 6(4), 4676–4697 (2018). DOI: 10.1016/j.jece.2018.06.060.
117. Eren, Z., and Acar, F. N. Adsorption of Reactive Black 5 from an aqueous solution: equilibrium and kinetic studies. *Desalination*, 194(1–3), 1–10 (2006).
118. Liu, L., Gao, Z. Y., Su, X. P., Chen, X., Jiang, L., and Yao, J. M. Adsorption removal of dyes from single and binary solutions using a cellulose-based bioadsorbent. *ACS Sustainable Chemistry & Engineering*, 3(3), 432–442 (2015). DOI: 10.1021/sc500848m.
119. Phoemphoonthanyakit, S., Seeharaj, P., Damrongsak, P., and Locharoenrat, K. Effect of adsorption characteristics of Rhodamine 6G dye solution in Fe_3O_4 magnetic nanoparticles on fluorescence quantum yield. *Journal of Spectroscopy*, 2019, 1–5 (2019).
120. Kousha, M., Daneshvar, E., Sohrabi, M. S., Jokar, M., and Bhatnagar, A. Adsorption of acid orange II dye by raw and chemically modified brown macroalga *Stoechospermum marginatum. Chemical Engineering Journal*, 192, 67–76 (2012). DOI: 10.1016/j.cej.2012.03.057.
121. Khan, T. A., and Nazir, M. Enhanced adsorptive removal of a model acid dye bromothymol blue from aqueous solution using magnetic chitosan-bamboo sawdust composite: batch and column studies. *Environmental Progress & Sustainable Energy*, 34(5), 1444–1454 (2015). DOI: 10.1002/ep.12147.
122. Crini, G. Non-conventional low-cost adsorbents for dye removal: a review. *Bioresource Technology*, 97(9), 1061–1085 (2006). DOI: 10.1016/j.biortech.2005.05.001.
123. Mazari, S. A., Ali, E., Abro, R., Khan, F. S. A., Ahmed, I., Ahmed, M., Nizamuddin, S., Siddiqui, T. H., Hossain, N., Mubarak, N. M., and Shah, A. Nanomaterials: applications, waste-handling, environmental toxicities, and future challenges – a review. *Journal of Environmental Chemical Engineering*, 9(2), 105028 (2021). DOI: 10.1016/j.jece.2021.105028.
124. Gong, M., Li, Y., Wang, H., Liang, Y., Wu, J. Z., Zhou, J., Wang, J., Regier, T., Wei, F., and Dai, H. An advanced Ni–Fe layered double hydroxide electrocatalyst for water oxidation. *Journal of the American Chemical Society*, 135(23), 8452–8455 (2013). DOI: 10.1021/ja4027715/.
125. Choy, J. H., Jung, J. S., Oh, J. M., Park, M., Jeong, J., Kang, Y. K., and Han, O. J. Layered double hydroxide as an efficient drug reservoir for folate derivatives. *Biomaterials*, 25(15), 3059–3064 (2004).
126. Ci, J., Cao, C., Kuga, S., Shen, J., Wu, M., and Huang, Y. Improved performance of microbial fuel cell using esterified corncob cellulose nanofibers to fabricate air-cathode gas diffusion layer. *ACS Sustainable Chemistry & Engineering*, 5(11), 9614–9618 (2017). DOI: 10.1021/acssuschemeng.7b01970.
127. Yan, H., Zhao, X. J., Zhu, Y. Q., Wei, M., Evans, D. G., and Duan, X. The periodic table as a guide to the construction and properties of layered double hydroxides.

In: *The Periodic Table II*. Structure and Bonding. Springer, pp. 89–120 (2019). DOI: 10.1007/430_2019_47.

128. Li, L., Gu, Z., Gu, W., Liu, J., and Xu, Z. P. Efficient drug delivery using SiO_2-layered double hydroxide nanocomposites. *Journal of Colloid and Interface Science*, 470, 47–55 (2016). DOI: 10.1016/j.apsusc.2022.155610.
129. Sun, J., Lei, Y., Dai, Z., Liu, X., Huang, T., Wu, J., Xu, Z. P., and Sun, X. Sustained release of brimonidine from a new composite drug delivery system for treatment of glaucoma. *ACS Applied Materials & Interfaces*, 9(9), 7990–7999 (2017). DOI: 10.1021/acsami.6b16509.

6 Recent Advances in Nanomaterials and Nanotechnology for Their Application in Dye Degradation from Wastewater

Shivani R. Pandya, Noble George, Srushti Jasani, Harjeet Singh, and Krishna Kumari Swain

6.1 INTRODUCTION

In the relentless pursuit of sustainable solutions for our ever-growing environmental challenges, recent advances in nanomaterials and nanotechnology have emerged as a beacon of hope. With wastewater pollution posing a significant threat to our ecosystems and public health, this field has taken centerstage in our quest for cleaner, safer water resources. Nanomaterials, with their minuscule dimensions and remarkable properties, offer a promising avenue for tackling one of the most pressing issues of our time: dye degradation from wastewater. In this realm of innovation, the alliance of nanotechnology and environmental science has birthed groundbreaking techniques and materials that not only combat pollution but also pave the way for a brighter, more sustainable future. In this exploration of recent advancements, we delve into the mesmerizing world of nanomaterials and nanotechnology, unveiling their potential to revolutionize the way we purify and protect our precious water resources.

Welcome to the frontier of progress, where science meets sustainability in the battle against wastewater pollution.

6.1.1 Background on Environmental Preservation

The concept of environmental preservation has garnered heightened attention in recent decades as a direct response to the escalating threats to the natural world that have been largely attributed to human activities. Environmental preservation, at its core, constitutes a multifaceted approach that encompasses responsible resource utilization, pollution mitigation, and the safeguarding of ecosystems, all with the

DOI: 10.1201/9781003441083-6

overarching goal of ensuring the long-term sustainability of planet Earth for the upcoming generations [1]. This imperative has been propelled to the forefront of global concerns due to the increasingly widespread acknowledgment of anthropogenic climate change and the depletion of critical natural resources.

To delve deeper into the scientific underpinnings of environmental preservation, it is crucial to recognize the interplay of various ecological and environmental processes. Human activities, such as industrialization and deforestation, have led to a surge in greenhouse gas emissions, primarily carbon dioxide (CO_2), methane (CH_4), and nitrous oxide (N_2O), which have collectively resulted in the phenomenon known as global warming [2]. This process intensifies the Earth's natural greenhouse effect, leading to a rise in average global temperatures, with profound consequences for climate patterns, sea levels, and the incidence and magnitude of severe weather occurrences.

Furthermore, unsustainable resource exploitation, including deforestation, overfishing, and the depletion of fossil fuels, has not only accelerated climate change but has also jeopardized biodiversity and ecosystem stability. The loss of biodiversity disrupts intricate ecological relationships, impeding the ability of ecosystems to provide vital services such as pollination, water purification, and carbon sequestration. Consequently, the depletion of natural resources exacerbates environmental degradation and threatens the resilience of ecosystems.

In response to these formidable challenges, environmental preservation advocates for a comprehensive array of strategies and measures. These include transitioning to renewable and low-carbon energy sources to mitigate greenhouse gas emissions, implementing rigorous pollution control actions to curtail the release of harmful pollutants into the environment, and establishing protected areas and conservation efforts to safeguard biodiversity and restore degraded ecosystems. Additionally, sustainable land and resource management practices, such as afforestation and sustainable agriculture, play a pivotal role in preserving natural resources and mitigating the impacts of human activities on the environment [3].

The concept of environmental preservation is not merely a matter of sentiment or ethics; it is firmly rooted in scientific understanding and evidence. Human-induced changes to the environment, notably climate change and resource depletion, pose tangible threats to the planet's ecological balance and the well-being of future generations. To address these challenges effectively, a scientifically informed approach to environmental preservation is essential, one that combines innovative technologies, sustainable practices, and global cooperation to safeguard the Earth's ecological integrity and ensure a sustainable future for all.

6.1.2 Impact of Industrial Activities on the Environment

Industrial activities, while pivotal for economic progress and elevating living standards, have brought forth a cascade of deleterious environmental ramifications. The onset of the industrial revolution heralded a surge in the discharge of pollutants and waste materials into the environment, with particular impacts on aqueous and atmospheric domains [4]. Industrial emissions have emerged as a substantial contributor to multiple forms of environmental degradation, including air pollution, the amplification of greenhouse gas concentrations, and the pollution of water reservoirs, culminating in pernicious repercussions for both human well-being and ecological systems.

The industrial sector has undeniably driven economic growth and technological advancement, but it has also ushered in a profusion of environmental challenges. Central to these challenges is the release of noxious substances into the atmosphere. Combustion processes, ubiquitous in industries, are a prominent source of air pollutants. These emissions encompass a spectrum of contaminants, including sulfur dioxide (SO_2), nitrogen oxides (NO_x), particulate matter (PM), and volatile organic compounds (VOCs) [5]. The release of such pollutants not only degrades air quality but also contributes to a litany of adverse health effects in human populations, including respiratory diseases, cardiovascular ailments, and even premature mortality.

In addition to atmospheric impacts, industrial operations have a profound influence on aquatic ecosystems. The contamination of water bodies through the discharge of industrial effluents containing heavy metals, toxic chemicals, and other contaminants poses a substantial threat to aquatic life and human health [6, 7]. The accumulation of pollutants in water systems disrupts the balance of ecosystems, impairs the quality of drinking water sources, and hampers aquatic biodiversity. This contamination is often accompanied by ecological disruptions, including the eutrophication of water bodies, the proliferation of harmful algal blooms, and the degradation of aquatic habitats [8].

Industrial activities have improved the economy and living standards but have also caused significant environmental damage. To mitigate harm, sustainable practices and technologies must be adopted in industrial processes.

6.1.3 Significance of Dye Degradation from Wastewater

The significance of dye degradation from wastewater arises as a critical environmental concern directly linked to industrial activities. Industries such as food, leather, textile, paper, cosmetics, and pharmaceuticals rely extensively on dyes for product coloration and enhancement, which, in turn, contributes to their widespread use. However, this practice leads to a substantial environmental issue when these dyes find their way into wastewater streams. Synthetic dyes, in particular, are often non-biodegradable and can persist in the environment over extended periods [6]. When these dyes are discharged into water bodies alongside industrial effluents, they pose significant risks to both human and animal health, disrupt aquatic ecosystems, and compromise overall water quality.

Addressing the degradation of dyes in wastewater represents a crucial facet of environmental preservation and pollution management. It involves the pressing necessity to develop efficient and cost-effective technologies for the removal and degradation of dyes from industrial effluents. Recent strides in nanomaterials and nanotechnology have furnished innovative solutions to confront this challenge. Nanomaterials, characterized by their exceptionally high surface area, modified surface properties, and distinctive electron conduction capabilities, have proven to be exceptionally effective in treating wastewater contaminated with dyes [9, 10].

This chapter seeks to investigate the synthesis and functionalization of nanoparticles in the context of eliminating dyes from industrial effluents. We will delve into the most current advancements in nanomaterials employed for dye removal via various mechanisms, encompassing biological processes, photocatalysis, and adsorption techniques. Additionally, we will underscore methodologies for enhancing the efficacy of nanomaterials in combatting dye pollution through tailored modifications. Lastly, we will identify gaps in our knowledge regarding the application of nanomaterials to environmental preservation and propose potential avenues for future research.

Through a comprehensive exploration of these subjects, this chapter endeavors to provide invaluable insights into the pivotal role of nanotechnology in mitigating the environmental ramifications of dye contamination while propelling the agenda of environmental conservation forward.

6.2 GROWTH OF DYE USAGE IN VARIOUS INDUSTRIES

The widespread and escalating utilization of dyes across diverse industrial sectors underscores a significant trend in contemporary manufacturing practices.

6.2.1 Food Industry

The food industry has undergone a substantial expansion in the utilization of dyes over the course of its development. Dyes constitute a fundamental component within the food sector, primarily harnessed for the enhancement of food products' visual appeal

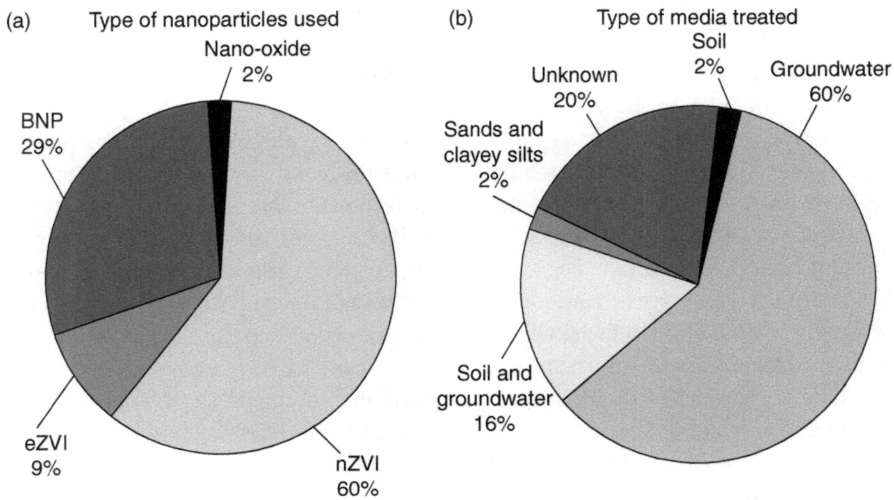

FIGURE 6.1 (a) Schematic representation of types of nanoparticles used for the remediation, with a predominant emphasis on zero-valent iron (ZVI) containing iron (Fe). (b) Illustrates the primary sources of treated or remediated media.

Source: **Reprinted from an open source [11].**

[12]. Their primary role revolves around the infusion of vibrant and enticing colors into various food items, thereby augmenting their esthetic allure for consumers. This application extends across a diverse spectrum of food products, ranging from candies and beverages to desserts and processed foods, where dyes are adeptly employed to achieve a diverse array of colors, spanning from vivid red hues to profound blues.

Despite their intended purpose of rendering food products more visually appealing, the proliferation of food dyes has concurrently elicited concerns pertaining to their safety and environmental implications. Certain synthetic food dyes have been associated with potential health hazards, including allergies and heightened levels of hyperactivity, particularly among children [12]. Furthermore, these dyes possess the propensity to leave residual traces in wastewater streams during food processing and manufacturing operations. Consequently, the efficacious removal of food dyes from industrial effluents emerges as an imperative endeavor, aimed at preventing their inadvertent discharge into aquatic ecosystems and safeguarding overall water quality.

In essence, the escalating prevalence of dyes within the food industry underscores their pivotal role in elevating the sensory attributes of food products. Nevertheless, this phenomenon also demands meticulous scrutiny regarding the safety of these dyes, particularly in light of potential health concerns, and necessitates robust wastewater treatment measures to mitigate their environmental footprint and ensure the preservation of water quality standards.

6.2.2 Leather Industry

The leather industry relies extensively on the application of dyes to impart coloration and finish to leather-based products, encompassing a wide spectrum of items such as shoes, bags, belts, and upholstery. The process of dyeing holds paramount importance within leather processing, as it not only serves to enhance the esthetic appeal of leather goods but also offers a diverse palette of color options to cater to the discerning preferences of consumers.

However, a consequential environmental challenge arises from the dyeing process in the leather industry, primarily linked to the substantial generation of wastewater replete with dyes and accompanying chemical constituents [13]. This wastewater, often laden with a complex cocktail of dyestuffs and auxiliary chemicals, presents a pressing ecological concern. The issue is exacerbated by the inherent characteristics of numerous leather dyes, many of which exhibit non-biodegradable properties and the proclivity to endure in the environment over extended durations. The discharge of such dye-laden effluents into natural ecosystems poses a formidable environmental threat, as it can lead to the pollution of aquatic environments and compromise the quality of soil in areas where wastewater is disposed of or inadvertently released [14].

Given these ecological challenges, the development and implementation of efficacious methodologies for the elimination and degradation of dyes from wastewater originating in leather manufacturing emerge as a pivotal imperative. Such endeavors are crucial not only for preserving environmental integrity but also for mitigating the potential consequences of dye-related pollution on aquatic ecosystems and soil ecosystems. Thus, the quest for innovative solutions in dye management within the leather sector aligns with broader sustainability goals, thereby striving to minimize the industry's ecological footprint and safeguard environmental equilibrium.

6.2.3 Textile Industry

The textile sector stands as one of the preeminent global consumers of dyes, with a pervasive reliance on these colorants for the purpose of fabric and garment coloring, as well as for various textile-related products [15]. The surging demand for vibrant, fashionable clothing and textiles has propelled the expansion of dye utilization within this industry. In the realm of textile manufacturing, the significance of dyes cannot be overstated. These compounds play a pivotal role in endowing fabrics and textile products with an expansive array of colors and esthetics to meet the ever-evolving preferences of consumers. As a result, dye usage has become synonymous with the creation of visually appealing and marketable textile items.

However, the textile dyeing processes, while indispensable for achieving aesthetic goals, are fraught with environmental consequences of substantial magnitude. Notably, these processes are renowned for their prodigious water consumption and the concurrent generation of wastewater laden with dyes, alongside auxiliary chemicals and heavy metals. This wastewater, a by-product of textile dyeing, is characterized by its complex composition and the potential to harbor a variety of environmentally deleterious constituents.

The ramifications of discharging untreated textile wastewater into natural water bodies are manifold and grave. Such actions engender severe pollution, posing a direct threat to aquatic ecosystems and the quality of receiving waters. The introduction of dyes into these environments can lead to ecological harm, affecting aquatic flora and fauna, impairing water quality, and disrupting the delicate balance of aquatic ecosystems [16].

In light of these pressing environmental challenges, the imperative to discover and deploy sustainable and efficacious methodologies for the eradication and treatment of textile dyes from wastewater assumes paramount significance. Addressing this critical concern not only aligns with the industry's commitment to environmental responsibility but also serves as a safeguard for the ecological integrity of our natural waterways. The pursuit of innovative, eco-friendly solutions for managing textile dye wastewater represents a pivotal stride toward harmonizing the textile industry's demand for color and style with the imperative of environmental preservation.

6.2.4 Paper Industry

Within the paper industry, dyes and pigments serve a pivotal role in bestowing coloration and aesthetic allure upon a myriad of paper-based products, encompassing newspapers, magazines, packaging materials, and decorative papers. The strategic application of dyes facilitates the production of visually captivating and informative printed materials, aligning with the industry's goal of creating engaging and informative paper products [17].

Nonetheless, the incorporation of dyes within the paper manufacturing process gives rise to a noteworthy environmental concern. This concern pertains to the potential release of wastewater tainted with residual dyes during the papermaking procedures. The discharge of such dye-laden effluents into natural watercourses, including rivers and streams, can engender detrimental consequences for aquatic ecosystems and exert adverse effects on overall water quality [18]. Given the extensive global consumption of paper and paper-based commodities, addressing the issue of dye pollution emanating from the paper industry is of paramount importance. It assumes a central role in the broader mission of conserving vital water resources and mitigating the industry's environmental footprint.

6.2.5 Cosmetic Industry

The cosmetic industry, renowned for its continuous pursuit of innovation and diversity in product formulations, heavily relies on the incorporation of dyes and pigments in the creation of a broad spectrum of makeup and personal care products. Dyes are prominently employed to infuse vibrant colors and esthetic allure into items such as lipsticks, eye shadows, nail polishes, and hair dyes. This relentless drive for novel product offerings and an expansive palette of colors has precipitated a consistent escalation in the utilization of dyes within the cosmetic sector [19].

The pivotal role played by dyes in cosmetics is manifest in their ability to enhance product visual appeal, ultimately catering to consumer preferences for vivid and diverse cosmetic selections. The application of dyes and pigments, therefore, constitutes an indispensable component of the cosmetics industry's quest to create enticing and fashionable products that resonate with a discerning clientele [20].

However, the employment of dyes in cosmetics concurrently engenders ecological concerns that manifest when these cosmetic products are removed and subsequently washed off, ultimately entering wastewater systems. The release of effluents from the cosmetic industry, laden with residual dyes, into environmental watercourses can potentially introduce a plethora of chemical compounds into the ecosystem. These compounds may include dye residues along with associated constituents found in cosmetic formulations. The discharge of such effluents raises apprehensions regarding the environmental fate of cosmetic dyes and the potential hazards they may pose to aquatic ecosystems and overall water quality [21]. The intricate mixture of chemical compounds present in cosmetic effluents, when introduced into natural environments, can contribute to adverse ecological effects, such as aquatic toxicity, bioaccumulation, and the disruption of aquatic life cycles [22].

Hence, the imperative to devise and implement successful approach for the elimination and degradation of cosmetic dyes from wastewater surfaces as a compelling necessity. Such measures are essential not only to preserve the integrity of water resources but also to mitigate the environmental repercussions stemming from the presence of cosmetic dye residues. In sum, addressing the intricate interplay between the cosmetic industry's reliance on dyes and their potential environmental consequences signifies a crucial facet of the broader endeavor to harmonize the cosmetic industry's pursuit of esthetics with the imperative of environmental protection.

6.2.6 Pharmaceutical Industry

The pharmaceutical industry, integral to the advancement of healthcare and therapeutic solutions, relies significantly on the application of dyes for a myriad of purposes. Dyes are instrumental in pharmaceutical processes, including drug formulation, tablet coating, and the visual identification of pharmaceutical products [23]. Their multifaceted utility encompasses distinguishing between various medications, augmenting product recognition, and enhancing patient adherence to prescribed treatment regimens.

In the context of drug formulation, dyes are often used to impart distinct colors to pharmaceutical compounds, allowing for easy differentiation between various drugs, dosages, or formulations. This plays a pivotal role in minimizing medication errors, ensuring patient safety, and facilitating accurate drug administration. Additionally, dyes are employed in tablet coating to enhance the aesthetic appeal of pills, making them more palatable and recognizable to patients. Such measures contribute to improved patient compliance, especially in cases where medication regimens are complex or long term.

However, in common with other industries, the pharmaceutical sector confronts challenges related to the generation of wastewater laden with dyes and associated chemical residues. The presence of pharmaceutical dyes in wastewater raises legitimate concerns, encompassing potential health risks and environmental ramifications [24]. These concerns stem from the fact that pharmaceutical dyes can include a range of chemical compounds, some of which may exhibit toxicity or other negative consequences on aquatic ecosystems and human health.

As the pharmaceutical industry continues its trajectory of growth and innovation, the need to address the environmental consequences of dye discharge becomes increasingly salient. Regulatory bodies and stakeholders within the pharmaceutical sector are increasingly recognizing the importance of minimizing the ecological footprint of pharmaceutical manufacturing processes. Consequently, exploring innovative methods for managing and mitigating the environmental impact of pharmaceutical dye effluents is of paramount importance.

In the forthcoming sections, we will delve into the distinct challenges posed by the usage of dyes investigate how advanced nanomaterials and nanotechnology can serve as instrumental tools in ameliorating the environmental impact. Specifically, we will examine how these cutting-edge technologies can facilitate the efficient removal and degradation of dyes from industrial effluents, thereby aligning manufacturing practices with the broader goals of environmental sustainability and preservation.

6.3 ENVIRONMENTAL CONSEQUENCES OF DYE DISPOSAL

The unregulated and unsystematic release of dyes, notably synthetic variants, into the natural environment gives rise to a myriad of ecological repercussions that necessitate urgent scrutiny. In this section, we will undertake an in-depth exploration of the precise challenges linked to dye disposal, underscoring the imperative of mitigating these issues through the application of cutting-edge technologies, such as nanomaterials and nanotechnology.

6.3.1 Dumping of Dyes into Water Bodies

Among the prevailing and disconcerting practices in the management of dyes, a prominent concern revolves around their unmediated discharge into aquatic ecosystems, encompassing rivers, lakes, and oceans [25]. This phenomenon is particularly prevalent within industrial contexts, where wastewater laden with dyes is often subjected to inadequate or, at times, absent treatment ahead of its discharge into these bodies of water.

The release of dyes into water bodies can entail severe repercussions on the aquatic ecosystem. These effects are multifaceted and can impact various aspects of the environment such as the following:

1. *Water pollution:* Stemming from the persistence of dye molecules in aquatic environments, water pollution presents a multifaceted ecological challenge with profound implications. Dyes, known for their vibrant and enduring colors, can persist in water bodies for protracted durations, thereby impinging on the natural equilibrium of aquatic ecosystems [26]. The consequences of this disruption extend across various ecological dimensions, warranting meticulous examination. The persistence of dyes in water bodies can lead to a notable consequence, namely the alteration of water coloration. The vibrant and long-lasting hues of dyes have the potential to mask or obscure the natural coloration of water, resulting in an optical transformation [27]. This transformation has significant implications for aquatic ecosystems, as it affects the visual cues that many aquatic organisms rely on for survival. The disruptions caused by the presence of dyes can hinder the ability of aquatic organisms to effectively detect their predators or prey. Essentially, the vivid colors of dyes create a perceptual distortion within the aquatic environment, blurring the distinction between concealment and exposure. This distortion undermines the fundamental mechanisms of predation and predation avoidance, potentially leading to imbalances within the ecosystem [28].

   The ramifications of these disruptions are manifold and ripple throughout the aquatic food web. For instance, predatory species may find it more challenging to locate their prey, resulting in potential imbalances in predator-prey dynamics. Conversely, prey species may struggle to recognize and evade their natural predators, rendering them more vulnerable to predation. These cascading effects can disrupt the intricate balance of the aquatic ecosystem, leading to shifts in species composition and abundance. Moreover, the persistence of dyes can hinder the photosynthetic processes of aquatic plants and algae by altering the light spectrum available for photosynthesis. This can further disrupt the base of the aquatic food chain, affecting herbivorous organisms that depend on these primary producers for sustenance [29, 30].
2. *Toxicity:* The toxicity associated with synthetic dyes poses a significant concern as it can have detrimental effects on aquatic ecosystems. Many synthetic dyes contain chemical constituents that are harmful to aquatic organisms, and their introduction into water bodies can lead to a cascade of adverse consequences, including the poisoning of these organisms [31]. The toxicity

of these dyes affects various aspects of aquatic life, impacting the well-being and reproductive capacities of the organisms.

The issue at the core of this concern is the potential harm caused by toxic compounds present in synthetic dyes when released into aquatic environments. These toxic chemicals, which are part of the dye formulations, can be detrimental to aquatic organisms. The repercussions of this toxicity are wide-ranging and complex. Aquatic organisms exposed to these harmful substances may experience acute or chronic health effects, ranging from physiological stress to mortality. Furthermore, their reproductive abilities may be compromised, leading to reduced population sizes or even localized extinctions [32].

The toxicity of synthetic dyes also disrupts aquatic food chains. As sensitive species succumb to the adverse effects of toxic dyes, the dynamics of predator–prey interactions are disturbed. This disruption can result in imbalances in population sizes and changes in species composition, ultimately affecting the structure and stability of the entire aquatic ecosystem [33].

3. *Reduced dissolved oxygen levels:* Reduced dissolved oxygen levels in aquatic ecosystems, induced by the decomposition of dyes and their associated by-products in water, represent a critical ecological concern. This process involves the consumption of substantial quantities of dissolved oxygen, a pivotal element for the sustenance of aquatic life [34]. The consequences of such oxygen depletion can manifest as the onset of hypoxic or even anoxic conditions within aquatic environments, both of which are highly detrimental to the well-being of fish and other aquatic organisms.

   The mechanism underlying this ecological challenge can be elucidated through the intricate processes of dye decomposition and subsequent oxygen utilization. When dyes and their associated by-products are introduced into water bodies, microbial communities may initiate the breakdown of these organic compounds. This microbial degradation process, akin to natural decomposition, requires oxygen as a vital component for respiration. Consequently, as microbes metabolize dye molecules and their by-products, they consume substantial amounts of dissolved oxygen from the aquatic environment [35].

The repercussions of reduced dissolved oxygen levels within aquatic ecosystems are profound and extend across multiple biological tiers. First, fish, being highly dependent on oxygen for respiration, are especially vulnerable to diminished oxygen availability. Under hypoxic conditions (lower than optimal oxygen levels) or anoxic conditions (complete absence of oxygen), fish may experience physiological stress, reduced growth rates, impaired reproductive capabilities, and even mortality [35]. Moreover, other aquatic organisms, including invertebrates and microbial communities, may also suffer adverse effects due to decreased oxygen concentrations. The consequences of oxygen depletion transcend individual species' vulnerabilities, impacting the entire aquatic ecosystem's structure and function. Hypoxic or anoxic conditions can disrupt the composition and abundance of species within the ecosystem, potentially leading to shifts in population dynamics and trophic interactions.

This, in turn, can compromise the overall ecological stability and resilience of the aquatic habitat [34].

6.3.2 Health and Environmental Risks

As we delve into the topic of releasing dyes into water, it becomes evident that the health and environmental risks associated with this action are significant and demand immediate attention. The potential risks associated with this practice highlight the need for comprehensive understanding and proactive measures to mitigate its impact.

The disposal of dyes into the environment carries significant health and environmental risks:

1. *Human health:* Some dye compounds are known to be harmful to human health. Exposure to certain dyes, either directly or through contaminated water and food, can lead to adverse health effects, including allergies, skin irritations, and, in extreme cases, carcinogenicity. The health risks associated

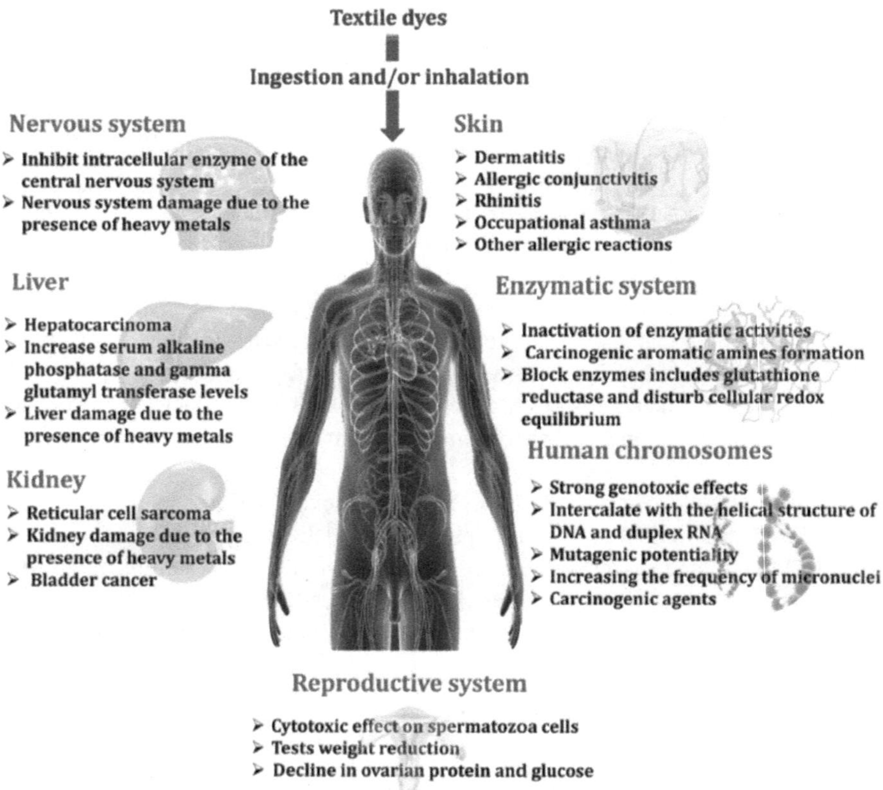

FIGURE 6.2 Depiction of the adverse impacts of textile dyes on human health.

Source: **Reprinted with permission from ref. 35.**

with dye exposure underscore the importance of preventing their release into the environment [35].

2. *Ecosystem disruption:* Dye pollution can disrupt ecosystems, leading to imbalances in species populations and biodiversity loss. As aquatic organisms are exposed to dye-contaminated environments, their habitats may become inhospitable, leading to the decline or extinction of sensitive species [34].
3. *Eutrophication:* The organic matter associated with dye compounds can contribute to eutrophication, a process in which water bodies become overly enriched with nutrients, leading to algal blooms and oxygen depletion. Eutrophication has disastrous repercussions on water quality and aquatic life [36].

6.4 NANOTECHNOLOGY AS A SOLUTION FOR DYE DEGRADATION

As the awareness of the environmental impacts of dye disposal grows, the utilization of nanotechnology in wastewater treatment has come to light as a possible strategy to tackle the challenges associated with dye pollution. This section aims to investigate the role of nanotechnology in the degradation of dyes, emphasizing its significance and the notable benefits of employing nanomaterials in this particular domain.

6.4.1 Overview of Nanotechnology in Wastewater Treatment

Nanotechnology has emerged as a pioneering paradigm in wastewater treatment, offering innovative solutions for the elimination of recalcitrant contaminants such as dyes. This burgeoning field harnesses the unique properties of nanomaterials to address the environmental challenges posed by dye pollutants. Various types of nanomaterials, including nanoparticles, nanocomposites, and nanotubes, have been employed with remarkable success. Their exceptional surface area-to-volume ratios, tailored surface properties, and distinctive electron conduction capabilities make them highly effective in the remediation of dye-contaminated wastewater [37]. Nanoparticles, for instance, facilitate dye degradation through photocatalysis, leveraging semiconductor materials like titanium dioxide or zinc oxide to catalyze the decomposition of dyes under ultraviolet (UV) or visible light irradiation. Alternatively, nanocomposites offer multifunctionality, combining properties such as adsorption and catalysis to synergistically remove and degrade dyes. Furthermore, nanotubes, with their porous structures, provide excellent adsorption capacities for dye molecules. These nanomaterials collectively underscore the transformative potential of nanotechnology in revolutionizing dye removal and degradation processes, thus advancing the cause of environmental preservation in wastewater treatment [38]. The integration of nanotechnology with conventional wastewater treatment methods represents a promising approach to enhance overall treatment efficiency while concurrently mitigating the dependence on chemical reagents and energy-intensive processes. Nanomaterials, owing to their unique physicochemical properties, can augment the performance of established treatment techniques. For instance, nanomaterials can serve as highly efficient adsorbents, facilitating the elimination of recalcitrant pollutants such as heavy metals or organic pollutants. Moreover, their catalytic prowess enables the degradation of persistent pollutants through advanced oxidation processes, reducing the need for extensive chemical dosing. This integration optimizes treatment outcomes, minimizes resource consumption, and advances the sustainability of wastewater treatment practices.

6.4.2 Advantages of Nanomaterials in Dye Degradation

The utilization of nanomaterials in dye degradation offers several noteworthy advantages, rendering it a promising approach in wastewater treatment. Primarily, nanomaterials possess an exceptionally high surface area-to-volume ratio, allowing for increased interaction with dye molecules present in wastewater. This heightened surface area facilitates efficient adsorption and catalytic reactions, leading to enhanced dye removal [39]. Owing to their small size and unique surface properties, nanomaterials exhibit enhanced reactivity. This elevated reactivity enables accelerated degradation of dyes and other contaminants, thereby improving the overall efficiency of dye removal processes. Moreover, nanomaterials offer customizability, as they can be synthesized and modified to suit specific wastewater treatment requirements. Properties such as size, shape, composition, and surface functionalization can be tailored to enhance the performance of nanomaterials in dye removal. Additionally, nanomaterial-based approaches have the potential to reduce chemical usage in wastewater treatment [38]. By relying on physical and catalytic processes, these approaches minimize the need for traditional chemical treatments, thereby reducing the production of chemical sludge and lowering operational costs. Also, nanomaterials can exhibit selectivity toward specific dyes or contaminants, enabling precise removal or degradation of targeted pollutants while leaving other constituents of wastewater largely unaffected [40]. This selectivity enhances the overall efficacy and specificity of dye removal processes. In conclusion, the utilization of nanomaterials in dye degradation offers a range of advantages that make it a promising and innovative approach in wastewater treatment.

6.5 SYNTHESIS OF NANOPARTICLES FOR DYE REMOVAL

In the realm of wastewater treatment for dye removal, the synthesis of nanoparticles assumes a pivotal role. This section will provide an in-depth exploration of the diverse methodologies employed in nanoparticle synthesis, emphasize the significance of tailoring nanoparticle attributes, and elucidate techniques aimed at optimizing nanomaterial efficacy.

6.5.1 Methods of Nanoparticle Synthesis

Nanoparticles can be fabricated through various methodologies, each possessing distinct merits and drawbacks. Several prevalent techniques employed for nanoparticle synthesis include:

TABLE 6.1
List of various methods employed for the synthesis of nanoparticles

Mode of Synthesis	Merits	Demerits	References
Chemical co-precipitation	• Simplicity • Cost-effectiveness • Controlled size and shape of nanomaterials • High yield • Synthesis of nanoparticles with homogeneous composition	• Unwanted impurities or by-products	[41, 42]
Sol–gel process	• Precise control over their size, shape, and composition of NPs. • Produce nanoparticles with high purity and homogeneity. • Good scalability and reproducibility.	• Time-consuming process • Use of hazardous chemicals and specialized equipment	[43]
Hydrothermal	• Precise control over particle size and morphology. • Purity and homogeneity of the nanoparticles. • Promote enhanced crystallinity. • Environmentally friendly	• The reaction time in hydrothermal synthesis can be relatively long.	[47]
Chemical vapour deposition	• Control over nanoparticle properties. • Good scalability • Versatility • Conformal coating	• Choice of precursor gases can be limited. • Reactor Design • Contamination from impurities • Temperature Sensitivity	[49]
Biological synthesis	• Reducing the reliance on harsh chemicals. • Mild reaction conditions • Excellent biocompatibility	• Low yield • Limited material range, • Process optimization challenges, • Contamination risks • Difficulties in scaling up production	[51]
Green synthesis	• Inherent sustainability • Simplicity, cost-effectiveness	• Choice of plant extract or other reagents may be limited. • Low yield • Contamination risks.	[52]

1. *Chemical co-precipitation:* This method is widely used in the synthesis of nanoparticles, particularly metal NPs. This technique involves the simultaneous precipitation of metal ions from a solution by the addition of a reducing agent or a precipitating agent [41]. One of the key advantages of chemical co-precipitation is its simplicity and cost-effectiveness. The materials required for this method are readily available and relatively inexpensive, making it an attractive option for enormous scale nanoparticle manufacturing. Additionally, the process can be easily scaled up to meet the desired quantities, making it suitable for industrial applications. Another merit of chemical co-precipitation is the ability to obtain nanoparticles with controlled size and shape. By carefully adjusting the reaction parameters such as the concentration of metal ions, the pH of the solution, and the reaction temperature, it is possible to achieve nanoparticles of specific sizes and morphologies. This control over particle size and shape is crucial, as it directly influences the nanoparticles' properties and applications. Chemical co-precipitation also offers a high yield of nanoparticles. The precipitation process can result in relatively high conversion of metal ions into nanoparticles, leading to a favorable yield. This efficiency is advantageous in terms of cost and resource utilization, as it minimizes waste and maximizes the production of nanoparticles. Additionally, chemical co-precipitation allows for the synthesis of nanoparticles with homogeneous composition. The simultaneous precipitation of metal ions ensures that the resulting nanoparticles have a uniform distribution of metal atoms, which is essential for achieving consistent properties and performance [42].

   However, it is important to note that chemical co-precipitation also has its limitations. One drawback is the potential for unwanted impurities or by-products to be incorporated into the nanoparticles during the precipitation process. These impurities can affect the nanoparticles' properties and hinder their desired applications. Careful purification steps may be required to remove these impurities and ensure the purity of the synthesized nanoparticles.
2. *Sol–gel process:* This is a versatile method for the controlled synthesis of nanoparticles, particularly metal oxide nanoparticles. This technique involves the transformation of a sol, which is a colloidal suspension of nanoparticles, into a gel-like material through a series of hydrolysis and condensation reactions. The gel is then subjected to heat treatment to form the desired nanoparticles.

   One of the key advantages of the sol–gel method is its ability to produce nanoparticles with precise control over their size, shape, and composition [43]. By adjusting the parameters such as the concentration of precursor materials, reaction temperature, and pH, the characteristics of the resultant nanoparticles can be tuned. This control is crucial for achieving desired functionalities and optimizing the performance of the nanoparticles in various applications.

   The sol–gel process also allows for the incorporation of dopants or additives into the nanoparticles, enabling the synthesis of composite or hybrid materials. This flexibility opens up opportunities for enhancing the properties of the nanoparticles, such as improved optical, electrical, or catalytic properties, by introducing suitable dopants or additives. Another advantage of the sol–gel method is the ability to produce nanoparticles with high purity and homogeneity. The precursor materials used in the process are typically in a highly pure form, and the controlled reaction conditions minimize the formation of impurities. This purity is essential for applications where the presence of impurities can adversely affect the performance or stability of the nanoparticles [44].

Furthermore, the sol–gel process offers good scalability and reproducibility. It can be easily scaled up to produce nanoparticles in larger quantities without significant changes in the synthesis procedure. This scalability is advantageous for industrial production and commercialization of nanoparticle-based products. Additionally, the sol–gel method is compatible with various deposition techniques, allowing for the direct integration of nanoparticles into thin films, coatings, or bulk materials. This versatility enables the fabrication of complex nanostructured materials with tailored properties and functionalities.

However, it is important to note that the sol–gel process also has some limitations. The synthesis of nanoparticles through the sol–gel method can be a time-consuming process, as it involves multiple reaction steps and requires careful control of reaction conditions. Furthermore, the sol–gel procedure may need the use of dangerous chemicals and specialized equipment, which might raise the synthesis's complexity and expense [45].

3. *Hydrothermal synthesis:* It is a widely utilized method for the synthesis of metal oxide nanoparticles and nanocomposites. This technique involves heating a reaction mixture under high-pressure conditions in an aqueous solution [46]. Its merits include precise control over particle size and morphology, resulting in tailored properties for specific applications. The process also ensures high purity and homogeneity of the nanoparticles, as impurities are minimized in the closed system. Moreover, the high-pressure and high-temperature conditions promote enhanced crystallinity, leading to nanoparticles with improved physical and chemical properties [47]. Hydrothermal synthesis is versatile and scalable, compatible with various precursor materials, and easily adaptable for large-scale production. It is considered environmentally friendly, employing water as a solvent and enabling lower reaction temperatures, reducing energy consumption and environmental impact. Additionally, the technique facilitates surface modification of nanoparticles during synthesis, allowing for the introduction of desired properties such as improved dispersibility, enhanced stability, or specific functional groups. Overall, hydrothermal synthesis is a valuable method for producing metal oxide nanoparticles and nanocomposites with tailored properties for diverse applications.
4. *Chemical vapor deposition (CVD):* It is a versatile technique used to produce thin films of nanoparticles. It involves introducing precursor gases into a reactor, where they undergo chemical reactions to form nanoparticles on a substrate surface. CVD offers excellent command of the composition, size, and morphology of the nanoparticles. By modifying the reaction conditions, such as temperature, pressure, and precursor concentrations, it is possible to

precisely tailor the properties of the synthesized nanoparticles. This control allows for the production of nanoparticles with specific characteristics suitable for various applications. This method is a highly scalable technique, making it suitable for large-scale production of thin films [48]. The process can be easily adapted to deposit nanoparticles on large substrate areas, enabling efficient and cost-effective manufacturing. CVD can be used to synthesize a broad range of nanoparticle materials, including metals, metal oxides, semiconductors, and carbon-based materials. This versatility makes CVD applicable to several fields, such as electronics, energy storage, catalysis, and optics. CVD enables the deposition of nanoparticles on substrates with complex geometries, including three-dimensional structures. This enables the construction of conformal coatings, where nanoparticles uniformly cover irregular surfaces, opening up new possibilities for advanced device fabrication and functional coatings [49].

The successful implementation of CVD relies on the availability and compatibility of suitable precursor gases. The choice of precursor gases can be limited, especially for certain compositions or complex materials, which can restrict the range of nanoparticles that can be synthesized using CVD. The design and configuration of the CVD reactor can influence the uniformity and quality of the deposited thin films. Achieving uniform coverage over a large substrate area can be challenging due to variations in gas flow, temperature distribution, and reactor geometry. This limitation can impact the scalability and reproducibility of the CVD process. Contamination from impurities in the precursor gases or the reactor chamber can affect the quality and purity of the synthesized nanoparticles. It is crucial to maintain a clean environment and carefully handle precursor gases to minimize contamination. CVD typically requires elevated temperatures to facilitate chemical reactions and nanoparticle formation. However, some substrates may be sensitive to high temperatures, limiting the choice of materials that can be used as substrates.

5. *Biological synthesis:* Also known as biofabrication, biological synthesis is an eco-friendly approach that utilizes living organisms such as bacteria and plants to produce nanoparticles [50]. This sustainable method aligns with the principles of green chemistry, reducing the reliance on harsh chemicals and energy-intensive processes [51]. It offers advantages such as mild reaction conditions, precise control over nanoparticle characteristics, and excellent biocompatibility. However, it also faces limitations including low yield, limited material range, process optimization challenges, contamination risks, and difficulties in scaling up production. Despite these limitations, biological synthesis holds promise for sustainable and tailored nanoparticle synthesis, with potential applications in various fields.
6. *Green synthesis:* Green synthesis methods, also known as environmentally friendly or sustainable synthesis methods, have gained significant attention in recent years due to their potential to create nanoparticles while minimizing the use of hazardous chemicals. These methods typically involve the utilization of plant extracts or other eco-friendly reagents as reducing and

stabilizing agents in nanoparticle synthesis [52]. One of the main merits of green synthesis is its inherent sustainability, as it reduces the environmental impact associated with conventional synthesis methods that often rely on toxic chemicals. Green synthesis also offers advantages such as simplicity, cost-effectiveness, and the ability to produce nanoparticles with controlled size, shape, and composition. Moreover, the use of plant extracts in synthesis processes can provide additional benefits, including the presence of bioactive compounds that can enhance the functionality of the resulting nanoparticles [53, 54]. However, green synthesis methods also have their limitations. One major limitation is the relatively low yield compared to traditional methods, which can hinder large-scale production. Additionally, the choice of plant extract or other reagents may be limited, restricting the range of materials that can be synthesized. Process optimization can also be challenging due to the variable nature of natural extracts, leading to inconsistencies in nanoparticle properties. Furthermore, contamination risks may arise from impurities present in the plant extracts. Despite these limitations, green synthesis methods hold great promise as environmentally sustainable alternatives for nanoparticle synthesis, with potential applications in various fields ranging from medicine to catalysis and beyond.

6.5.2 Tailoring Nanoparticle Characteristics

The characteristics of nanoparticles play a pivotal role in their efficacy for dye removal. Tailoring these characteristics to meet specific requirements is essential. Tailoring nanoparticle characteristics is a critical aspect of nanoparticle synthesis, as it allows for the precise control and customization of their properties to meet specific application requirements [55]. Numerous methods and techniques can be employed to achieve this goal. One approach involves manipulating the size of nanoparticles, which can be accomplished through variations in reaction conditions such as temperature, pH, and concentration of reactants. Controlling the size of nanoparticles is crucial, as it directly influences their optical, electronic, and catalytic properties. Another important characteristic that can be tailored is the shape of nanoparticles. By carefully selecting the reaction conditions, such as the choice of surfactants or solvents, it is possible to produce nanoparticles with specific shapes, such as spheres, rods, or cubes. Shape control is advantageous as it affects the nanoparticle's surface area, surface plasmon resonance, and catalytic activity. Additionally, the composition of nanoparticles can be customized by using different precursor materials or by doping the nanoparticles with specific elements. This enables the fine-tuning of their chemical reactivity, magnetic properties, or optical behavior. Surface functionalization is yet another method to modify nanoparticle characteristics [56]. By attaching various functional groups or molecules to the nanoparticle surface, it is possible to enhance their stability, biocompatibility, or targeting capabilities. Finally, the aggregation state of nanoparticles can be controlled to influence their behavior. For instance, controlling the degree of aggregation can affect the nanoparticle's optical properties or drug release kinetics. Overall, tailoring nanoparticle characteristics through precise control over size, shape, composition, surface functionalization, and aggregation state is paramount in creating nanoparticles with desired properties for applications ranging from drug delivery and imaging to energy storage and catalysis [57].

6.5.3 Enhancing Nanomaterial Efficiency

Efforts to enhance nanomaterial efficiency in dye removal involve surface functionalization, incorporating dopants or specific elements, and optimizing size and morphology. Functionalizing nanomaterial surfaces with specific groups or molecules improves their affinity for dye molecules, enhancing adsorption. Incorporating dopants or elements enhances catalytic activity and surface reactivity, increasing dye degradation efficiency. Optimizing size and morphology, such as using smaller nanoparticles or specific shapes, improves dye adsorption and photocatalytic degradation capabilities.

6.5.3.1 Modification Techniques

1. *Doping:* It is a technique that involves introducing foreign atoms or ions into the lattice structure of nanoparticles, which can alter their electronic structure and enhance their photocatalytic activity. By selectively incorporating dopants, such as transition metal ions, into the nanoparticle lattice, the band structure of the material can be modified, resulting in improved photocatalytic properties [58]. The introduced dopants can create localized energy levels within the band gap of the nanoparticles, allowing for efficient charge separation and transfer. This enhanced charge separation reduces the recombination rate of electron–hole pairs, thereby increasing the overall efficiency of the photocatalytic process [59]. Additionally, doping can also introduce defect sites or surface states that serve as active sites for dye molecule adsorption and reaction, further enhancing the dye removal efficiency. The choice of dopants and their concentration play critical roles in determining the extent of electronic structure modification and subsequent photocatalytic activity enhancement. Proper optimization of these factors is necessary to achieve the desired improvements in dye removal efficiency using doped nanoparticles [60].
2. *Composite materials:* Formed by combining nanoparticles with other materials like polymers or nanotubes, composite materials offer a promising avenue for achieving improved dye adsorption and degradation properties. The incorporation of nanoparticles into these composites can enhance their surface area and provide additional active sites for dye molecule interaction. Moreover, the synergistic effects between the nanoparticles and the host material can lead to enhanced dye adsorption capacity and increased surface reactivity [61]. The presence of nanoparticles in the composite can significantly increase the surface area available for dye adsorption due to their high surface-to-volume ratio. This enlarged surface area allows for more dye molecules to come into contact with the composite material, facilitating efficient adsorption. Additionally, the nanoparticles can possess unique surface

properties and functional groups, which can further enhance the affinity and selectivity of the composite towards specific dye molecules [62].

Furthermore, the combination of nanoparticles with polymers or nanotubes can create a hierarchical structure within the composite material [63]. This hierarchical structure promotes effective mass transport of dye molecules toward the active sites, facilitating their adsorption and subsequent degradation. The polymer or nanotube matrix can also provide mechanical stability to the composite, preventing the aggregation or loss of nanoparticles during the dye removal process.

The composite material can also exhibit enhanced degradation properties due to the synergistic effects between the nanoparticles and the host material. For example, the nanoparticles can act as photocatalysts, generating reactive species upon exposure to light, while the polymer or nanotube matrix can act as a support, ensuring the stability and efficient utilization of the nanoparticles' catalytic properties [64]. This cooperative behavior can enhance the photocatalytic degradation of dye molecules, leading to improved dye removal efficiency.

Overall, the combination of nanoparticles with polymers or nanotubes in composite materials offers a versatile and effective approach for enhancing dye adsorption and degradation properties. The synergistic effects and unique characteristics of these composites provide opportunities for developing efficient and sustainable solutions for dye removal applications.

6.5.3.2 Surface Functionalization

Functionalization of nanomaterials has emerged as a promising strategy for enhancing their efficiency in dye degradation. Through the introduction of specific functional groups onto the surface of nanomaterials, such as metal oxides or carbon-based nanomaterials, the affinity and reactivity toward dye molecules can be significantly improved. These functional groups can act as active sites for dye adsorption and provide additional catalytic functionality, such as electron transfer or reactive oxygen species generation, to facilitate the degradation process. Furthermore, functionalization allows for better control over the surface properties, morphology, and stability of nanomaterials, enabling tailored and efficient dye degradation. This approach holds great potential for the development of advanced nanomaterial-based systems for environmental remediation and wastewater treatment applications Figure 6.3 [65].

Ion-exchange processes offer a versatile and effective means to modify nanoparticle surfaces for the purpose of removing specific dye ions from wastewater. Through this process, ions present on the surface of nanoparticles are exchanged with target ions in the surrounding solution, resulting in the selective removal of the desired dye ions. The surface modification of nanoparticles can be achieved by introducing functional groups, such as cationic or anionic exchange sites, which have a high affinity for the target dye ions. The exchanged ions can then be removed from the system through methods like filtration or sedimentation. This approach allows for the efficient removal of dye ions from wastewater, as the modified nanoparticles act as highly selective adsorbents. Additionally, the exchange capacity of the nanoparticles can be tailored by adjusting the surface functionalization, providing control over the

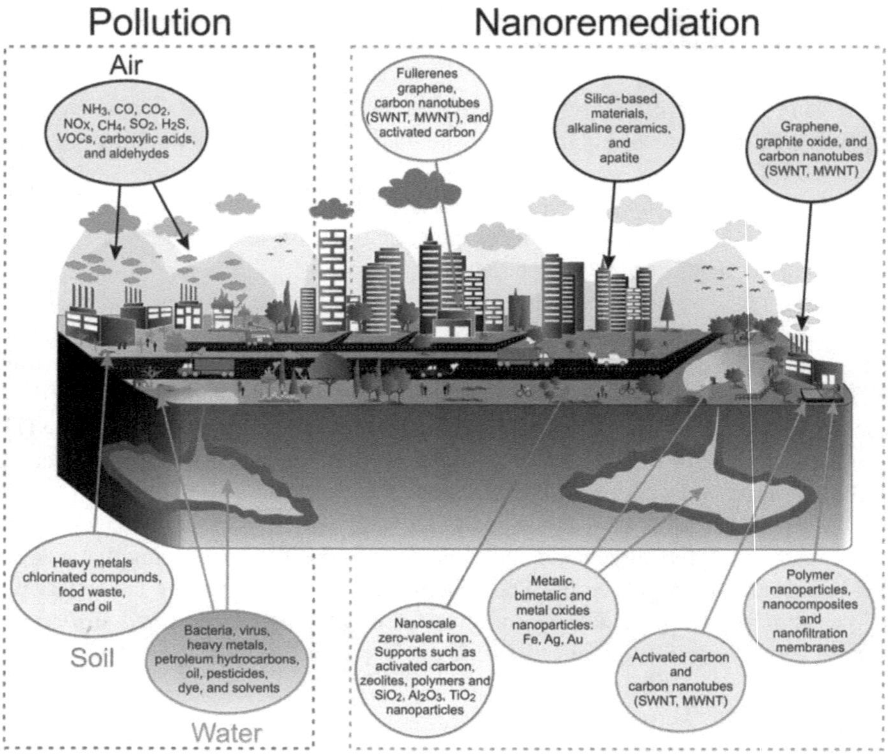

FIGURE 6.3 Various kinds of nanomaterials are used in nanoremediation.

Source: **Reprinted from an open source [66].**

efficiency and capacity of the ion-exchange process. Overall, ion-exchange processes utilizing modified nanoparticles offer a promising avenue for the development of advanced wastewater treatment technologies with enhanced selectivity and efficiency in dye ion removal [67, 68].

Coating nanoparticles with materials such as graphene oxide or silica has emerged as a valuable approach to safeguard against aggregation, enhance stability, and augment their adsorption capacity. By incorporating a protective layer around the nanoparticle surface, these coatings effectively prevent the undesired aggregation of nanoparticles, which can occur due to various factors such as van der Waals forces or surface charge interactions. The presence of the coating not only acts as a physical barrier but also provides additional functional groups or active sites that can enhance the adsorption capacity of the nanoparticles Figure 6.4 [10]. Furthermore, the coating materials themselves often possess high stability and excellent dispersibility, contributing to the overall stability of the coated nanoparticles. The controlled deposition of materials like graphene oxide or silica onto the nanoparticle surface allows for precise control over the coating thickness and composition, facilitating the optimization of the coating's protective and adsorptive properties. Overall, the coating of nanoparticles with materials like graphene oxide or silica represents a promising

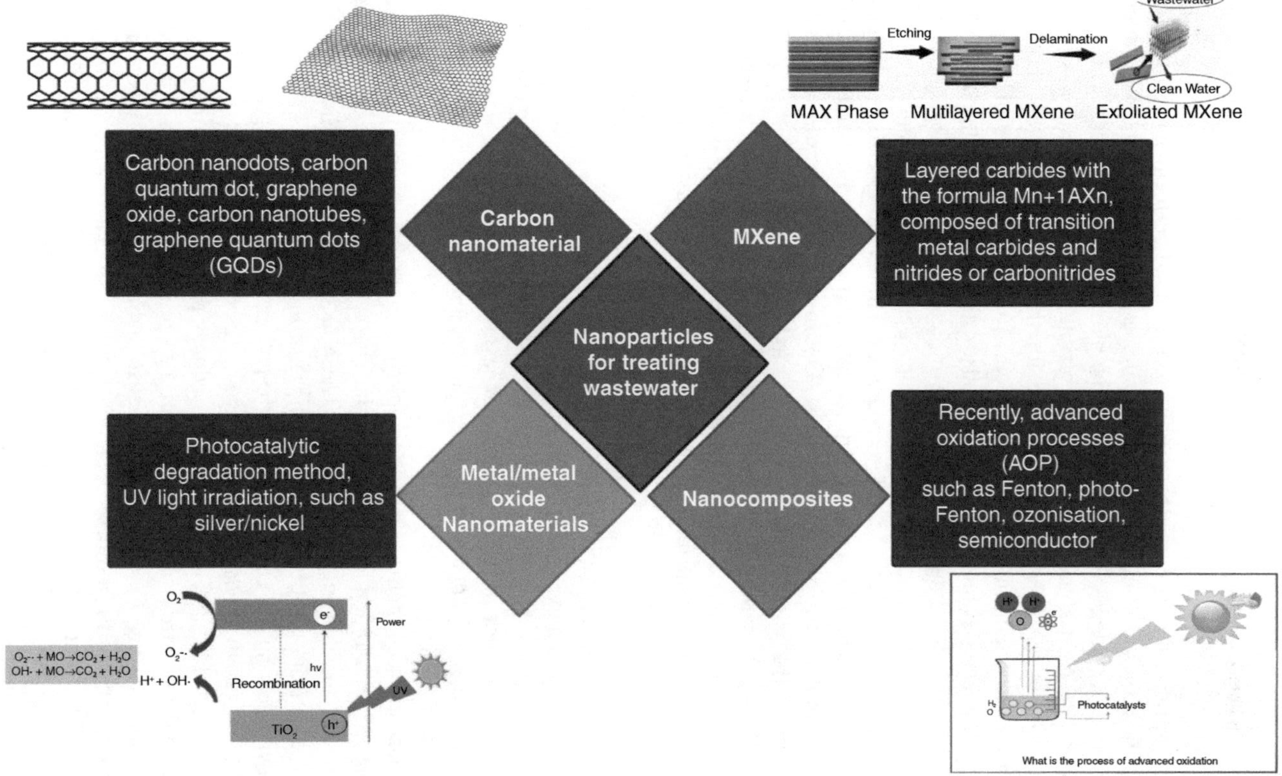

FIGURE 6.4 Different nanoparticles to remediate wastewater.

strategy to improve stability, prevent aggregation, and enhance the adsorption capacity of nanoparticles, enabling their effective utilization in various applications, including catalysis, sensing, and environmental remediation.

6.5.3.3 Increasing Reactivity

Photocatalytic enhancement strategies play a crucial role in improving the photocatalytic activity of nanoparticles, leading to enhanced performance in dye degradation applications. Optimization of factors such as light source, pH, and temperature can significantly impact the efficiency of the photocatalytic process. The choice of an appropriate light source, such as UV, visible, or solar irradiation, is essential as it determines the energy level required for the excitation of the photocatalyst and subsequent generation of reactive species [30]. Adjusting the pH of the solution can influence the surface charge and adsorption behavior of the nanoparticles, thereby affecting the interaction with dye molecules and the subsequent degradation process. Moreover, controlling the temperature can influence the reaction kinetics and the stability of the photocatalyst. Higher temperatures can promote faster reactions, while lower temperatures can help maintain the stability and prevent the degradation of the photocatalyst. Optimizing these factors allows for the fine-tuning of the photocatalytic system, maximizing the efficiency of dye degradation. By understanding and manipulating these parameters, researchers can develop advanced photocatalytic systems that exhibit enhanced performance in the degradation of dyes, contributing to the development of sustainable and efficient wastewater treatment technologies.

Reusability of nanoparticles in dye removal processes is a crucial aspect that can significantly enhance their efficiency and reduce operational costs. Developing methods for the recovery and subsequent reuse of nanoparticles offers several advantages in terms of sustainability and cost-effectiveness. By implementing suitable recovery techniques, nanoparticles that have been utilized for dye removal can be efficiently separated from the treated wastewater, allowing for their subsequent reuse in subsequent cycles [69].

Various recovery methods can be employed, including centrifugation, filtration, and magnetic separation, depending on the characteristics of the nanoparticles and the nature of the dye removal process. These techniques enable the separation of nanoparticles from the treated wastewater, ensuring their efficient recovery without loss or degradation [70]. Once recovered, the nanoparticles can undergo a regeneration process to restore their adsorption capacity and remove any absorbed dye molecules.

Reusability of nanoparticles not only reduces the need for continuous synthesis or procurement of fresh nanoparticles but also minimizes the generation of waste, thereby contributing to environmental sustainability. Additionally, the reuse of nanoparticles helps to optimize operational costs associated with the dye removal process, as it eliminates the need for frequent replacement of nanoparticles, reducing overall expenses. Furthermore, the ability to recover and reuse nanoparticles promotes a more efficient use of resources and supports the development of a circular economy. It allows for the utilization of nanoparticles over multiple cycles, maximizing their lifespan and minimizing their environmental impact [71].

Through the implementation of these techniques and strategies, scientists and engineers are capable of customizing nanomaterials to achieve effective and sustainable removal of dyes from wastewater, thereby making significant contributions toward environmental preservation and the mitigation of dye pollution.

6.6 MECHANISMS OF DYE REMOVAL USING NANOMATERIALS

Dye removal using nanomaterials involves various versatile mechanisms that contribute to the efficient elimination of dyes from wastewater. Biological processes employ enzymes or microorganisms immobilized on nanomaterials to break down dye molecules through enzymatic degradation or microbial activity. Photocatalytic processes utilize nanomaterials as catalysts to generate reactive species upon exposure to light, which subsequently degrade dyes through oxidation or reduction reactions. Adsorption processes involve the physical or chemical interaction between nanomaterials' surfaces and dye molecules, leading to their attachment and subsequent removal from the wastewater. These mechanisms collectively provide effective and sustainable approaches for dye removal, offering potential solutions to mitigate dye pollution in the environment.

6.6.1 Biological Processes

Biological processes for dye removal using nanomaterials involve the use of microorganisms or enzymes immobilized on nanomaterial surfaces. Here's a detailed scientific explanation of this mechanism:

1. *Microbial degradation:* Microbial degradation of dye molecules through enzymatic reactions is a significant biological process utilized in dye removal. Certain microorganisms, such as bacteria and fungi, possess the capability to produce enzymes that can break down complex dye molecules into simpler, less harmful substances [72]. In biological processes, nanomaterials can be employed as a support matrix for immobilizing these microorganisms, providing a suitable environment for their growth and enzymatic activity. The nanomaterials not only enhance the stability and activity of the immobilized microorganisms but also facilitate the contact between the microorganisms and the dye molecules in the wastewater. This immobilization technique ensures the prolonged exposure of the microorganisms to the dyes, allowing for efficient degradation and removal. Furthermore, the nanomaterials' large surface area and porous structure promote the diffusion of the dye molecules toward the immobilized microorganisms, enhancing the overall dye degradation efficiency [73]. This innovative approach utilizing nanomaterials as support matrices for microbial degradation offers a promising avenue for sustainable and effective dye removal from wastewater.
2. *Enzymatic pathways:* Enzymes immobilized on nanomaterials play a crucial role in catalyzing the breakdown of dye molecules through the initiation of chemical reactions [74]. These enzymes, including peroxidases and

laccases, exhibit specific catalytic properties that enable the oxidation of dye compounds, resulting in the fragmentation of the dye molecules into smaller, less toxic by-products. The immobilization of enzymes on nanomaterials offers several advantages, particularly in terms of enhancing enzyme stability and activity. Nanomaterials provide a suitable microenvironment for the enzymes, shielding them from denaturation and maintaining their structural integrity, which is essential for their catalytic function. Additionally, the high surface area and unique physicochemical properties of nanomaterials facilitate efficient enzyme-substrate interactions, ensuring optimal contact between the immobilized enzymes and the dye molecules. This enhanced interaction promotes the effective breakdown of dyes, leading to their degradation into less harmful substances [75]. Overall, the utilization of nanomaterials for enzyme immobilization represents a promising strategy for enhancing enzyme stability and activity, ultimately contributing to the efficient removal of dyes from wastewater.

6.6.2 Photocatalytic Processes

Photocatalytic processes utilize nanomaterials to facilitate the degradation of dyes under light irradiation. The mechanism or chemistry behind the photocatalytic degradation of dyes using nanoparticles is explained below:

1. *Band gap excitation:* When nanomaterials like titanium dioxide (TiO_2) are exposed to light, they undergo a fascinating process known as photoexcitation. This phenomenon occurs due to the unique electronic structure of the nanomaterial, specifically its band gap [76]. The band gap is the energy difference between the valence band, which contains the electrons in their ground state, and the conduction band, which represents the energy levels that electrons can occupy when excited. When photons of light, either UV or visible, interact with the nanomaterial, they can be absorbed if their energy matches or exceeds the band gap energy [77]. This absorption initiates a series of events that lead to the excitation of electrons from the valence band to the conduction band, generating electron–hole pairs. The process begins with the photon transferring its energy to an electron in the valence band, elevating it to a higher energy level within the conduction band. This excitation is possible because the absorbed photon's energy is equivalent to the energy difference between the valence and conduction bands. Once in the conduction band, the excited electron becomes mobile, gaining the ability to move freely throughout the nanomaterial. Simultaneously, the loss of an electron from the valence band creates a positively charged vacancy called a hole. This hole can also move freely within the nanomaterial. These electron–hole pairs are short-lived and highly reactive species. The electron in the conduction band and the hole in the valence band possess opposite charges, leading to an attractive force between them. However, due to their mobility, they can quickly recombine and return to their ground state, resulting in the dissipation of the absorbed energy as heat. To harness the photoexcited

electron–hole pairs for various applications, such as photocatalysis, it is crucial to prevent or minimize their recombination. This is achieved by utilizing suitable nanomaterial structures, doping techniques, or surface modifications that can trap or separate the electron and hole effectively. By controlling the recombination processes, nanomaterials like TiO_2 can exploit the photoexcited electron–hole pairs to facilitate chemical reactions [76]. For instance, in photocatalytic processes, the photoexcited electrons can participate in reduction reactions, while the holes can engage in oxidation reactions, promoting the degradation of various organic compounds, including dyes [78].

2. *Generation of reactive oxygen species:* When exposed to light, the nanomaterial absorbs photons, generating electron–hole pairs in its structure. The excited electrons in the conduction band and the holes in the valence band of the nanomaterial possess high reactivity. In the presence of water or oxygen, the photogenerated holes (h^+) can react with water molecules, leading to the formation of hydroxyl radicals (•OH). These hydroxyl radicals are highly reactive and can oxidize the dye molecules, breaking them down into smaller, less complex compounds. Additionally, the photogenerated electrons (e^-) can reduce oxygen molecules, producing superoxide radicals (•O^{2-}), which also contribute to the degradation process (Figure 6.5). The large surface area and

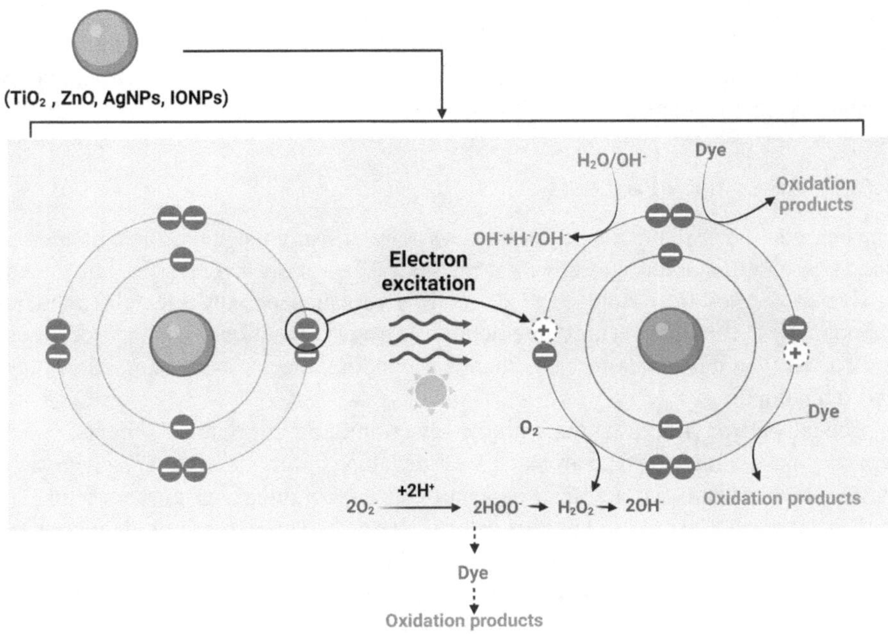

FIGURE 6.5 Mechanism of photocatalytic degradation of dyes in wastewater using nanoparticles.

Source: **Adapted and modified from an open source [81].**

unique physicochemical properties of nanomaterials enhance the adsorption of dye molecules onto their surface, increasing the contact between the dye and the photocatalyst. This promotes the efficiency of the photocatalytic reaction by facilitating the transfer of electrons and holes to the adsorbed dye molecules [79, 80].

Furthermore, the band gap energy of the nanomaterial plays a crucial role in determining its photocatalytic activity. Nanomaterials with appropriate band gap energies, such as TiO_2, can absorb visible light, enabling the utilization of solar energy for dye degradation. However, the band gap of TiO_2 restricts its activity to the UV region, necessitating the development of strategies to extend its absorption range into the visible light region. Overall, photocatalytic processes involving nanomaterials exploit the generation of reactive species, such as hydroxyl radicals and superoxide radicals, to initiate oxidation and reduction reactions, respectively, leading to the degradation of dye molecules. The unique properties of nanomaterials, combined with their ability to harness light energy, make them promising candidates for efficient and sustainable dye removal from wastewater.

Photocatalytic processes utilizing nanomaterials offer a promising and eco-friendly solution for dye removal and water treatment. By harnessing renewable solar energy and producing non-toxic end products, these processes eliminate the need for additional energy sources and reduce the environmental impact associated with traditional methods. Nanomaterials, such as titanium dioxide, play a crucial role in driving the degradation of dyes through their unique properties. This sustainable approach not only addresses dye removal but also shows potential for treating various organic pollutants. Overall, photocatalytic processes contribute to a cleaner and healthier environment by minimizing energy consumption and reducing overall environmental impact.

6.6.3 Adsorption Processes

The degradation or removal of dyes from wastewater using the mechanism of adsorption is a widely studied and effective method. Adsorption involves the attachment of dye molecules to a solid surface, such as activated carbon, biochar, or metal nanoparticles, through various interactions. These interactions can include physical forces (van der Waals forces), chemical bonding, electrostatic interactions, and hydrogen bonding.

The adsorption process starts with the selection of appropriate adsorbents, which typically have a high surface area and well-developed pore structure [77]. Activated carbon, biochar, and certain metal nanoparticles are commonly used adsorbents due to their large surface area and porous nature. These characteristics provide more sites for dye molecules to attach, increasing the adsorption capacity.

The adsorption of dye molecules onto the adsorbent surface occurs through different types of interactions Dye molecules often carry a net charge, while nanomaterials may possess opposite charges or exhibit dipole moments. Electrostatic attractions between dye molecules and nanomaterial surfaces can promote adsorption. Physical adsorption involves weak van der Waals forces between the adsorbent surface and the dye molecules. It is a reversible process and can be influenced by factors such as temperature and concentration. On the other hand, chemical adsorption involves the formation of chemical bonds between the adsorbent surface and the dye molecules. This type of adsorption is stronger and more stable compared to physical adsorption [82, 83].

The relationship between the amount of dye adsorbed and its concentration in the wastewater is described by adsorption isotherms. Commonly used isotherms include the Langmuir and Freundlich isotherms. The Langmuir isotherm assumes monolayer adsorption, while the Freundlich isotherm accounts for multilayer adsorption. The rate at which dye molecules are adsorbed onto the adsorbent surface is described by adsorption kinetics. The pseudo-first-order and pseudo-second-order kinetics are commonly used models to describe the adsorption process. The pseudo-second-order kinetics model is often found to provide a better fit to experimental data [84, 85].

The pH of the wastewater plays a significant role in the adsorption process. It can affect the surface charge of the adsorbent and the ionization state of the dye molecules, thereby influencing the adsorption capacity. Additionally, temperature can also impact adsorption. Higher temperatures can enhance the adsorption process.

After adsorption, the adsorbent may become saturated with dye molecules. Regeneration techniques, such as desorption using appropriate solvents or thermal treatment, can be employed to recover the adsorbent and reuse it for subsequent adsorption cycles. While the adsorption mechanism for the degradation or removal of dyes from wastewater offers several advantages, including high efficiency, simplicity, and cost-effectiveness, there are some limitations to consider. Adsorption may not be effective for certain types of dyes or complex dye mixtures. The adsorption capacity of the adsorbent may decrease over time due to fouling or saturation [71]. The presence of other contaminants in wastewater can compete with dyes for adsorption sites, reducing the overall efficiency.

Furthermore, the disposal of spent adsorbents and the potential release of adsorbed dyes during regeneration should be carefully managed to avoid environmental contamination. Understanding these mechanisms of dye removal using nanomaterials is crucial for designing effective and efficient dye remediation systems, contributing to cleaner water and a more sustainable environment.

6.7 RECENT DEVELOPMENTS IN NANOMATERIALS FOR DYE REMOVAL

As the demand for efficient and sustainable wastewater treatment methods continues to grow, recent developments in nanomaterial-based technologies for dye removal have seen significant advancements. In this section, we will explore these developments as an author, focusing on innovations and case studies that highlight the effectiveness of nanomaterials in addressing dye pollution in wastewater.

6.7.1 Innovations in Nanomaterial-Based Technologies

Considerable progress has been made in the field of nanocomposite development through the combination of various nanomaterials such as metal oxides, carbon-based materials, and polymers. These innovative nanocomposites demonstrate synergistic effects, resulting in improved abilities for dye adsorption and catalytic degradation.

6.7.1.1 Metal Oxide-Based Nanocomposites

Metal oxide nanoparticles, such as zinc oxide (ZnO), titanium dioxide (TiO_2), and iron oxide (Fe_2O_3), have been widely incorporated into nanocomposites for improved dye adsorption and catalytic degradation (Figure 6.6). The high surface area and unique properties of metal oxides contribute to their enhanced performance. For example, ZnO-based nanocomposites have shown excellent photocatalytic activity and can effectively degrade various dyes under visible light irradiation. The combination of metal oxides with other nanomaterials further enhances their adsorption and degradation capabilities [86].

6.7.1.2 Carbon-Based Nanocomposites

Carbon-based nanomaterials, such as carbon nanotubes (CNTs) and graphene, have also been extensively used in the development of advanced nanocomposites for dye adsorption and catalytic degradation. CNTs, with their high surface area and unique structural properties, offer excellent adsorption capacity for dyes. The incorporation of CNTs into nanocomposites enhances their stability and provides additional active sites for dye adsorption. Graphene-based nanocomposites have shown remarkable

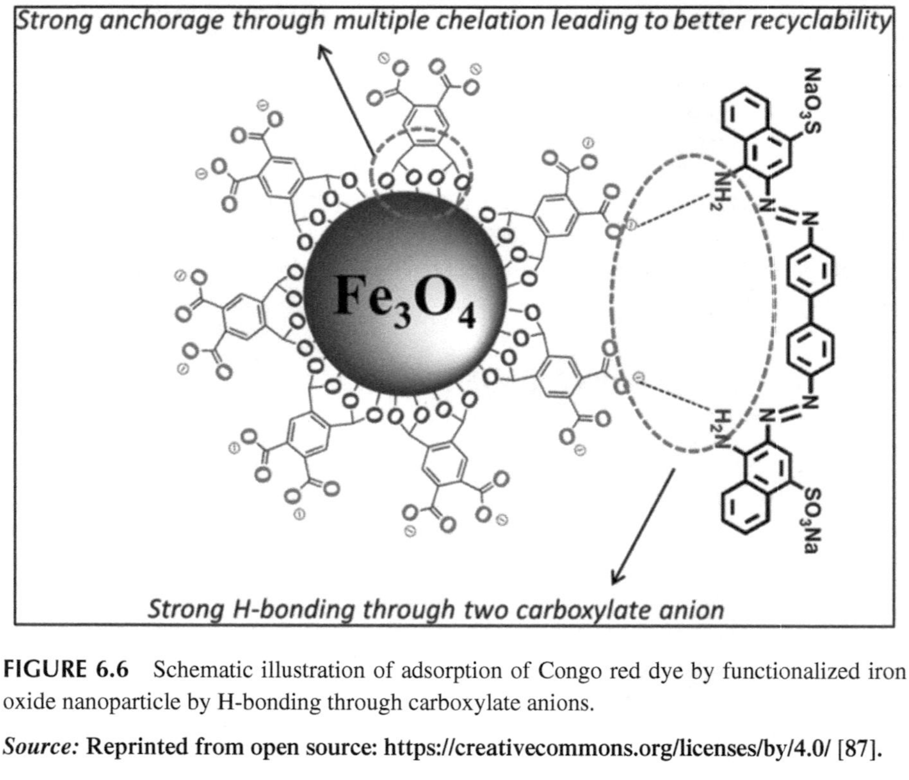

FIGURE 6.6 Schematic illustration of adsorption of Congo red dye by functionalized iron oxide nanoparticle by H-bonding through carboxylate anions.

Source: **Reprinted from open source: https://creativecommons.org/licenses/by/4.0/** [87].

catalytic activity and can efficiently degrade dyes through various mechanisms, including adsorption and photocatalysis [88, 89].

6.7.1.3 Polymer-Based Nanocomposites

Polymer-based nanocomposites have garnered significant attention due to their versatility and tunable properties. Conducting polymers, such as polyaniline (PANI) and polypyrrole (PPy), have been widely used in nanocomposites for enhanced dye adsorption and catalytic degradation. These polymers possess excellent electrical conductivity and can act as efficient catalysts for dye degradation. The combination of conducting polymers with other nanomaterials, such as metal oxides or carbon-based materials, further enhances their performance and stability [63].

6.7.1.4 Synergistic Effects and Mechanisms

The combination of different nanomaterials in advanced nanocomposites leads to synergistic effects, where the overall performance exceeds the sum of individual components. These synergistic effects arise from the complementary properties and interactions between the nanomaterials [90]. For example, the incorporation of metal oxides into carbon-based nanocomposites can enhance the adsorption capacity and photocatalytic activity, resulting in improved dye degradation. Similarly, the combination of conducting polymers with metal oxides or carbon-based materials can enhance electrical conductivity and catalytic activity, leading to enhanced dye degradation. The mechanisms involved in the enhanced dye adsorption and catalytic degradation of these advanced nanocomposites are multifaceted [91]. They can include physical adsorption, chemical reactions, photocatalysis, and electrochemical processes. The specific mechanisms depend on the nanocomposite composition, dye properties, and environmental conditions.

6.7.1.5 Smart Nanomaterials

The incorporation of responsive nanomaterials that exhibit changes in their properties in response to external stimuli has garnered significant attention in scientific research. One prominent example is the use of stimuli-responsive polymers, which have the ability to selectively adsorb dyes under specific pH or temperature conditions, thereby simplifying the dye removal process. Stimuli-responsive polymers are designed to undergo reversible changes in their physical or chemical properties in response to external stimuli such as pH, temperature, light, or magnetic fields. These polymers possess unique characteristics that enable them to respond to specific environmental cues, making them highly versatile and adaptable for various applications [92].

In the context of dye adsorption, stimuli-responsive polymers can be engineered to have specific functional groups or side chains that interact with dyes in a selective manner. For instance, by adjusting the pH of the solution, the polymer can undergo conformational changes, exposing or hiding the functional groups responsible for dye adsorption. This pH-responsive behavior allows for the selective capture and removal of dyes from a solution, as the polymer only adsorbs dyes under specific pH conditions [93, 94].

The incorporation of responsive nanomaterials, such as stimuli-responsive polymers, in nanocomposites offers several advantages. First, it allows for the development of materials with tailored properties that can be precisely controlled by external stimuli. This tunability enables the optimization of adsorption and degradation capabilities for specific applications. Second, the synergistic effects resulting from the combination of different nanomaterials in the nanocomposite can further enhance the overall performance, leading to improved dye adsorption and catalytic degradation capabilities.

6.7.1.6 Nanostructured Membranes and Adsorbents

The membranes composed of nanomaterials like graphene oxide or zeolites have shown great potential in the selective removal of dyes from wastewater. These membranes possess unique structural characteristics at the nanoscale, which enable them to exhibit high permeability and selectivity, making them highly effective in dye separation processes [95].

Graphene oxide, a two-dimensional nanomaterial derived from graphene, offers several advantageous properties for membrane applications. Its layered structure with abundant oxygen-containing functional groups provides a large surface area and enhanced interactions with dye molecules. This enables efficient adsorption and separation of dyes based on size, charge, or other specific interactions. The mechanical strength and chemical stability of graphene oxide also contribute to the durability and long-term performance of these membranes [96].

Zeolites, on the other hand, are crystalline aluminosilicate materials with well-defined nanoporous structures. The nanopores in zeolites can be precisely engineered to have specific sizes and shapes, allowing for the selective adsorption and separation of molecules based on size and polarity. By tailoring the composition and structure of zeolite membranes, high selectivity for specific dye molecules can be achieved while maintaining reasonable permeability for efficient wastewater treatment [97].

Nanofiltration membranes and nano adsorbents have also played a significant role in the selective removal of specific dye molecules. Nanofiltration membranes are designed with pore sizes in the range of 1–10 nm, enabling the separation of dyes based on their molecular size and charge. The precise engineering of the membrane structure allows for the selective rejection of larger dye molecules while allowing smaller water molecules to pass through, resulting in effective dye removal (Figure 6.7).

Nano adsorbents, on the other hand, are nanomaterials with high adsorption capacities and specific functional groups that can selectively bind with dye molecules. These functional groups can be tailored to exhibit affinity toward specific dyes, enabling the targeted removal of particular dye molecules from complex mixtures. By controlling the pore size and functional group composition of nano adsorbents, high selectivity and efficiency in dye removal processes can be achieved [99].

The development of these nanostructured membranes, nanofiltration membranes, and nano adsorbents has significantly advanced the field of selective dye removal. Their precise control over pore sizes, surface chemistry, and functional groups allows for the selective separation and removal of specific dye molecules from wastewater. These technologies offer high permeability, selectivity, and capacity, making them

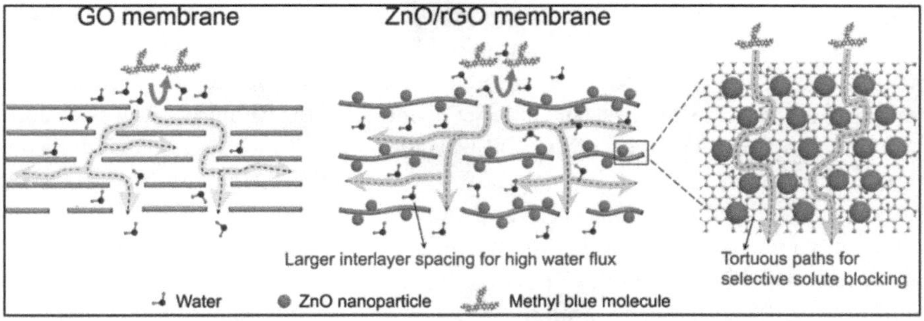

FIGURE 6.7 Mechanism of metal oxide/reduced graphene oxide nanocomposites for ultrahigh-flux nanofiltration membrane.

Source: **Reprinted from an open source: https://creativecommons.org/licenses/by/4.0/ [98].**

valuable tools in treating complex dye mixtures and addressing the challenges associated with dye pollution in various industries [100].

6.8 CASE STUDIES

Nanomaterial-based technologies have emerged as promising solutions for addressing dye contamination in wastewater due to their unique physicochemical properties and high surface area-to-volume ratio. The real-world applicability and effectiveness of these technologies have been demonstrated through a multitude of case studies and success stories. By leveraging the enhanced adsorption capacities and catalytic activities of nanomaterials, such as metal oxides, carbon-based nanomaterials, and composite materials, significant advancements have been achieved in the efficient removal of dyes from various industries, including textiles, pharmaceuticals, and printing. This section aims to elucidate the commercially available nanomaterial-based technologies for dye removal.

The nanomembrane market is divided into polymers, metal, hybrid, and other categories. Polymer nanomembranes are further segmented into spiral, tubular, and hollow fiber types, each with specific applications. Helical polymers are cost-effective and provide efficient membrane area, making them suitable for high-volume use. Tubular membranes are highly resistant to plugging and excel at filtering fibrous compounds. Hollow fiber membranes are ideal for filtering low solids and fluid streams. The versatility of polymer-based nanomembranes, with their varying pore sizes, has led to increased demand and market growth. Metal-based nanomembranes, known for their rough nature, are primarily used in challenging filtration applications.

Various nanomembranes are commercially available for wastewater treatment. NF200 and NF270 membranes achieved over 90% removal of Everzol Black, Everzol Blue, and Everzol Red dyes at an initial concentration of 600 mg/L and a pressure range of 3–12 bars. PMIA membrane exhibited excellent removal efficiency of Eriochrome Black T dye, exceeding 99% at an initial concentration of 1 mg/L, a pressure of 0.4 MPa, and a concentration of 1 g/L. Acrylic grafted Poly sulfone membranes effectively removed 9 different textile dyes, with removal percentages ranging from 86% to 99%, at an initial concentration of 50 mg/L. Thin-film composite membranes, such as CMC-Na/PP and poly-sulfone polyamide, achieved removal percentages of 82.2% to 99.9% for Sunset Yellow, Methyl blue, and Congo Red dyes at various conditions including an initial concentration of 100 mg/L, a pH of 6.8, and a pressure range of 6.2–6.9 L/m^2 h. The CMC-Na/PP thin film composite membrane also exhibited high removal efficiency of Reactive Black 5 dye, ranging from 60% to 97%, at concentrations of 0.4–2 g/L and pressures of 5–25 psi. UV grafting on PPSU membranes achieved removal percentages of 99.98% and 86.76% for Safranine O and Orang II dyes, respectively, at an initial concentration of 50 mg/L, a duration of 30 minutes, and a pressure of 5 bars [101].

Thin-film composite/nanocomposite membranes were manufactured at a pilot scale using innovative materials. The membranes demonstrated improved water/wastewater fluxes and removal efficiencies. The use of sulfonic acid groups in the S-DADPS monomer and the addition of halloysite nanotubes (HNTs) accelerated the membrane performance. The pilot-scale membranes performed well with synthetic and textile wastewater, although there was a slight decrease in performance with real textile wastewater due to higher fluxes. The 60% s-DADPS membrane showed significant improvement in wastewater flux without compromising other parameters. It was also cost-effective at the pilot scale [102].

6.9 FUTURE DIRECTIONS AND RESEARCH GAPS

The field of nanomaterial applications for dye removal in wastewater treatment is continuously evolving. As we strive for more effective and sustainable solutions, several unexplored areas and potential research avenues emerge. In this section, we will discuss these future directions and research gaps in detail.

6.9.1 Unexplored Areas in Nanomaterial Applications

6.9.1.1 Nanomaterials for Emerging Dye Types

Nanomaterials have been widely investigated for their effectiveness in removing traditional dyes from wastewater. However, there is a growing need to explore their efficacy in treating emerging dye types, including novel organic dyes, nanomaterial-based dyes, and dyes used in advanced technologies like quantum dots and organic photovoltaics. To address this, research is being conducted to investigate the adsorption and degradation capabilities of nanomaterials for these dyes. Studies have shown that various nanomaterials, such as nano-membranes, ZnO, and zero-valent metal and metal oxide nanoparticles, exhibit promising potential for the removal of different types of dyes from wastewater [21, 103]. Additionally, the use of nanocarriers, such as superparamagnetic iron oxide nanoparticles, in combination with external stimuli like magnetic fields, ultrasound, heat, and light, has shown controlled release capabilities, which can be beneficial for targeted drug delivery systems. The photocatalytic degradation of dyes using nanomaterials has also emerged as an effective and eco-friendly method for wastewater treatment. As the industrial landscape evolves and new dye types emerge, further research is needed to explore the effectiveness of nanomaterials in treating these dyes and to develop sustainable solutions for wastewater management.

6.9.1.2 Nanomaterials in Multi-Pollutant Scenarios

The treatment of real-world wastewater poses a significant challenge due to the presence of multiple pollutants, including dyes, heavy metals, pharmaceuticals, and organic compounds. While research on the individual removal of these pollutants using nanomaterials has made significant progress, the simultaneous removal of multiple pollutants using nanomaterials remains largely unexplored. Developing nanomaterial-based systems that can selectively adsorb or degrade different pollutants within a single treatment process would be a significant advancement in wastewater treatment technology [104, 105]. For instance, studies have shown that functionalized CNT and graphene oxide-based nanocomposites exhibit excellent adsorption capabilities for heavy metals and organic compounds. Similarly, the combination of nanomaterials, such as zero-valent iron nanoparticles and titanium dioxide nanoparticles, has been investigated for their photocatalytic degradation potential against dyes and pharmaceuticals. However, further research is needed to explore the simultaneous removal of multiple pollutants using nanomaterials, including the design of multifunctional nanomaterials and the optimization of treatment processes to ensure high selectivity and efficiency.

6.9.1.3 Long-Term Stability and Regeneration

The long-term stability and regeneration potential of nanomaterials used in dye removal are crucial aspects that require further attention. Investigating the reusability and durability of nanomaterials under continuous operation conditions is essential for practical applications and cost-effectiveness in wastewater treatment [69]. While nanomaterials have shown promising adsorption and degradation capabilities for dye removal, their performance over an extended period of time and under repeated cycles of operation needs to be thoroughly evaluated. Factors such as material degradation, loss of active sites, and potential leaching of nanoparticles into the treated water need to be considered. Studies have demonstrated successful regeneration methods for certain nanomaterials, including thermal regeneration, desorption using solvents, and photocatalytic regeneration. However, it is necessary to assess the efficiency and effectiveness of these regeneration methods in maintaining the performance and stability of nanomaterials over multiple cycles [106]. Additionally, understanding the impact of various operating conditions, such as pH, temperature, and the presence of coexisting pollutants, on the reusability and durability of nanomaterials is crucial for optimizing their practical application in wastewater treatment. Overall, comprehensive investigations are required to address the long-term stability and regeneration potential of nanomaterials, ensuring their reliable and cost-effective use in dye removal processes.

6.9.1.4 Nanomaterials in Low-Resource Settings

Adapting nanomaterial-based technologies for use in low-resource settings and developing regions is a crucial area of research. The development of affordable and user-friendly systems that can be deployed in areas with limited advanced infrastructure holds great potential for addressing various challenges. For instance, in the field of healthcare, the application of nanomaterials in point-of-care diagnostics can enable rapid and cost-effective disease detection in resource-limited settings. Additionally, the use of nanomaterials in water treatment can provide efficient and affordable solutions for addressing water pollution and scarcity issues. The development of nanomaterial-based systems that are easy to operate, require minimal maintenance and can function without the need for complex infrastructure is essential for their successful implementation in low-resource settings. Furthermore, research should focus on understanding the specific needs and constraints of these regions to ensure that the developed technologies are tailored to their requirements. Collaborative efforts between researchers, policymakers, and local communities are crucial for the successful adaptation and deployment of nanomaterial-based technologies in low-resource settings and developing regions.

6.9.2 Potential Research Avenues

6.9.2.1 Tailoring Nanomaterial Properties

Researchers should continue to explore methods for precisely tailoring the properties of nanomaterials, including size, shape, composition, and surface functionalization. Fine-tuning these parameters can enhance the selectivity and efficiency of nanomaterials in dye removal.

6.9.2.2 Mechanistic Studies

In-depth mechanistic studies are essential to gain a fundamental understanding of how nanomaterials interact with different dye molecules and the kinetics of adsorption and degradation processes. This knowledge will inform the rational design of nanomaterials for specific dye types.

6.9.2.3 Integration with Conventional Processes

Further research is needed to optimize the integration of nanomaterial-based technologies with conventional wastewater treatment processes. Developing hybrid systems that combine the strengths of both nanomaterials and traditional methods can improve overall treatment efficiency.

6.9.2.4 Environmental Impact Assessment

Evaluating the environmental impact of nanomaterial-based dye removal processes is crucial. Research should focus on assessing the fate and toxicity of nanomaterials and their byproducts in treated water and sludge, ensuring that the overall environmental footprint remains low.

6.9.2.5 Policy and Regulation

Researchers can contribute to the development of policies and regulations governing the use of nanomaterials in wastewater treatment. Collaborations with regulatory bodies can help establish guidelines for safe and responsible nanomaterial use.

6.10 CONCLUSIONS

In this comprehensive exploration of nanomaterials and nanotechnology for dye degradation in wastewater, we have gained valuable insights into a field of critical importance for environmental preservation. In this concluding section, we will summarize the key takeaways and insights from the preceding chapters and emphasize the vital role of nanotechnology in safeguarding our environment.

6.10.1 Key Takeaways and Insights

Throughout this book chapter, we have uncovered several key takeaways and insights:

Environmental preservation: The industrial revolution has led to the widespread use of dyes across various industries, contributing to the pollution of air and water bodies. The improper disposal of dyes poses significant risks to the environment, aquatic life, and human health.

Nanomaterial advantages: Nanomaterials offer a promising solution to address dye pollution in wastewater due to their high surface area, reactivity, and customizability. They can effectively remove or degrade dyes through adsorption, photocatalysis, and biological processes.

Synthesis and modification: The synthesis of nanomaterials and the modification of their characteristics are critical aspects of designing efficient dye removal systems. Tailoring size, shape, composition, and surface properties can optimize their performance.

Mechanisms of dye removal: Dye removal using nanomaterials operates through various mechanisms, including biological processes, photocatalytic processes, and adsorption processes. Understanding these mechanisms is essential for designing effective treatment systems.

Recent developments: Recent innovations in nanomaterial-based technologies have expanded their capabilities. Advanced nanocomposites, smart nanomaterials, and hybrid systems have emerged, demonstrating improved efficiency and sustainability.

Future directions: Future research should explore uncharted areas, such as the application of nanomaterials to emerging dye types, multi-pollutant scenarios, and eco-friendly synthesis methods. Long-term stability, adaptation to low-resource settings, and mechanistic studies are also crucial research avenues.

6.10.2 Importance of Nanotechnology in Environmental Preservation

Nanotechnology plays a pivotal role in environmental preservation, particularly in the context of dye removal from wastewater. Its significance lies in its ability to provide sustainable and efficient solutions to combat dye pollution and safeguard our environment:

Efficiency: Nanomaterials offer unparalleled efficiency in dye removal and degradation, reducing the environmental impact of dye disposal.

Sustainability: Green synthesis methods and biodegradable nanomaterials contribute to sustainable dye removal practices.

Selectivity: Nanomaterials can be tailored to selectively target specific dye types, minimizing the use of chemicals and reducing waste.

Innovation: Nanotechnology continues to drive innovation in the field of wastewater treatment, addressing evolving challenges and emerging pollutants.

Global impact: Nanomaterial-based dye removal technologies can have a global impact by improving water quality, protecting aquatic ecosystems, and ensuring access to clean water for communities worldwide.

In summary, the utilization of nanomaterials and nanotechnology in the context of dye removal represents not only a scientific pursuit but also a pivotal measure in safeguarding our environment and upholding the long-term viability of our planet. Thus, through collaborative efforts between researchers and policymakers, we can anticipate the realization of a more pristine, robust, and sustainable future for all stakeholders involved.

REFERENCES

1. R. Sharma and P. Malaviya, "Ecosystem services and climate action from a circular bioeconomy perspective," *Renew. Sustain. Energy Rev.*, vol. 175, p. 113164, Apr. 2023. doi: 10.1016/j.rser.2023.113164.
2. Committee on Methods for Estimating Greenhouse Gas Emissions By National Research Council, Division on Earth and Life Studies, Board on Atmospheric Sciences and Climate, *Verifying Greenhouse Gas Emissions: Methods to Support International Climate*, National Academies Press, Washington, DC, 2010. Accessed: Oct. 6, 2023. [Online]. Available: https://books.google.co.in/books?hl=en&lr=&id=5jJkAgAAQBAJ&oi=fnd&pg=PP1&dq=Human+activities,+such+as+industrialization+and+deforestation,+have+led+to+a+surge+in+greenhouse+gas+emissions,+primarily+carbon+dioxide+(CO2),+methane+(CH4),+and+nitrous+oxide+(N
3. A.L. Cowie, T.D. Penman, L. Gorissen, M.D. Winslow, J. Lehmann, T.D. Tyrrell, S. Twomlow, A. Wilkes, R. Lal, J.W. Jonesand A. Paulsch,"Towards sustainable land management in the drylands: Scientific connections in monitoring and assessing dryland degradation, climate change and biodiversity," *L. Degrad. Dev.*, vol. 22, no. 2, pp. 248–260, Mar. 2011. doi: 10.1002/ldr.1086.
4. J. O. Unuofin, "Garbage in garbage out: the contribution of our industrial advancement to wastewater degeneration," *Environ. Sci. Pollut. Res.*, vol. 27, no. 18, pp. 22319–22335, Jun. 01, 2020. doi: 10.1007/s11356-020-08944-5.

5. A. L. Robinson, A. P. Grieshop, N. M. Donahue, and S. W. Hunt, "Updating the conceptual model for fine particle mass emissions from combustion systems," *J. Air Waste Manage. Assoc.*, vol. 60, no. 10, pp. 1204–1222, 2010. doi: 10.3155/1047-3289.60.10.1204.
6. L. Pereira and M. Alves, "Dyes-environmental impact and remediation," in *Environmental Protection Strategies for Sustainable Development*, Springer Netherlands, pp. 111–162, 2012. doi: 10.1007/978-94-007-1591-2_4.
7. G. M. Sandeepa, B. Lakshmanna, and M. Madakka, "Recent advancements in the bioremediation of heavy metals from the polluted environment by novel microorganisms," in *Microbiology for Cleaner Production and Environmental Sustainability*, CRC Press, pp. 383–394, 2023. doi: 10.1201/9781003394600-20.
8. O. A. Oyewole, D. Gana, B. B. Adamu, A. O. Ayanwale, and E. C. Egwim, "Bioremediation of dye," in *Microbiology for Cleaner Production and Environmental Sustainability*, CRC Press, pp. 363–382, 2023. doi: 10.1201/9781003394600-19.
9. S. Zahmatkesh, M. Hajiaghaei-Keshteli, A. Bokhari, S. Sundaramurthy, B. Panneerselvam, and Y. Rezakhani, "Wastewater treatment with nanomaterials for the future: A state-of-the-art review," *Environ. Res.*, vol. 216, p. 114652, Jan. 2023. doi: 10.1016/j.envres.2022.114652.
10. A. Maqbool, A. Shahid, Z. Jahan, M.B.K. Niazi, M.A. Inam, A.M. Tawfeek, E.M. Kamel and M.S. "Development of ZnO-GO-NiO membrane for removal of lead and cadmium heavy metal ions from wastewater," *Chemosphere*, vol. 338, Oct. 2023. doi: 10.1016/j.chemosphere.2023.139622.
11. B. Karn, T. Kuiken, and M. Otto, "Nanotechnology and in situ remediation: A review of the benefits and potential risks," *Environ. Health Perspect.*, vol. 117, no. 12, pp. 1823–1831, Dec. 2009. doi: 10.1289/ehp.0900793.
12. M. Carocho, M. F. Barreiro, P. Morales, and I. C. F. R. Ferreira, "Adding molecules to food, pros and cons: A review on synthetic and natural food additives," *Compr. Rev. Food Sci. Food Safety*, vol. 13, no. 4, pp. 377–399, Jul. 01, 2014. doi: 10.1111/1541-4337.12065.
13. Arshid Mahmood Ali, Arslan Khan, Muhammad Shahbaz, Muhammad Imtiaz Rashid, Muhammad Imran, Khurram Shahzad and Aishah Binti Mahpudz., "A renewable and sustainable framework for clean fuel towards circular economy for solid waste generation in leather tanneries," *Fuel*, vol. 351, Nov. 2023. doi: 10.1016/j.fuel.2023.128962.
14. J. Kanagaraj, T. Senthilvelan, R. C. Panda, and S. Kavitha, "Eco-friendly waste management strategies for greener environment towards sustainable development in leather industry: a comprehensive review," *J. Cleaner Prod.*, vol. 89, pp. 1–17, Feb. 15, 2015. doi: 10.1016/j.jclepro.2014.11.013.
15. P. M. Dellamatrice, M. E. Silva-Stenico, L. A. B. de Moraes, M. F. Fiore, and R. T. R. Monteiro, "Degradation of textile dyes by cyanobacteria," *Brazilian J. Microbiol.*, vol. 48, no. 1, pp. 25–31, Jan. 2017. doi: 10.1016/j.bjm.2016.09.012.
16. F. F. Brites, V. S. Santana, and N. R. C. Fernandes-Machado, "Effect of support on the photocatalytic degradation of textile effluents using Nb_2O_5 and ZnO: photocatalytic degradation of textile dye," *Topics Catal*, Mar. 2011, pp. 264–269. doi: 10.1007/s11244-011-9657-2.
17. T. Shindhal, R. Parita, V. Sunita, A. Pandey, H.H. Ngo, W. Guo, H.Y. Ng, and Mohammad J. Taherzadeh "A critical review on advances in the practices and perspectives for the treatment of dye industry wastewater," *Bioengineered*, vol. 12, no. 1, pp. 70–87, Jan. 01, 2021. doi: 10.1080/21655979.2020.1863034.
18. L. G. Covinich, D. I. Bengoechea, R. J. Fenoglio, and M. C. Area, "Advanced oxidation processes for wastewater treatment in the pulp and paper industry: a

review," *Am. J. Environ. Eng.*, vol. 4, no. 3, pp. 56–70, Jun. 2017. doi: 10.5923/J.AJEE.20140403.03.
19. K. G. Pavithra, S. K. P., V. Jaikumar, and S. R. P., "Removal of colorants from wastewater: A review on sources and treatment strategies," *J. Indust. Eng. Chem.*, vol. 75, pp. 1–19, Jul. 25, 2019. doi: 10.1016/j.jiec.2019.02.011.
20. S. Nayak, S. R. Prasad, D. Mandal, and P. Das, "Carbon dot cross-linked polyvinylpyrrolidone hybrid hydrogel for simultaneous dye adsorption, photodegradation and bacterial elimination from waste water," *J. Hazard. Mater.,* vol. 392, p. 122287, Jun. 2020. doi: 10.1016/j.jhazmat.2020.122287.
21. M. Chandhru, S. K. Rani, and N. Vasimalai, "Reductive degradation of toxic six dyes in industrial wastewater using diaminobenzoic acid capped silver nanoparticles," *J. Environ. Chem. Eng.*, vol. 8, no. 5, p. 104225, Oct. 2020. doi: 10.1016/j.jece.2020.104225.
22. M. Roy and R. Saha, "Dyes and their removal technologies from wastewater: a critical review," in *Intelligent Environmental Data Monitoring for Pollution Management*, Academic Press, pp. 127–160, 2020. doi: 10.1016/B978-0-12-819671-7.00006-3.
23. L. Liu, Z. Chen, J. Zhang, D. Shan, Y. Wu, L. Bai, and B. Wang, "Treatment of industrial dye wastewater and pharmaceutical residue wastewater by advanced oxidation processes and its combination with nanocatalysts: a review," *J. Water Proc. Eng.*, vol. 42, p. 102122, Aug. 01, 2021. doi: 10.1016/j.jwpe.2021.102122.
24. P. O. Oladoye, T. O. Ajiboye, E. O. Omotola, and O. J. Oyewola, "Methylene blue dye: toxicity and potential elimination technology from wastewater," *Results Eng.*, vol. 16, p. 100678, Dec. 01, 2022. doi: 10.1016/j.rineng.2022.100678.
25. A. Tkaczyk, K. Mitrowska, and A. Posyniak, "Synthetic organic dyes as contaminants of the aquatic environment and their implications for ecosystems: a review," *Sci. Total Environ.*, vol. 717, p. 137222, May 15, 2020. doi: 10.1016/j.scitotenv.2020.137222.
26. B. S. Rathi, P. S. Kumar, and D. V. N. Vo, "Critical review on hazardous pollutants in water environment: occurrence, monitoring, fate, removal technologies and risk assessment," *Sci. Total Environ.*, vol. 797, p. 149134, Nov. 2021. doi: 10.1016/j.scitotenv.2021.149134.
27. O. Sacco, M. Matarangolo, V. Vaiano, G. Libralato, M. Guida, G. Lofrano, and M. Carotenuto, "Crystal violet and toxicity removal by adsorption and simultaneous photocatalysis in a continuous flow micro-reactor," *Sci. Total Environ.*, vol. 644, pp. 430–438, Dec. 2018. doi: 10.1016/j.scitotenv.2018.06.388.
28. P. Franco, W. Navarra, O. Sacco, I. De Marco, A. Mancuso, V. Vaiano and V. Venditto, "Photocatalytic degradation of atrazine under visible light using Gd-doped ZnO prepared by supercritical antisolvent precipitation route," *Catal. Today*, vol. 397–399, pp. 240–248, Aug. 2022. doi: 10.1016/j.cattod.2021.09.025.
29. Z. Balta and E. B. Simsek, "Discovering of the photocatalytic performance of $BiFeO_3$/BNQDs immobilized polyester filters for efficient continuous-flow elimination of recalcitrant antibiotic via PMS activated process," *Opt. Mater. (Amst).*, vol. 133, Nov. 2022. doi: 10.1016/j.optmat.2022.113015.
30. K. Tanji, J. A. Navio, A. Chaqroune, J. Naja, F. Puga, M. C. Hidalgo and A. Kherbeche "Fast photodegradation of rhodamine B and caffeine using ZnO-hydroxyapatite composites under UV-light illumination," *Catal. Today*, vol. 388–389, pp. 176–186, Apr. 2022. doi: 10.1016/j.cattod.2020.07.044.
31. K. Singha, P. Pandit, S. Maity, and S. R. Sharma, "Harmful environmental effects for textile chemical dyeing practice," in *Green Chemistry for Sustainable Textiles: Modern Design and Approaches*, Woodhead Publishing, pp. 153–164, 2021. doi: 10.1016/B978-0-323-85204-3.00005-1.

32. S. M. A. G. Ulson de Souza, E. Forgiarini, and A. A. Ulson de Souza, "Toxicity of textile dyes and their degradation by the enzyme horseradish peroxidase (HRP)," *J. Hazard. Mater.*, vol. 147, no. 3, pp. 1073–1078, Aug. 2007. doi: 10.1016/j.jhazmat.2007.06.003.
33. S. Khan and A. Malik, "Toxicity evaluation of textile effluents and role of native soil bacterium in biodegradation of a textile dye," *Environ. Sci. Pollut. Res.*, vol. 25, no. 5, pp. 4446–4458, Feb. 2018. doi: 10.1007/s11356-017-0783-7.
34. R. Kishor, D. Purchase, G. D. Saratale, R.G. Saratale, L. F. R. Ferreira, M. Bilal, R. Chandra and R.N. Bharagava, "Ecotoxicological and health concerns of persistent coloring pollutants of textile industry wastewater and treatment approaches for environmental safety," *J. Environ. Chem. Eng.*, vol. 9, no. 2, p. 105012, Apr. 2021. doi: 10.1016/j.jece.2020.105012.
35. R. Al-Tohamy, S.S. Ali, F. Li, K.M. Okasha, Yehia A-G. Mahmoud, T. Elsamahy, H. Jiao, Y. Fu and J. Sun, "A critical review on the treatment of dye-containing wastewater: ecotoxicological and health concerns of textile dyes and possible remediation approaches for environmental safety," *Ecotoxicol. Environ. Safety*, vol. 231, p. 113160, Feb. 01, 2022. doi: 10.1016/j.ecoenv.2021.113160.
36. D. W. Schindler, "Eutrophication and recovery in experimental lakes: implications for lake management," *Science*, vol. 184, no. 4139, pp. 897–899, May 1974. doi: 10.1126/science.184.4139.897.
37. Y. Xiong, H. Wan, M. Islam, W. Wang, L. Xie, S. Lü, S.M. Fijul Kabir, H. Liu and S. Mahmud, "Hyaluronate macromolecules assist bioreduction (AuIII to Au0) and stabilization of catalytically active gold nanoparticles for azo contaminated wastewater treatment," *Environ. Technol. Innov.*, vol. 24, p. 102053, Nov. 2021. doi: 10.1016/j.eti.2021.102053.
38. A. Jawed, R. Verma, V. Saxen, and L. M. Pandey, "Photocatalytic metal nanoparticles: a green approach for degradation of dyes," in *Photocatalytic Degradation of Dyes: Current Trends and Future Perspectives*, Elsevier, pp. 251–275, 2021. doi: 10.1016/B978-0-12-823876-9.00003-2.
39. N.N. Mohammad Jafri, J. Jaafar, N.H. Alias, S. Samitsu, F. Aziz, W.N. Wan Salleh, M.Z. Mohd Yusop, M.H. Othman, M.A. Rahman, A.F. Ismail, T. Matsuura, "Synthesis and characterization of titanium dioxide hollow nanofiber for photocatalytic degradation of methylene blue dye," *Membranes (Basel)*, vol. 11, no. 8, p. 581, Jul. 2021. doi: 10.3390/membranes11080581.
40. M. E. El-Naggar, E. K. Radwan, and S. T. El-Wakeel, "Functionalized nanofibers for remediation of organic pollutants and catalytic applications," in *Functionalized Nanofibers: Synthesis and Industrial Applications*, Elsevier, pp. 483–501, 2023. doi: 10.1016/B978-0-323-99461-3.00028-5.
41. S. R. Pandya, S. Patel, S. Bakshi, and M. Singh, "In vitro DNA binding, antioxidant, antimicrobial and anticancer assessment of amino acid functionalized magnetic nanoparticles," *Appl. Surf. Sci.*, vol. 451, pp. 1–19, Sep. 2018. doi: 10.1016/J.APSUSC.2018.04.190.
42. S. R. Pandya and M. Singh, "Preparation and characterization of magnetic nanoparticles and their impact on anticancer drug binding and release processes moderated through a 1st tier dendrimer," *RSC Adv.*, vol. 6, no. 44, pp. 37391–37402, Apr. 2016. doi: 10.1039/C6RA02139E.
43. M. Parashar, V. K. Shukla, and R. Singh, "Metal oxides nanoparticles via sol–gel method: a review on synthesis, characterization and applications," *J. Mater. Sci.: Mater. Electron.*, vol. 31, no. 5, pp. 3729–3749, Mar. 01, 2020. doi: 10.1007/s10854-020-02994-8.

44. M. Epifani, C. Giannini, L. Tapfer, and L. Vasanelli, "Sol–gel synthesis and characterization of Ag and Au nanoparticles in SiO_2, TiO_2, and ZrO_2 thin films," *J. Am. Ceram. Soc.*, vol. 83, no. 10, pp. 2385–2393, Oct. 2000. doi: 10.1111/j.1151-2916.2000.tb01566.x.
45. D. Bokov, A. Turki Jalil, S. Chupradit, W. Suksatan, M. Javed Ansari, I.H. Shewael, G.H. Valiev and E. Kianfar, "Nanomaterial by sol–gel method: synthesis and application," *Adv Mater. Sci. Eng.*, vol. 2021, 2021. doi: 10.1155/2021/5102014.
46. S. Suthakaran, S. Dhanapandian, N. Krishnakumar, and N. Ponpandian, "Hydrothermal synthesis of surfactant assisted Zn doped SnO_2 nanoparticles with enhanced photocatalytic performance and energy storage performance," *J. Phys. Chem. Solids*, vol. 141, p. 109407, Jun. 2020. doi: 10.1016/j.jpcs.2020.109407.
47. M. M. Sajid, N. Amin, N. A. Shad, S. B. Khan, Y. Javed, and Z. Zhang, "Hydrothermal fabrication of monoclinic bismuth vanadate (m-$BiVO_4$) nanoparticles for photocatalytic degradation of toxic organic dyes," *Mater. Sci. Eng. B*, vol. 242, pp. 83–89, Mar. 2019. doi: 10.1016/j.mseb.2019.03.012.
48. J. Zhang, T. Liu, L. Fu, and G. Ye, "Synthesis of nanosized ultrathin MoS_2 on montmorillonite nanosheets by CVD method," *Chem. Phys. Lett.*, vol. 781, p. 138972, Oct. 2021. doi: 10.1016/j.cplett.2021.138972.
49. A. M. Ramesh, A. Gangadhar, M. Chikkamadaiah, J. Krishnegowda, and S. Shivanna, "Synthesis of graphene nanosheets by emitted black carbon and its sustainable applications," *J. Environ. Chem. Eng.*, vol. 8, no. 5, p. 104071, Oct. 2020. doi: 10.1016/j.jece.2020.104071.
50. R. R. El-Behery, E. S. R. El-Sayed, and G. S. El-Sayyad, "Gamma rays-assisted bacterial synthesis of bimetallic silver-selenium nanoparticles: powerful antimicrobial, antibiofilm, antioxidant, and photocatalytic activities," *BMC Microbiol.*, vol. 23, no. 1, pp. 1–18, Dec. 2023. doi: 10.1186/s12866-023-02971-1.
51. D. Jain, A.A. Shivani, Bhojiya, H. Singh, H.K. Daima, M. Singh, S.R. Mohanty, B.J. Stephen and A. Singh, "Microbial fabrication of zinc oxide nanoparticles and evaluation of their antimicrobial and photocatalytic properties," *Front. Chem.*, vol. 8, p. 559994, Sep. 2020. doi: 10.3389/fchem.2020.00778.
52. H. Singh, M.F. Desimone, S. Pandya, S. Jasani, N. George, M. Adnan, A. Aldarhami, A.S. Bazaid and S.A. Alderhami, "Revisiting the green synthesis of nanoparticles: uncovering influences of plant extracts as reducing agents for enhanced synthesis efficiency and its biomedical applications," *Int. J. Nanomed.*, vol. 18, pp. 4727–4750, Aug. 2023. doi: 10.2147/IJN.S419369.
53. S. Qasim, A. Zafar, M.S. Saif, Z. Ali, M. Nazar, M. Waqas, A.U. Haq, T. Tariq, S.G. Hassan, F. Iqbal and X.G. Shu, "Green synthesis of iron oxide nanorods using Withania coagulans extract improved photocatalytic degradation and antimicrobial activity," *J. Photochem. Photobiol. B Biol.*, vol. 204, p. 111784, Mar. 2020. doi: 10.1016/j.jphotobiol.2020.111784.
54. M. Aravind, A. Ahmad, I. Ahmad, M. Amalanathan, K. Naseem, S.M.M. Mary, C. Parvathiraja, S. Hussain, T.S. Algarni, M. Pervaiz and M. Zuber, "Critical green routing synthesis of silver NPs using jasmine flower extract for biological activities and photocatalytical degradation of methylene blue," *J. Environ. Chem. Eng.*, vol. 9, no. 1, p. 104877, Feb. 2021. doi: 10.1016/j.jece.2020.104877.
55. S. R. Pandya, "Surface-tailored iron oxide magnetic nanomaterials for biomedical applications," pp. 1–40, Mar. 2023. doi: 10.21741/9781644902332-1.
56. V. Harish, M.M. Ansari, D. Tewari, A.B. Yadav, N. Sharma, S. Bawarig, M.L. García-Betancourt, A. Karatutlu, M. Bechelany and A. Barhoum, "Cutting-edge advances in tailoring size, shape, and functionality of nanoparticles and nanostructures: a

review," *J. Taiwan Inst. Chem. Eng.*, vol. 149, p. 105010, Aug. 01, 2023. doi: 10.1016/j.jtice.2023.105010.

57. M. D. Nguyen, H. V. Tran, S. Xu, and T. R. Lee, "Fe_3O_4 nanoparticles: structures, synthesis, magnetic properties, surface functionalization, and emerging applications," *Appl. Sci. (Switzerland)*, vol. 11, no. 23, p. 11301, Nov. 29, 2021. doi: 10.3390/app112311301.
58. R. Akram, A. Fatima, Z. M. Almohaimeed, Z. Farooq, K. W. Qadir, and Q. Zafar, "Photocatalytic degradation of methyl green dye mediated by pure and Mn-doped zinc oxide nanoparticles under solar light irradiation," *Adsorpt. Sci. Technol.*, vol. 2023, 2023. doi: 10.1155/2023/5069872.
59. I. Maryam, T. Iqbal, S. Afsheen, and A. M. Ali, "Synthesis and characterization of Ta-doped WO_3 nanomaterials for their application as an efficient photocatalyst," *J. Inorg. Organomet. Polym. Mater.*, pp. 1–14, Jun. 2023. doi: 10.1007/s10904-023-02776-9.
60. I. Y. Jeon, H. J. Noh, and J. B. Baek, "Nitrogen-doped carbon nanomaterials: synthesis, characteristics and applications," *Chem. Asian J.*, vol. 15, no. 15, pp. 2282–2293, Aug. 03, 2020. doi: 10.1002/asia.201901318.
61. F. S. Razavi, D. Ghanbari, and M. Salavati-Niasari, "Comparative study on the role of noble metal nanoparticles (Pt and Pd) on the photocatalytic performance of the $BaFe_{12}O_{19}/TiO_2$ magnetic nanocomposite: green synthesis, characterization, and removal of organic dyes under visible light," *Ind. Eng. Chem. Res.*, 2022. doi: 10.1021/acs.iecr.2c01066.
62. M. Ahmaruzzaman and S. R. Mishra, "Photocatalytic performance of g-C_3N_4 based nanocomposites for effective degradation/removal of dyes from water and wastewater," *Mater. Res. Bull.*, vol. 143, p. 111417, Nov. 01, 2021. doi: 10.1016/j.materresbull.2021.111417.
63. V. Melinte, L. Stroea, and A. L. Chibac-Scutaru, "Polymer nanocomposites for photocatalytic applications," *Catalysts*, vol. 9, no. 12, p. 986, Nov. 24, 2019. doi: 10.3390/catal9120986.
64. P. Jadhav, S. Shinde, S.S. Suryawanshi, B. Teli, P.S. Patil, A.A. Ramteke, N.G. Hiremathand N.R. Prasad, "Green AgNPs decorated ZnO nanocomposites for dye degradation and antimicrobial applications," *Eng. Sci.*, vol. 12, pp. 79–94, 2020. doi: 10.30919/es8d1138.
65. L. Huang, S. Yang, J. Chen, J. Tian, Q. Huang, H. Huang, Y. Wen, F. Deng, X. Zhang and Y. Wei, "A facile surface modification strategy for fabrication of fluorescent silica nanoparticles with the aggregation-induced emission dye through surface-initiated cationic ring opening polymerization," *Mater. Sci. Eng. C*, vol. 94, pp. 270–278, Jan. 2019. doi: 10.1016/j.msec.2018.09.042.
66. M. L. Del Prado-Audelo, I. García Kerdan, L. Escutia-Guadarrama, J. M. Reyna-González, J. J. Magaña, and G. Leyva-Gómez, "Nanoremediation: nanomaterials and nanotechnologies for environmental cleanup," *Front. Environ. Sci.*, vol. 9, p. 793765, Dec. 24, 2021. doi: 10.3389/fenvs.2021.793765.
67. S.K Panda, I. Aggarwal, H. Kumar, L. Prasad, A. Kumar, A. Sharma, D.V.N. Vo, D. Van Thuan and V. Mishra, "Magnetite nanoparticles as sorbents for dye removal: a review," *Environ. Chem. Lett.*, vol. 19, no. 3, pp. 2487–2525, Jan. 2021. doi: 10.1007/S10311-020-01173-9.
68. M. E. Mahmoud, G. M. Nabil, M. A. Khalifa, N. M. El-Mallah, and H. M. Hassouba, "Effective removal of crystal violet and methylene blue dyes from water by surface functionalized zirconium silicate nanocomposite," *J. Environ. Chem. Eng.*, vol. 7, no. 2, p. 103009, Apr. 2019. doi: 10.1016/j.jece.2019.103009.

69. X. Ma, S. Zhao, Z. Tian, G. Duan, H. Pan, Y. Yue, S. Li, S. Jian, W. Yang, K. Liu, S. He, "MOFs meet wood: reusable magnetic hydrophilic composites toward efficient water treatment with super-high dye adsorption capacity at high dye concentration," *Chem. Eng. J.*, vol. 446, p. 136851, Oct. 2022. doi: 10.1016/j.cej.2022.136851.
70. S. Joshi, V. K. Garg, N. Kataria, and K. Kadirvelu, "Applications of Fe_3O_4@AC nanoparticles for dye removal from simulated wastewater," *Chemosphere*, vol. 236, p. 124280, Dec. 2019. doi: 10.1016/j.chemosphere.2019.07.011.
71. Kiran, R. K. Rathour, R. K. Bhatia, D. S. Rana, A. K. Bhatt, and N. Thakur, "Fabrication of thermostable and reusable nanobiocatalyst for dye decolourization by immobilization of lignin peroxidase on graphene oxide functionalized $MnFe_2O_4$ superparamagnetic nanoparticles," *Bioresour. Technol.*, vol. 317, p. 124020, Dec. 2020. doi: 10.1016/j.biortech.2020.124020.
72. S. Varjani, P. Rakholiya, H. Y. Ng, S. You, and J. A. Teixeira, "Microbial degradation of dyes: an overview," *Bioresour. Technol.*, vol. 314, p. 123728, Oct. 01, 2020. doi: 10.1016/j.biortech.2020.123728.
73. M. B. Ceretta, Y. Vieira, E. A. Wolski, E. L. Foletto, and S. Silvestri, "Biological degradation coupled to photocatalysis by ZnO/polypyrrole composite for the treatment of real textile wastewater," *J. Water Process Eng.*, vol. 35, p. 101230, Jun. 2020. doi: 10.1016/j.jwpe.2020.101230.
74. N.S. Alsaiari, A. Amari, K.M. Katubi, F.M. Alzahrani, H.N. Harharah, F.B. Rebahand M.A. Tahoon, "The biocatalytic degradation of organic dyes using laccase immobilized magnetic nanoparticles," *Appl. Sci.*, vol. 11, no. 17, p. 8216, Sep. 2021. doi: 10.3390/app11178216.
75. J. K. H. Wong, H. K. Tan, S. Y. Lau, P. S. Yap, and M. K. Danquah, "Potential and challenges of enzyme incorporated nanotechnology in dye wastewater treatment: a review," *J. Environ. Chem. Eng.*, vol. 7, no. 4, p. 103261, Aug. 01, 2019. doi: 10.1016/j.jece.2019.103261.
76. M. Ikram, E. Umar, A. Raza, A. Haider, S. Naz, D.A. Ul-Hamid, J. Haider, I. Shahzadi, J. Hassan and S. Ali, "Dye degradation performance, bactericidal behavior and molecular docking analysis of Cu-doped TiO_2 nanoparticles," *RSC Adv.*, vol. 10, no. 41, pp. 24215–24233, Jun. 2020. doi: 10.1039/d0ra04851h.
77. V. A. Tran, A. N. Kadam, and S. W. Lee, "Adsorption-assisted photocatalytic degradation of methyl orange dye by zeolite-imidazole-framework-derived nanoparticles," *J. Alloys Compd.*, vol. 835, p. 155414, Sep. 2020. doi: 10.1016/j.jallcom.2020.155414.
78. M. S. Nadeem, T. Munawar, F. Mukhtar, M. Naveed ur Rahman, M. Riaz, and F. Iqbal, "Enhancement in the photocatalytic and antimicrobial properties of ZnO nanoparticles by structural variations and energy bandgap tuning through Fe and Co co-doping," *Ceram. Int.*, vol. 47, no. 8, pp. 11109–11121, Apr. 2021. doi: 10.1016/j.ceramint.2020.12.234.
79. F. Ameen, T. Dawoud, and S. AlNadhari, "Ecofriendly and low-cost synthesis of ZnO nanoparticles from Acremonium potronii for the photocatalytic degradation of azo dyes," *Environ. Res.*, vol. 202, p. 111700, Nov. 2021. doi: 10.1016/j.envres.2021.111700.
80. M. A. Albo Hay Allah and H. A. Alshamsi, "Green synthesis of AC/ZnO nanocomposites for adsorptive removal of organic dyes from aqueous solution," *Inorg. Chem. Commun.*, vol. 157, p. 111415, Nov. 2023. doi: 10.1016/j.inoche.2023.111415.
81. M. B. Sumi, A. Devadiga, K. V. Shetty, and M. B. Saidutta, "Solar photocatalytically active, engineered silver nanoparticle synthesis using aqueous extract of mesocarp

of *Cocos nucifera* (Red Spicata Dwarf)," *J. Exp. Nanosci.*, vol. 12, no. 1, pp. 14–32, Jan. 2017. doi: 10.1080/17458080.2016.1251622.

82. K. K. Chenab, B. Sohrabi, A. Jafari, and S. Ramakrishna, "Water treatment: functional nanomaterials and applications from adsorption to photodegradation," *Mater. Today Chem.*, vol. 16, p. 100262, Jun. 01, 2020. doi: 10.1016/j.mtchem.2020.100262.
83. D.T.C. Nguyen, H.T. Le, T.T. Nguyen, T.T.T. Nguyen, L.G. Bach, T.D. Nguyen and T. Van Tran, "Multifunctional ZnO nanoparticles bio-fabricated from *Canna indica* L. flowers for seed germination, adsorption, and photocatalytic degradation of organic dyes," *J. Hazard. Mater.*, vol. 420, p. 126586, Oct. 2021. doi: 10.1016/j.jhazmat.2021.126586.
84. M. Sharma, M. Poddar, Y. Gupta, S. Nigam, D.K. Avasthi, R. Adelung, R. Abolhassani, J. Fiutowski, M. Joshi and Y.K. Mishra, "Solar light assisted degradation of dyes and adsorption of heavy metal ions from water by CuO–ZnO tetrapodal hybrid nanocomposite," *Mater. Today Chem.*, vol. 17, p. 100336, Sep. 2020. doi: 10.1016/j.mtchem.2020.100336.
85. V. K. Mrunal, A. K. Vishnu, N. Momin, and J. Manjanna, "Cu_2O nanoparticles for adsorption and photocatalytic degradation of methylene blue dye from aqueous medium," *Environ. Nanotechnol. Monit. Manag.*, vol. 12, p. 100265, Dec. 2019. doi: 10.1016/j.enmm.2019.100265.
86. C. H. Nguyen and R. S. Juang, "Efficient removal of cationic dyes from water by a combined adsorption-photocatalysis process using platinum-doped titanate nanomaterials," *J. Taiwan Inst. Chem. Eng.*, vol. 99, pp. 166–179, Jun. 2019. doi: 10.1016/j.jtice.2019.03.017.
87. S. Chatterjee, N. Guha, S. Krishnan, A. K. Singh, P. Mathur, and D. K. Rai, "Selective and recyclable Congo red dye adsorption by spherical Fe_3O_4 nanoparticles functionalized with 1,2,4,5-benzenetetracarboxylic acid," *Sci. Rep.*, vol. 10, no. 1, pp. 1–11, Jan. 2020. doi: 10.1038/s41598-019-57017-2.
88. M. Nasrollahzadeh, M. Sajjadi, S. Iravani, and R. S. Varma, "Carbon-based sustainable nanomaterials for water treatment: state-of-art and future perspectives," *Chemosphere*, vol. 263, p. 128005, Jan. 01, 2021. doi: 10.1016/j.chemosphere.2020.128005.
89. N. Madima, S. B. Mishra, I. Inamuddin, and A. K. Mishra, "Carbon-based nanomaterials for remediation of organic and inorganic pollutants from wastewater. A review," *Environ. Chem. Lett.*, vol. 18, no. 4, pp. 1169–1191, Apr. 15, 2020. doi: 10.1007/s10311-020-01001-0.
90. Rachna, M. Rani, and U. Shanker, "Synergistic effects of zinc oxide coupled copper hexacyanoferrate nanocomposite: robust visible-light driven dye degradation," *J. Colloid Interface Sci.*, vol. 584, pp. 67–79, Feb. 2021. doi: 10.1016/j.jcis.2020.09.079.
91. M. Dhanalakshmi, K. Saravanakumar, S. L. Prabavathi, and V. Muthuraj, "Iridium doped ZnO nanocomposites: synergistic effect induced photocatalytic degradation of methylene blue and crystal violet," *Inorg. Chem. Commun.*, vol. 111, p. 107601, Jan. 2020. doi: 10.1016/j.inoche.2019.107601.
92. T. Senasu, T. Chankhanittha, K. Hemavibool, and S. Nanan, "Visible-light-responsive photocatalyst based on ZnO/CdS nanocomposite for photodegradation of reactive red azo dye and ofloxacin antibiotic," *Mater. Sci. Semicond. Process.*, vol. 123, p. 105558, Mar. 2021. doi: 10.1016/j.mssp.2020.105558.
93. H. B. Ahmed, M. M. Mikhail, S. El-Sherbiny, K. S. Nagy, and H. E. Emam, "pH responsive intelligent nano-engineer of nanostructures applicable for discoloration of reactive dyes," *J. Colloid Interface Sci.*, vol. 561, pp. 147–161, Mar. 2020. doi: 10.1016/j.jcis.2019.11.060.

94. D. Majhi and B. N. Patra, "Polyaniline and sodium alginate nanocomposite: a pH-responsive adsorbent for the removal of organic dyes from water," *RSC Adv.*, vol. 10, no. 71, pp. 43904–43914, Dec. 2020. doi: 10.1039/d0ra08125f.
95. N. Puri, A. Gupta, and A. Mishra, "Recent advances on nano-adsorbents and nanomembranes for the remediation of water," *J. Cleaner Product.*, vol. 322 p. 129051, Nov. 01, 2021. doi: 10.1016/j.jclepro.2021.129051.
96. N. Kumari and B. Meena, "Graphene-based materials for water treatment and purification." In *Handbook of Research on Water Sciences and Society*. IGI Global Scientific Publishing, 2022, pp. 375–399.doi: 10.4018/978-1-7998-7356-3.ch016.
97. R. Pachaiappan, S. Rajendran, and L. C. Ponce, *Nanoparticles in Industrial Wastewater Treatment: An Overview*, Springer, Cham, pp. 133–186, 2022. doi: 10.1007/978-3-030-98202-7_6.
98. W. Zhang, H. Xu, F. Xie, X. Ma, B. Niu, M. Chen, H. Zhang, Y. Zhang and D. Long, "General synthesis of ultrafine metal oxide/reduced graphene oxide nanocomposites for ultrahigh-flux nanofiltration membrane," *Nat. Commun.*, vol. 13, no. 1, pp. 1–10, Jan. 2022. doi: 10.1038/s41467-022-28180-4.
99. R. Suresh, S. Rajendran, L. Gnanasekaran, P. L. Show, W. H. Chen, and M. Soto-Moscoso, "Modified poly(vinylidene fluoride) nanomembranes for dye removal from water – a review," *Chemosphere*, vol. 322, p. 138152, May 2023. doi: 10.1016/j.chemosphere.2023.138152.
100. S. Manikandan, R. Subbaiya, M. Saravanan, M. Ponraj, M. Selvam, and A. Pugazhendhi, "A critical review of advanced nanotechnology and hybrid membrane based water recycling, reuse, and wastewater treatment processes," *Chemosphere*, vol. 289, p. 132867, Feb. 2022. doi: 10.1016/j.chemosphere.2021.132867.
101. M. A. Abdel-Fatah, "Nanofiltration systems and applications in wastewater treatment: review article," *Ain Shams Eng. J.*, vol. 9, no. 4, pp. 3077–3092, Dec. 01, 2018. doi: 10.1016/j.asej.2018.08.001.
102. B. Keskin, S. Korkut, T. Ormancı-Acar, T. Turken, C.E. Tas, Y.Z. Menceloglu, S. Unal and I. Koyuncu, "Pilot scale nanofiltration membrane fabrication containing ionic co-monomers and halloysite nanotubes for textile dye filtration," *Water Sci. Technol.*, vol. 87, no. 6, pp. 1529–1541, Mar. 2023. doi: 10.2166/wst.2023.081.
103. S. Verma, B. Tirumala Rao, R. Singh, and R. Kaul, "Photocatalytic degradation kinetics of cationic and anionic dyes using Au–ZnO nanorods: role of pH for selective and simultaneous degradation of binary dye mixtures," *Ceram. Int.*, vol. 47, no. 24, pp. 34751–34764, Dec. 2021. doi: 10.1016/j.ceramint.2021.09.014.
104. S. Gokul Eswaran, P. Shahid Afridi, and N. Vasimalai, "Effective multi toxic dyes degradation using bio-fabricated silver nanoparticles as a green catalyst," *Appl. Biochem. Biotechnol.*, vol. 195, no. 6, pp. 3872–3887, Jun. 2023. doi: 10.1007/s12010-022-03902-y.
105. S. Marimuthu, A.J. Antonisamy, S. Malayandi, K. Rajendran, P.C. Tsai, A. Pugazhendhi and V.K. Ponnusamy, "Silver nanoparticles in dye effluent treatment: a review on synthesis, treatment methods, mechanisms, photocatalytic degradation, toxic effects and mitigation of toxicity," *J. Photochem. Photobiol. B Biol.*, vol. 205, p. 111823, Apr. 2020. doi: 10.1016/j.jphotobiol.2020.111823.
106. H. He, T. C. Zhang, L. Ouyang, and S. Yuan, "Superwetting and photocatalytic $Ag_2O/TiO_2@CuC_2O_4$ nanocomposite-coated mesh membranes for oil/water separation and soluble dye removal," *Mater. Today Chem.*, vol. 23, p. 100717, Mar. 2022. doi: 10.1016/j.mtchem.2021.100717.

7 Environmental Concern to the Dye Pollution

Malabika Borah

7.1 INTRODUCTION

Dyes are a group of soluble colored organic compounds which have the ability to impart color to a given substrate. It is because of the presence of chromophoric groups in its molecular structures. The application of these synthetic dyes makes our clothing colorful and inexpensive and lasts for a long time [1]. However, the synthetic dyes can lead to several problems. It is known that the dyeing process requires a lot of water and every place does have effective ways of cleaning before their disposal into the environment. Nowadays, wastewater released from textile dyeing is considered a huge pollutant around the world as some dyes do not ever degrade in water, whereas the others that can degrade produce harmful substances. Some additives used in the dyeing process also may be composed of harmful substances such as alkalies and acids. It can affect plant life in the water too as most of the dyes consist of substances that have the ability to decrease the rate of photosynthesis, the process by which plants get nutrients.

In recent years, the dye industries have been increasingly developed. There are more than 10,000 dyes used in textile manufacturing industries alone. A major source of color released into the environment is associated with the disposal of untreated dye effluents from textile dyeing processes and so there is a huge need for the reduction of the percentage of these residual dyes. Consequently, dyes have become a common industrial environmental pollutant, and it became essential for innovations and changes in the processes to develop appropriate and environment-friendly treatment technologies for the residues.

7.2 HISTORY OF DYE

Dyes are used primarily in the production of consumer products, including paints, textiles, printing inks, paper, and plastics. They add color and patterns to materials. Natural dyes extracted from vegetables, fruit, and flowers have been used since 3500 BC to color fabrics and other materials.[1] These dyes were replaced by chemical dyes later on that bond with the fabric, providing and retaining richer color throughout washing and exposure [1].

DOI: 10.1201/9781003441083-7

The first pigments were probably used to mark the skin for ritual purposes or for sun protection which were prepared from natural sources such as plants, berries, roots, or animals like mollusks and insects and mixtures of soil or other materials with water or saliva. The blue color was produced from a plant called indigo and several shades of red were prepared from smashing insects (bugs) such as kermis and cochineal. Similarly, a very rare natural purple dye came from crushed snails. Some natural dyes gave strong coloring, whereas many of them were found to fade over time. The extensive prehistoric record of pigments' use indicates that red and black pigments derived from natural rocks or other geological components. With the development of civilization, the pigments began to be used in paints made on temple walls, tombs, ceramics, or homes and also to dye textile fibers [2, 3].

Synthetic dyes were introduced in 1856 by William Perkin, a young British chemist, who had synthesized a synthetic pale purple color while trying to create synthetic quinine for medicinal use and realized its applicability as a dye. Following his route, several workers started to artificially synthesize dyes with a variety of colors. Many dyes were also prepared from coal tar [4]. This awareness in the development of synthetic dyes leads to a variety of chemical dye production where Germany evolved as a leader. By World War I, the Germans manufactured most of the synthetic dyes used in the textile industry, and from then on natural dyes were largely forgotten effective synthetic dyes were eagerly accepted in the expanding industries except in places where the synthetic dyes were unavailable or where people kept traditional ways of coloring textiles alive [5, 6].

7.3 PATHWAYS OF EXPOSURE

Wastewater discharged from a huge number of industries like textile, leather, paint, food, pharmaceutical, etc. is a key pathway for exposure of the dyes into the environment. In most of the pollution sites, wastewater from the dye industry is directly dumped into surface waters without treatment, thus deteriorating the aquatic environment and posing a threat to living organisms. Wastewater consists of a large number of different chemicals from the processing of dyes and the presence of dye molecules in water channels is an emerging alarm to an environmental scientist. The majority of pollution exposure comes from the ingestion of contaminated water and ingestion of food, which has been irrigated with contaminated water. It is estimated that textile dyeing and treatments contribute up to 17–20% of total industrial water pollution [1, 7].

7.3.1 Effects on Environment

The dye industries are responsible for an extensive list of environmental impacts even in low concentrations. The scraps of textile fabrics and discarded packaging contribute as the primary solid waste responsible for air pollution involving the release of substances with unwanted composition. It results in high loads of organic matter, micronutrients, heavy metal cations, and pathogenic microorganisms (Figure 7.1) [8].

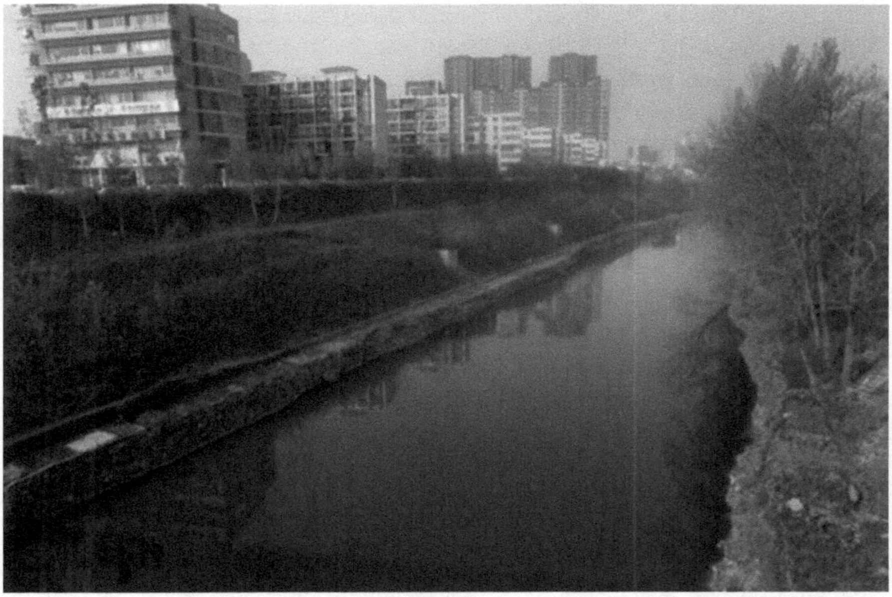

FIGURE 7.1 Jian River in Luoyang, North China turned red as a result of dumping a red dye into the city's storm water pipe network in 2011.

***Source:* STR/AFP/Getty Images.**

The main damage caused by the textile industries is from the discharge of untreated effluents into the water bodies [8], which normally constitute about 80% of the total emissions produced by these industries [9]. Most of the residual waters of the textile industry have relatively high levels of biochemical oxygen demand (BOD) and chemical oxygen demand (COD) [10]. However, the presence of large amounts of nonbiodegradable organic compounds in the wastewater is known to be the major problem [11, 12].

The color from the textile dyes in wastewater (< 1 ppm) is highly visible and causes aesthetic damage in terms of transparency and gas solubility of the water bodies. Most processes performed in textile mills produce atmospheric emissions. Gaseous emissions have been identified as one of the greatest pollution problems for the textile industry. Textile mills usually generate nitrogen and sulfur oxides from boilers and hydrocarbons from drying ovens and from mineral oils in high-temperature drying or curing. Processes like finishing and drying operations, printing, dyeing, fabric preparation, and wastewater treatment plants can emit formaldehyde, acids, softeners, and other volatile compounds. Residues from fiber preparation sometimes emit pollutants during heat-setting processes too. Among all pollutants, acetic acid and formaldehyde are two major emissions of concern in textiles [6, 10] which results in a reduction in the penetration of light through water, hampering the rate of photosynthesis and dissolved oxygen (DO) levels [13, 14]. Textile dyes are also toxic, have mutagenic and carcinogenic activities, and can cross entire food chains, affecting the entire aquatic life. In this context, special mention should be made to azo-type textile dyes, which retain around 15–50% of the wastewater that remains unreacted during the dyeing process. This wastewater containing azo compounds is generally used for irrigation in agriculture, particularly in developing countries, but it acts as a retardant for the germination and growth of plants (Figure 7.2) [15, 16].

The removal of color from dye-containing wastewater is the first and major concern, but the point of degrading dyes is not only to remove color but to eliminate or substantially decrease its toxicity. The conventional treatment plants are responsible for the bioaccumulation of the dyes in sediments and soil, as well as in the public water supply systems [17]. In general, dyes have low toxicity in mammals and aquatic organisms, but they can be partially degraded or transformed into toxic products, mainly aromatic amines formed by the reduction of the azo-type compounds into dangerous aromatic amines [18]. Assessment of the toxicity of dyes is therefore of utmost importance. Various short-term screening methods have been developed to detect mutagenic or carcinogenic substances. Azo dyes, which constitute the largest group of synthetic colorants, are found to have been linked to bladder cancer, splenic sarcomas, and hepatocarcinomas [18].

Another possibility involves the combination of dyes with intermediate synthetic compounds or their degradation products, leading to the generation of other mutagenic and carcinogenic substances. Long-term exposures, in particular, may have a profound impact on aquatic biota and human health in a similar way as in the case of metal complex dyes [19]. This type of dye, consisting of nickel, copper, cobalt, and

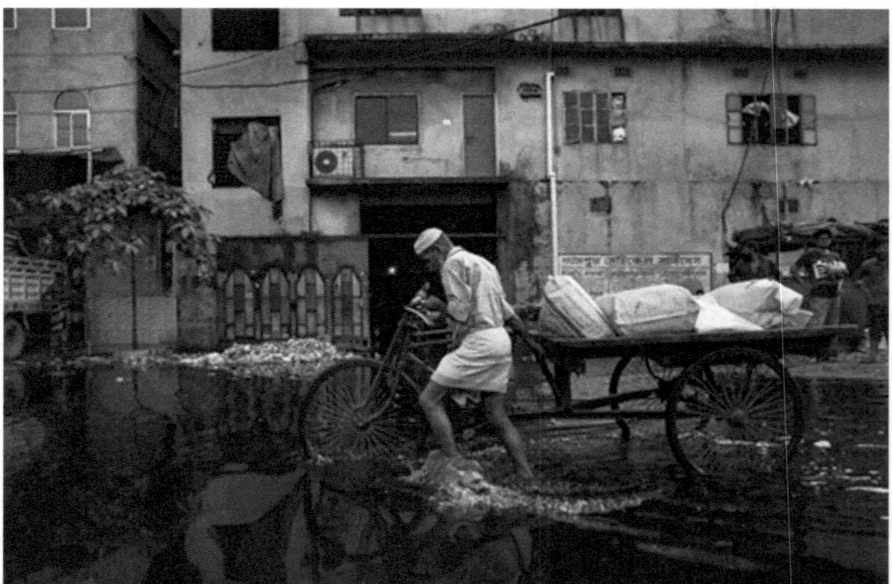

FIGURE 7.2 Flooded colored water from Buriganga River in Dhaka, Bangladesh in 2018.

Source: **Allison Joyce/Getty Images.**

chromium, is widely used in textile industries [20, 21]. Once released into the aquatic environment, the metal cations may be assimilated by the fish gills, resulting in their accumulation in certain tissues. They can, therefore, reach the human organs through the food chain, causing a series of pathological effects. In addition, they may result in considerable damage to the growth and development of plants, especially in photosynthesis and carbon dioxide assimilation [22].

One of the most important impacts of the dye industry is that affects the soil quality. As we know, the soil is composed of several mineral and organic constituents and it is the basis for agriculture. However, when different effluents from different industries somehow reach the fields, they block the pores of the soil resulting in the loss of agricultural yield [1, 6].

7.3.2 Monitoring Parameters for Effluents from the Dye Industries

Dye effluents mainly wastewater are characterized by strong color, high turbidity, broadly fluctuating pH, high COD, and BOD concentration, and large amounts of total suspended solids and total dissolved solids (TDS and TSS) due to the presence of different pollutants within the water environment. Among all these parameters, the most visible indicator is the color, and thus it plays a very important role in the collective awareness of an industry. The presence of color results in a decrease in the photosynthetic activity of aquatic life affecting the other parameters. However, it is very difficult to remove the color by conventional methods. Similarly, the value of pH affects the rate of biological reaction associated with the survival of various microorganisms as well as the permeability of the soil. The presence of divalent metallic cations such as Ca^{2+}, Mg^{2+}, Sr^{2+}, Fe^{2+}, etc. results in highly turbid and polluted water as a result of their precipitation, that is why water softening methods should be carried out before discharge.

BOD is the measure of the amount of oxygen required for the degradation of organic components present in the wastewater by bacteria, whereas COD is the measure of the amount of oxygen required for the oxidation of all inorganic and organic chemicals. DO also gives information on the amount of gaseous oxygen present indicating the extent of circulation of oxygen from the surrounding air. BOD, COD, and DO are interrelated as an increase in BOD leads to a decrease in DO which may induce hypoxia conditions within the aquatic organisms. Similarly, an increase in COD indicates the presence of high levels of chemicals in the wastewater which may result in toxic conditions making the effluents incompatible with the survival of water-living organisms [15].

Total dissolved solutes (TDS) value is also an important parameter to check the quality of water. Water with a high TDS value is not recommended for drinking and irrigation purposes. Again, the high total suspended solids (TSS) level results from the higher amount of suspended particles resulting in high turbidity of the water bodies which in turn disturbs the process of the food chain in aquatic media [6]. Electrical conductivity is another factor whose increased value indicates the presence of a higher concentration of the dissolved salts or ions which means that water is not suitable for irrigation.

During the various processes like bleaching and disinfecting, a number of chlorine-containing compounds are used such as hydrochloric acid, hypochloric acid, etc. This results in high chloride concentration in water leading to destruction of the different food chains in aquatic microorganisms as well as in the abnormal rise in the TDS and TSS values. In addition, the presence of oil or grease in the water also hampers the photosynthetic processes in the microorganisms resulting in decreased DO and thereby disturbs the food chain. Detergents, however, can remove the oil but create foaming.

7.4 REMOVAL TECHNIQUES

Generally, dyes are designed to resist very harsh conditions; therefore, they are retained in the dye effluents to a large extent and difficulties arise in their removal by conventional wastewater treatments. Other criteria when designing dyes are their fixation degree to fiber and fastness and resistance to microbial attack though the degree of fixation varies with the types of fiber, shade, and dyeing parameters. Dye fixation rate values are useful in giving an approximate idea of the amount released which are found to be below 2–10% for basic, dispersed, and direct dyes, but can reach 50% for reactive dyes [23, 24] Nowadays, reactive dyes are the most commonly used in the textile industries and there is a need for finding an efficient method of dye removal with special attention to this class.

While designing the removal techniques, it has to be particularly kept in mind that the wastewater is devoid of harmful substances, especially mutagenic, carcinogenic, and allergenic chemicals. However, the removal techniques are not only associated with the removal of color but also are involved with the nature of degradation and mineralization of the dye molecules. There are mainly three broad methods for dye removal: physical, chemical, and biological methods. Exclusive treatment by one of these three methods has proved to be insufficient for the removal of color and other effluents from textile industry wastewater. Some dyes are difficult to biodegrade, whereas some, particularly the hydrolyzed reactive and certain acidic dyes, are not readily absorbed and hence difficult to remove (Figure 7.3) [1].

7.4.1 Physical Methods

Basically, physical methods are often used as pretreatment methods of dye wastewater to facilitate the recovery of dye molecules from wastewater as their salt content further reduces the biodegradability [25]. It is found that physical methods can effectively remove color, but the molecules are not degraded and so require proper disposal. In addition, these methods involve excessive chemicals which themselves can create another problem of pollution. Different physical methods such as membrane separation technology including reverse osmosis, ultrafiltration, microfiltration, magnetic separation as well as adsorption techniques have been widely used in dye removal [26] with very high efficiency from 85% to 99% [27]. Reverse osmosis permits the removal of all mineral salts, hydrolyzed reactive dyes, and chemical auxiliaries, but the problem has been higher energy consumption [28]. Ultrafiltration has been used

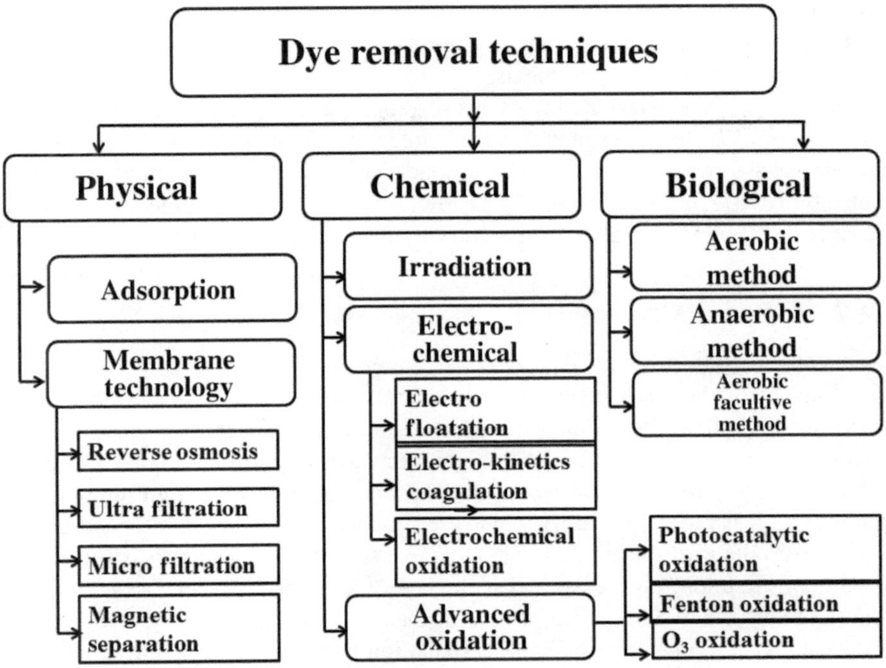

FIGURE 7.3 Schematic diagram of dye removal techniques.

for the removal of hydrophobic compounds and, similarly, microfiltration is found to be suitable for treating dye baths containing pigment dyes [29].

The adsorption technique also serves as a non-useful method for the treatment of contaminated waters, particularly if the adsorbent does not require any pre-treatment process before its application. It can be considered superior to other techniques from the viewpoint of cost, simplicity, flexibility, and ease of operation. Several adsorbents such as zeolites, alumina, silica gel, and activated carbon have been extensively used for dye removal, among which activated charcoal is the most highly used adsorbent in the industrial sector [30]. Decolorization occurs by this method, generally through two mechanisms – sorption and ion exchange – and is affected by several physico-chemical parameters such as dye–sorbent interaction, surface area, particle size, temperature, pH, and time of contact. In the case of activated carbon as a sorbent, the pH of the solution plays an important role in the sorption process as it is amphoteric in nature.

Biosorption is another method where the accumulation of pollutants can be done with the help of biological materials, thus allowing the recovery and environmentally acceptable disposal of pollutants. The mechanism of biosorption is not completely understood yet, but it is thought to take place on the cell wall. Textile dyes vary greatly in their chemistries, so their interaction with biomaterials depends on the nature of the dye as well as the specific chemistry within the biomaterial. However, this technique has gained importance because of its effectiveness and low cost. In addition, the use of dead rather than live biomaterials eliminates also the problems of toxic waste and nutrient requirements.

These different physical methods have several advantages such as a simple design, ease of operation, low cost, and fewer chemical requirements, but these have several drawbacks too such as toxic by-products and sludge production and limited applicability [31, 32]. In addition, COD, BOD, pH, color, high temperature, and the presence of heavy metals also hamper the usefulness of these methods.

7.4.2 Chemical Methods

Chemical methods used for dye removal are mainly coagulation or flocculation including electro-flotation, electro-kinetic coagulation; irradiation or electrochemical processes; and advanced oxidation methods. The basic principle of these methods is to remove the dye effluents by applying an electric current through electrodes resulting in different chemical reactions. These methods involve high removal efficiency as well as pollution control which are applicable for a variety of contaminants.

However, the electrochemical methods have some drawbacks also, such as high energy consumption, high cost, and incidence of side reactions like oxygen evolution and hydrogen evolution [33]. Some of the chemical treatment methods such as electrochemical oxidation and Fenton's oxidation have been reported to have a very high rate of color removal with the disadvantage of forming iron oxide sludge [34]. Ozonation has been found to be the most effective method for reactive dye decolorization with around 98–99% efficiency, but its installation requires additional costs [28]. Advanced oxidation technology is a new water treatment technology in recent years [26]. During this treatment, hydroxyl radicals are produced which can stabilize many structures making them difficult to decompose by microorganisms, and they are converted into nontoxic biodegradable substances without any excess sludge formation [35]. However, sometimes there may be the production of some undesirable toxic products that may release harmful aromatic amines.

7.4.3 Biological Methods

Biological treatment has been the most favored economical alternative for many industrial wastewater treatment processes as compared to physical and chemical processes involving high energy consumption and high cost. These methods involve biochemical reactions which are carried out in living cells or via enzymes. These methods of treatment are generally preferred for dye treatment due to their high efficiency and environmentally friendly nature.

Biological methods include aerobic, anaerobic, and aerobic facultative treatment methods. In aerobic pathways, the mechanism involves the oxidative degradation of dyes without the cleavage of azo bond avoiding the formation of toxic aromatic amines. But some essential components also get oxidized in this method reducing its efficiency. Aerobic bacteria and fungi such as *Phanerochaete chrysosporium*, *Trametes* species, and *Aspergillus* species have been described to oxidatively decolorize many dyes including azo dyes. However, anaerobic biological treatment methods using bacteria such as *Bacteroides* species, *Eubacterium* species, *Clostridium* species, etc. are able to decolorize azo dye solutions, but giving toxic aromatic amines as products, [28] although they occur with non-specificity depending on the organism involved and the dyes converted. Thus, the anaerobic pathway is generally more satisfactory than the aerobic one but requires the complete degradation of the intermediate products.

Therefore, for the most effective removal of dye effluents, aerobic facultative methods are introduced where an aerobic treatment is followed just after the initial anaerobic reduction of the azo bond where the balance between anaerobic and aerobic stages must be carefully controlled for the complete safe degradation of dyes. These two-stage treatment methods may be of different combinations such as of two biological processes or a mixture of biological and physicochemical processes. The choice of the processes depends on the type of effluents, availability of the methods, and the locality of the application. However, one of the main drawbacks reported for the biological approaches is that they are less effective and should be administered over a long period of time for better performance.

7.5 CASE STUDIES

The textile industry is one of the largest industries in the world which provides employment to a large extent in poor countries like India, Bangladesh, Pakistan, Sri Lanka, and Vietnam. However, the effluents released from these textile dyeing industries are responsible for environmental pollution, especially polluting the water bodies.

Islam and his co-worker studied and reported the different types of textile dyes used in different industries in South Asian countries and their contribution to environmental pollution where they found that the physicochemical parameters involved in those dye effluents such as COD, TDS, and BOD exceeded their standard limits affecting the aquaculture, agriculture, ecology, environment, and public health in these countries [36]. Malir and Lyari are major rivers in Pakistan receiving effluents from different industries and draining these into the Arabian Sea. Studies reported that the water bases of Faisalabad in the same country are polluted due to the discharge of untreated effluents which further flow into a much larger water body Chenab. The pH of effluents for discharges was found to be slightly alkaline because of the extensive use of salts in dyeing processes [37].

In Sri Lanka, The Kelani River emerges as the most highly polluted river [36] loaded with pollutants, including Zn, Cd, and Pb at ~52.5, ~2.7, and ~7.4 ppb, respectively [38]. It is because of the discharging of organic dye waste into the river from several nearby textile industries. Water pollution due to the textile industry in Sri Lanka was reported at ~43.56% in 2006, according to the World Bank collection of development indicators.

Textile effluent pollutes the soil which is the basis for agriculture. These effluents present in the fields obstruct the pores of the soil causing in loss of yield due to the prohibition of permeability of roots. Several reports stated that the effluent of Modi Textile Factory Ltd. in Modinagar, Uttar Pradesh in India was alkaline and reddish brown in color, deficient in DO containing a huge amount of dissolved, suspended, and volatile solids. Textile processing industries in Pali, Jodhpur, and Barmer districts release a huge amount of effluents to nearby rivers Bandy, Jojri, and Luni respectively, causing serious geo-environmental contamination, health and agricultural hazards. A study on the effect of textile dyeing effluents on soils collected from the agricultural fields in Jojripur River showed higher accumulations of Na, P, and K [39].

The application of dyestuffs and pigments in textile and dyeing industries may cause a number of health effects such as disturbances in normal functions like respiration, osmoregulation, and reproduction. The toxic nature of the textile dyeing effluent may also cause an increased rate of mortality. In addition, it has been found that textile materials can cause dermatitis, asthma, nasal problems, and rhinitis after prolonged exposure. Such types of effects were observed in the people in the Noyyal River basin in Tamil Nadu in India due to the injection of contaminated wastewater [40].

Islam and Mostafa [36] reported the effect of discharging untreated textile dyeing effluents in Bangladesh where most of these textile industries are situated along the bank of the rivers. A complex mixture of dangerous organic and inorganic chemicals from these industries is generally discharged into the aquatic bodies without treatment or after partial treatment. Factories and industries at Tongi close to Dhaka regularly dispose of their effluents in the nearby river, thus polluting the water of the Turag giving it a dark color and a strong smell. Researchers found the values of pH, TDS, DO, and BOD in the range of 7.24–7.61 ppm, 239–1349 ppm, 1.22–3.66 ppm, and 2.44–0.86 ppm, respectively [36].

Saver is the leading manufacturing belt near Dhaka in Bangladesh having several textile and dyeing industries where a huge amount of effluents are produced every day and are discharged into the neighboring land, farming fields, and irrigation networks which lastly enter into the river. Researchers analyzed water samples of Saver for pH, temperatures, DO, BOD, COD, and TDS and found that most of the parameters exceeded their permissible limits [41].

The industrial effluents are regularly dumped into Dhalai Beel, which then enters into the Bansal River without any treatment. Therefore, the water becomes unsafe for fish and microorganisms of the Dhalai Beel [42]. There are several industrial units at Fatulla, Panchabatee, Kachpur, Rupashi, Tarabo, Hotabo, Sonargaon, Araihazar, Rupganj, and Gopaldee which discharge effluents directly into the river Shitalakkhya. The Bangladesh Center for Advanced Studies (BCAS) analyzed that the TDS value in this river increased from 216 to 446 mg/L within the period 1980–1998. Several researchers have analyzed polluted water collected from different water bodies in these areas and found that these are highly alkaline and highly polluted due to huge TDS content in effluents [42, 43].

Due to the unavailability of canal water and subsoil water, farmers near Bhatinda, Punjab in India have to irrigate their fields with toxic sludge flowing into a drain through their villages which carries sludge from factories located in Barnala district. Farmers of Kot Bhara, Kot Bakhtu, Kot Fatta, Ramgarh Bhunder, Chathewala, Jeewan Singh Wala, Shergah, Mallwala, Kaile Bander, Chak Ruldu Singh Wala, Pathrala, Manak Khana and other villages along the banks of the Lisada drain near Bhatinda have been using this toxic black water for 20 years for irrigation. The effect on crops irrigated with sludge can be observed through symptoms like plaque in teeth, joint pain, and grey hair of villagers there [1].

Dass and his coworkers have studied and reported the impact of Tirupur garment industrial effluent discharges on agriculture at the Noyyal River basin in Tamil Nadu, India [44]. Their study observed that the majority of the rural communities did not depend on the river water for drinking, irrigation, fishing, washing clothes, or bathing the livestock. The results suggested that the water in the river was polluted and not good for agriculture. However, if remedial action and prevention steps are not taken, in due course, then agriculture will disappear soon. Although the people were aware of water pollution, their awareness was not yet translated into action, which was mainly because of a lack of awareness among them [44].

A large number of people are engaged in the dyeing process at Shantipur in the district of Nadia, West Bengal, India. Samples of wastewater were collected from 11 textile dyeing units in this area for physiochemical analysis, whose results showed that most of the parameters, including conductivity, chloride, COD, and BOD, have crossed the maximum permissible limit. The result of the BOD/COD ratio also indicates that those effluents have a large percentage of nonbiodegradable materials [45]. The colors of the discharge of all the factories have indicated the presence of dye residue, which is toxic, carcinogenic, and destroying the local ecosystem. Avian populations of Nadia district are in a decline phase, as observed from the active nests and bird counts.

Contrary to all the above studies, several research groups have gone through different environmental audits too in different industries [46–60]. An environmental audit was reported in the garment manufacturing industries from the perspective of human factors in Bengaluru, Karnataka, India, where they monitored several environmental parameters such as noise level, illumination, and temperature using instruments like sound level meter, lux meter, and handheld thermometer and compared the values against Occupational Safety and Health Administration (OSHA) standards. During

TABLE 7.1
Physicochemical parameters of textile effluents collected from different areas

Area	pH	TDS (mg/L)	BOD (mg/L)	COD (mg/L)	References
Punjab, India	4.30–11.90	430–49440	108–790	120–3000	[52]
Nadia, West Bengal, India	7–7.9	-	210–350	550–1140	[46]
Maharashtra, India	7.9–9.5	-	158–226	548–816	[53]
Gujarat, India	4–13	8–20	72–93	32–58	[54]
Karachi, Pakistan	7.5–11.55	2469–7295	85–653	115–705	[55]
Faisalabad, Pakistan	8–14	2700–4200	211–487	590–880	[56]
Dhaka, Bangladesh	8.7–10	460–5981	90–460	508	[57]
Chittagong, Bangladesh	8.9–11	685–1338	140–420	487–1120	[58, 59]
Gazipur, Bangladesh	8.9–10	531–1006	560–965	-	[59–61]

their study, medical record investigation and interactions with the employees were also performed, which indicate that the workers are exposed to health-related illnesses such as heat stress, heat stroke, eye strain, headache, dizziness, etc. [48].

7.6 CONCLUSIONS

The environment is the basis of life for all living organisms. Several dye effluents in different forms are found to pollute the environment, covering all of its dimensions. Particularly toxic dye-containing wastewater is a major problem because textile mills all over the world regularly discharge millions of gallons of wastewater into natural water resources, which poses serious environmental and public health risks in many countries in recent years. The treatment of this wastewater, on the other hand, represents a significant challenge as there is no specific and economically viable technique for its removal. Hence, more research is required to establish a more advanced zero-waste process that can minimize environmental as well as public health hazards.

To protect the environment, every industry should regularly monitor the different parameters related to environmental safety. The management as well as the workers should be well aware of all the environmental safety measures to be taken in case of the incidence of exceeded value of the parameters than the permitted levels. It is to be kept in mind that the production area of the textile industry should be at a distant place to avoid the consumption of chemicals by air as well, and the wastes from the industries should ensure and adopt effective removal techniques before disposal into the environment.

Above all, there is a huge need to design and produce luxurious and sensuous fabric in such a way that is nontoxic, ethical, and sustainable. Environmentally benign technologies should be developed for mainstream manufacturers, and efforts are needed to raise peoples' awareness about the far-reaching implications of their textile choices and choose the use of eco-friendly products.

REFERENCES

1. Kant, R. Textile Dyeing Industry and Environmental Hazard. *Natural Science*, 4(1), 22–26 (2012). DOI: 10.4236/ns.2012.41004.
2. Abel, A. The History of Dyes and Pigments: From Natural Dyes to High Performance Pigments. In *Theories and Applications*. London, UK: Wood Head Publishing Series in Textiles; DCC (Europe) Ltd. (2012).
3. Pugh, T. W., and Cecil, L. G. The Contact Period of Central Petén, Guatemala in Color. *Res: Anthropology and Aesthetics*, 61, 315–329 (2012). DOI: 10.1086/RESvn1ms23647838.
4. Ardila-Leal, L. D., Poutou-Pinales, R. A., Pedroza-Rodriguez, A. M., and Quevedo-Hidalgo B. E. A Brief History of Colour, the Environmental Impact of Synthetic Dyes and Removal by Using Laccases. *Molecules*, 26, 3813 (2021). DOI: 10.3390/molecules26133813.
5. Mangal, V. P. The Future of Indian Dyes & Dye Intermediates. *Textile Review*, 23 (2010). www.indiantextilejournal.com/articles/FAdetails.asp?id=2420

6. Chokalingam, P., Maruthavanan, T., and Prakash, C. Environmental Impacts of Textile Industries. *The Indian Textile Journal*, 4 (2009).
7. Dye Manufacturing. *Pollution Prevent and Abatement Handbook.* Washington, DC: World Bank Group (1998). https://documents1.worldbank.org/curated/en/758631468314701365/pdf/multi0page.pdf
8. Bhatia, S. C. *Pollution Control in Textile Industry.* WPI Publishing (2017). DOI: 10.1201/9781315148588.
9. Wang, D. M. Environmental Protection in Clothing Industry. In: *Sustainable Development: Proceedings of the International Conference on Sustainable Development (ICSD2015).* Singapore: World Scientific Publishing, pp. 729–735 (2016). DOI: 10.1142/9789814749916_0076.
10. Setiadi, T., Andriani, Y., and Erlania, M. Treatment of Textile Wastewater by a Combination of Anaerobic and Aerobic Processes: A Denim Processing Plant Case. In: S. Ohgaki, K. Fukushi, H. Katayama, S. Takizawa, and C. Polprasert (Eds.), *Southeast Asian Water Environment: Selected Papers from the First International Symposium on Southeast Asian Water Environment (Biodiversity and Water Environment), Bangkok, Thailand, October 2003.* Oxford: IWA Publishingpp. 159–166 (2006).
11. Orts, F., del Rio, A. I., Molina, J., Bonastre, J., and Cases, F. Electrochemical Treatment of real Textile Wastewater: Trichomy Procian HEXL. *Journal of Electroanalytical Chemistry*, 808, 387–394 (2017). DOI: 10.1016/j.jelechem.2017.06.051.
12. Lellis, B., Favaro-Polonio, C. Z., Pamphile, J. A., and Polonio, J. C. Effects of Textile Dyes on Health and the Environment and Bioremediation Potential of Living Organisms. *Biotechnology Research and Innovation*, 3, 275–290 (2019).
13. Hassan, M. M., and Carr, C. M. A Critical Review on Recent Advancements of the Removal of Reactive Dyes from Dye House Effluent by Ion-Exchange Adsorbents. *Chemosphere*, 209, 1, 201–219 (2018). DOI: 10.1016/j.chemosphere.2018.06.043.
14. Imran, M., Crowley, D. E., Khalid, A., Hussain, S., Mumtaz, M. W., and Arshad, M. Microbial Biotechnology for Decolorization of Textile Wastewaters. *Reviews in Environmental Science and Biotechnology*, 14(1), 73–92 (2015). DOI: 10.1007/s11157-014-9344-4.
15. Newman, M. C. *Fundamentals of Ecotoxicology: The Science of Pollution.* Boca Raton: CRC Press (2015).
16. Sandhya, S. Biodegradation of Azo Dyes under Anaerobic Condition: Role of Azoreductase. In: H. A. Erkurt (Ed.), *Biodegradation of Azo Dyes. The handbook of Environmental Chemistry.* Berlin, Heidelberg: Springer, vol. 9, pp. 39–57 (2010). DOI: 10.1007/698_2009_43.
17. Pereira, L. and Alves, M. Dyes – Environmental Impact and Remediation. In: A. Malik, E. Grohmann (Ed.), *Environmental Protection Strategies for Sustainable Development, Strategies for Sustainability.* Springer Science Business Media, pp. 111–162 (2012).
18. Puvaneswari, N., Muthukrishnan, J., and Gunasekaran, P. Toxicity Assessment and Microbial Degradation of Azo Dyes. *Indian Journal of Experimental Biology*, 44, 618–626 (2006).
19. Ito, T., Adachi, Y., Yamanashi, Y., and Shimada, Y. Long-Term Natural Remediation Process in Textile Dye-Polluted River Sediment Driven by Bacterial Community Changes. *Water Research*, 100, 458–465 (2016). DOI: 10.1016/j.watres.2016.05.050.
20. Brock, T., Groteklaes, M., and Mischke, P. *European Coatings Handbook.* Vincentz Netwark GmbH & Co. KG (2000).

21. Christie, R. M. *Colour Chemistry*. United Kingdom: Royal Society of Chemistry (2001).
22. Copaciu, F., Opris, O., Coman, V., Ristoiu, D., Niinemets, U., and Copolovici, L. Diffuse Water Pollution by Anthraquinone and Azo Dyes in Environment Importantly alters Foliage Volatiles, Carotenoids and Physiology in Wheat (*Triticum aestivum*). *Water, Air, and Soil Pollution* 224(3), 1478 (2013). DOI: 10.1007/s11270-013-1478-4.
23. Al-Degs, Y. S., Khraishen, M. A. M., Allen, S. J., and Ahmad, M. N. Effect of Carbon Surface Chemistry on the Removal of Reactive Dyes from Textile Effluent. *Water Research*, 34, 927–935 (2000). DOI: 10.1016/S0043-1354(99)00200-6.
24. Hao, O. J., Kim, H., and Chiang, P.-C. Decolourization of Wastewater. *Critical Review in Environmental Science and Technology*, 30, 449–505 (2000). DOI: 10.1080/10643380091184237.
25. Liana, V. Application of Membrane Technology in Printing and Dyeing Waste-Water Treatment. *Guangxi Textile Technology*, 39(1), 59–60 (2010).
26. Liu, Q. Pollution and Treatment of Dye Wastewater. In: *4th International Symposium on Resource Exploration and Environmental Science*. IOP Conference Series: Earth and Environmental Science. IOP Publishing Ltd, vol. 514, p. 052001 (2020). DOI: 10.1088/1755-1315/514/5/052001.
27. Samsami, S., Mohamadi, M., Sarrafzadeh, M. H., Rene, E. R., and Firoozbahr, M. Recent Advances in the Treatment of Dye-Containing Wastewater from Textile Industries: Overview and Perspectives. *Process Safety and Environment Protection*, 143, 138–163 (2020). DOI: 10.1016/j.psep.2020.05.034.
28. Archna, Lokesh, K. N., and Siva Kiran, R. R. Biological Methods of Dye Removal from Textile Effluents – A Review. *Journal of Biochemistry and Technology*, 3(5), S177–S180 (2012). https://jbiochemtech.com/storage/models/article/Jy7St8mZxoKVFB3CvHnLP0XRJR1KigoOvIGKCq3vtozVJ9QaB74Zn1JVzFr0/biological-methods-of-dye-removal-from-textile-effluents-a-review.pdf
29. Van der Bruggen, B., Comelis, G., and Vandecasteele, C. Fouling of Nanofiltration and Ultra-Filtration Membranes Applied for Wastewater Regeneration in Textile Industry. *Desalination* 175, 111–119 (2005). DOI: 10.1016/j.desal.2004.09.025.
30. Jadhav, A. and Jadhav, N. C. Treatment of Textile Wastewater using Adsorption and Adsorbents. In: *Sustainable Technologies for Textile Wastewater Treatments*. Wood Head Publishing, pp. 235–273 (2021). DOI: 10.1016/B978-0-323-85829-8.00008-0.
31. Cao, G., Wang, R., Ju, Y., Jing, B., Duan, X., Ao, Z., Jiang, J., Li, F., and Ho, S. H. Synchronous Removal of Emulsions and Soluble Organic Contaminants via a Microalgae-Based Membrane System: Performance and Mechanisms. *Water Research*, 206, 117741 (2021). DOI: 10.1016/j.watres.2021.117741.
32. Akpomie, K. G., and Conradie, J. Advances in Application of Cotton-Based Adsorbents for Heavy Metals Trapping, Surface Modifications and Future Perspectives. *Ecotoxicology Environment Safety*, 201, 110825 (2020). DOI: 10.1016/j.ecoenv.2020.110825.
33. Kishor, R., Purchase, D., Saratale, G. D., Saratale, R. G., Ferreira, L. F. R., Bilal, M., Chandra, R., and Bharagava, R. N. Ecotoxicological and Health Concerns of Persistent Colouring Pollutants of Textile Industry Wastewater and Treatment Approaches for Environmental Safety. *Journal of Environment Chemical Engineering*, 9, 105012 (2021). DOI: 10.1016/j.jece.2020.105012.
34. Saxe, J. P., Lubenow, B. L., Chiu P. C., Huang, C.-P., and Cha D. K. Enhanced Biodegradation of Azo Dyes Using an Integrated Elemental Iron-Activated Sludge System: I. Evaluation of System Performance. *Water Environment Research*, 78, 19–25 (2006). DOI: 10.2175/106143005x84477.

35. Al-Tohamy, R., Ali, S. S., Li, F., Okasha, K. M., Mahmoud, Y. A.-G., Elsamahy, T., Jiao, H., Fu, Y., and Sun, J. A Critical Review on the Treatment of Dye-Containing Wastewater: Ecotoxicological and Health Concerns of Textile Dyes and Possible Remediation Approaches for Environmental Safety. *Ecotoxicology and Environmental Safety*, 231, 113160 (2022). DOI: 10.1016/j.ecoenv.2021.113160.
36. Islam, M. R., and Mostafa, M. G. Textile Dyeing Effluents and Environmental Concerns – A Review. *Journal of Environment Science & Natural Resources*, 11(1–2), 131–144 (2019). DOI: 10.3329/jesnr.v11i1-2.43380.
37. Nergis, Y. M., Sharif, M., Akhatar, N. A., and Hussain, A. Quality Characterization and Magnitude of Pollution Implications in Textile Mills Effluents. *Journal of Quality and Technology Management*, 5, 27–40 (2009).
38. Ileperuma, O. Environmental Pollution in Sri Lanka – A Review. *Journal of National Science Foundation Sri Lanka*, 28(4), 310–315 (2010). DOI: 10.4038/jnsfsr.v28i4.2644.
39. Chhokor, P. K., Datta, S., Joshi, H. C., and Pathak, S. Impact of Industrial Effluents on Soil Health and Agriculture-Indian Experience, Part-II – Tannery and Textile Industrial Effluents. *Journal of Scientific and Industrial Research*, 59, 446–454 (2000).
40. Elango, R. G., and Elango, S. Physico-Chemical Parameters of Textile Dyeing Effluent and Its Impacts with Case Study. *International Journal of Research in Chemistry and Environment*, 7(1), 17–22 (2016).
41. Mia, C. M. Assessment of Effluent Quality of Dhaka Export Processing Zone (DEPZ Old) with Special Emphasis on Textile and Dye Industries. M.Sc. Thesis, Department of Chemistry, JU (2001).
42. Sultana, M. Analysis of Some Trace Elements in the Uncultivated Soil of Saver by ICP M. *Bangladesh Journal of environmental Science*, 1, 57–62 (2003).
43. Hannan, M. A., Rahman, M. A., and Haque, M. F. An Investigation on the Effects of Bleaching Powder with Dyeing Industries Effluents. *Research Journal of Environmental Protection*, 4, 301–308 (2011).
44. Dass, I. M., and Muniyandi, B. Impact of Tirupur Garment Industrial Effluents Discharges on Agriculture at Noyyal River Basin. *Shanlax International Journal of Economics*, 1(4), 21–29 (2013).
45. Mondal, M., Biswas, G., and Bhattacharya, R. Environmental Stresses from Dye Factories: A Case Study at Nadia, West Bengal. *International Journal of Environmental Sciences*, 6 (4), 467–471 (2016). DOI: 10.6088/ijes.6052.
46. Parsons, K. C. Environmental Ergonomics: A Review of Principles, Methods and Models. *Applied Ergonomics*, 31(6), 581–594 (2000). DOI: 10.1016/s0003-6870(00)00044-2.
47. Sarder, B., Imrhan, S. N., and Mandahawi, N. Ergonomic Workplace Evaluation of an Asian Garment Factory. *Journal of Human Ergology*, 35, 45–51 (2006).
48. Calvin, S., and Joseph, B. Occupation Related Accidents in Selected Garment Industries in Bangalore City. *Indian Journal of Community Medicine*, 31(3), 103–144 (2006).
49. Parimalam, P., Kamalamma, N., and Ganguli, A. K. Ergonomic Interventions to Improve Work Environment in Garment Manufacturing Units. *Indian Journal of Occupational and Environmental Medicine*, 10(2), 74–77 (2006). DOI: 10.4103/0019-5278.27304.
50. Padmini, D. S., and Venmathi, A. Unsafe Work Environment in Garment Industries, Tirupur, India, Department of Resource Management, Faculty of Home Science. *Journal of Environmental Research and Development*, 7(1A), 569–575 (2012).

51. Kaur, H., and Sharma, G. Removal of Dyes from Textile Industry Effluent: A Review. *International Journal of Humanities and Social Science*, 59–60 (2015).
52. Amte, G. K., and Mahaska, T. V. Studies on Textile-Dyeing Effluent from Bhiwandi City Dist.: Thane, Maharashtra, India. *Journal of Industrial Pollution Control*, 28(2), 197–199 (2012). www.icontrolpollution.com/articles/studies-on-textiledyeing-effluent-from-bhiwandi-citydist-thane-maharashtra-india-.pdf
53. Patel, R., Tajddin K., Patel A., and Patel B. Physico-Chemical Analysis of Textile Effluent. *International Journal of Research and Scientific Innovation*, II(V), 33–36 (2005).
54. Imtiazuddin S. M., Mumtaz M., and Mallick K. A. Pollutants of Wastewater Characteristics in Textile Industries. *Journal of Basic & Applied Sciences*, 8, 554–556 (2012). DOI: 10.6000/1927-5129.2012.08.02.47.
55. Nosheen S., Nawaz H., and Rehman K. U. Physico-Chemical Characterization of Effluents of Local Textile Industries of Faisalabad-Pakistan. *International Journal of Agriculture Biology*, 2(3): 231–233 (2000).
56. Kamal A. K. I., Ahmed F., Hassan M., Uddin M. K., and Hossain S. M. Characterization of Textile Effluents from Dhaka Export Processing Zone (DEPZ) Area in Dhaka. *Bangladesh Pollution*, 2(2), 153–161 (2016). DOI: 10.7508/pj.2016.02.005.
57. Sultana Z., Ali M. E., Uddin M. S., and Haque M. M. Implementation of Effluent Treatment Plants for Waste Water Treatment. *Journal of Environmental Protection*, 4(3), 301–308 (2013). DOI: 10.4236/jep.2013.43035.
58. Sultana Z., Ali M. E., Uddin M. S., and Haque M. M. Study on Implementation of Effluent Treatment Plants for Safe Environment from Textile Waste. *Journal of Research in Environmental Science and Toxicology*, 2(1), 9–16 (2014). www.interesjournals.org/articles/study-on-implementation-of-effluent-treatment-plants-for-safe-environment-from-textile-waste.pdf
59. Hannan M. A., Rahman M. A., and Haque M. F. An Investigation on the Effects of Bleaching Powder with Dyeing Industries Effluents. *Journal of Environmental Protection*, 4, 301–308 (2011).
60. Hannan M. A., Rahman M. A., and Haque M. F. An Investigation on Quality Characterization and Magnitude of Pollution Implications with Textile Dyeing Industries Effluent using Bleaching Powder. *DUET Journal*, 1(2), 49–59 (2011).

8 Dyes and Dyeing Processes

Environmental, Social and Economical Aspects

Tarun Parangi

8.1 INTRODUCTION: THE PROBLEM

The word "Dye" is now very familiar to the world as is being used primarily in the production of daily consumer products including plastics, papers, paints, textiles, printing inks, etc. They add color and patterns to materials. Natural dyes extracted from vegetables, fruit, and flowers have been used since 3500 BC to color fabrics and coatings in the building sector and leather products [1–4]. These dyes were replaced by chemical dyes that bond with the fabric, thereby providing and retaining richer color throughout washing and exposure [1]. The existing source of natural dyes contributes only 1% of global demand around 1000 tons [5].

A dye which is a colored substance has an affinity to the substrate to which it is being applied. The dye is generally applied in an aqueous solution, and may require a mordant to improve the fastness of the dye on the fiber. On the other hand, pigment is a coloring matter, usually in the form of an insoluble powder that is mixed with oil, water, etc. to make paint. The pigment lays on the surface and becomes part of the dry film.

Today, color and colored systems have become part of fashion life called "Fast Fashion" and, therefore, dyes and dyeing processes are getting interest, and this trend has been accelerating through modern textile industries [7]. However, it has a huge impact on the environment, economy, and society as well. Thus, many scientific communities are studying the global economy along with sustainable development promoting the concept of forming an economic design for control of potentially destructive compounds used in various dye industries.

The conceptual framework for this chapter is based on a consideration of existing literature in developing a new perspective that participates sustainability into textile dyeing processes. The strategy we used to collect and analyze the data was the qualitative methodology, following the line of reasoning that begins with an understanding of the fundamentals and issues related to the impacts of dyeing processes and, consequently, a search for solutions.

DOI: 10.1201/9781003441083-8

8.2 DYE INDUSTRIALISM

The manufacturing and utility of dyestuffs is an antique art in the world. Archaeological indication shows that in India dyeing was an extensive activity as early as the third millennium BCE. The dyes manufactured in factory/industries started to enter the market at an early time of mid-19th century. The German chemical industry was a first beginner in the business of synthesizing the coloring agents of natural dyes. Over time, the industrialism of synthetic dyes has come across the business of natural dyes. Particularly, in case of indigo, the transition from natural to artificial/synthetic dyes totaled a setback of earlier trade structures [1, 2].

The development of dye industrialism has an important role in the economic growth of Asian countries like India, China, Korea, Taiwan, and Indonesia [10–12]. Along with accelerated growth, poverty rates have declined in many countries. Some countries have managed to achieve growth with equity, whereas in others inequality has remained high. The main emphasis is on describing their growth processes and strategies, the role of industrial development, the contribution of a range of policies to growth performance, and the impact of growth on poverty and income inequality. The study begins with a short theoretical discussion of the impact of industrial development on growth and the impact of growth on poverty and income inequality and then proceeds to the country examples.

The dyestuff industry has recently seen a movement toward association and as a result, organized players are now controlled to take a lead in the global market. Small units about ~1000 that exist today still compete in the sectors where cost realization is lower and the competition severe. Large and organized players about ~50 are moving up for global competitiveness by leveraging technology, product novelty and brand forming. Increased focus is being laid on environmental friendliness and at the same time the industry is ensuring greater customer focus through technical facilities and marketing competences, to look global rivalry [13].

The dyestuffs industry has ~1000 divisions manufacturing dyes, dyestuffs, and pigments with a capacity to produce ~75,000 to ~80,000 tonnes per annum (tpa) of textile dyes and organic pigments [14]. The capacity for production of pigments is estimated to be 40k tpa, half of which is in the small-scale sector. The number of units is the largest in a single country worldwide and is a case of too little being produced by too many. In this large spread of units, there are only about 146 units in the organized sector with an installed capacity of 58k tpa, covering over 75% of the total installed capacity in the country. Of these, 40 are fairly large in size. In terms of production, the organized sector contributes about two-thirds.

The total market is estimated at over Rs. 50 billion, of which the market for organic pigments is estimated at Rs. 3 billion [14–16]. The market in quantitative terms is made up of basic dyes, azo acid and direct dyes, disperse dyes, fast color bases, reactive dyes, sulfur dyes, vat dyes, organic pigments, naphthols, optical brighteners, and others. Nearly 80,000 tonnes of the materials are imported and a quarter of the domestic production is exported annually. The overall market is expanding at around 6.5% as of now. The dye markets are mostly dominated by reactive and dispersed dyes. The demand for reactive and dispersed dyes is expected to grow in the future as these two dyes are dominant in all regions.

India is the sixth-largest chemical-producing country in the world and the third-largest producer in Asia [17, 18]. It is also among the top three basic chemical-producing countries globally. India's dye manufacturing industry is growing rapidly now. The migration of the pigments business to Asia, particularly mainland China and India, continues. Since the mid-1990s, production in mainland China and India has rapidly increased, and mainland China is now the world's largest organic color pigment producer, especially for commodity-type pigments. Additional medium-tier to higher-value organic pigments are also migrating to mainland China from North America, Europe, and Japan, as the large multinational producers no longer have patent protection over many of their products. Production in Europe, the United States, and Japan continues on a downward trend as the market has become globalized and gross margins have been squeezed, leading to plant shutdowns and restructuring. The volume of unfinished pigments imported to North America, Western Europe, and Japan for finishing continues to decrease as more finished pigment is imported from mainland China (Figure 8.1) [8].

The industry has a blend of Indian enterprises and the millions existing side by side. Atul Products, Sudarshan Chemical Industries, Jay Synth Dye Chem., Mardia Chemicals, and several others have secured a niche in the marketplace among the Indian enterprises. The million companies have also come to play a dominant role such as IDI (formerly ICI), Ciba Speciality Chemicals (India), and Clariant India.

The industry experts are now looking forward to becoming a capable association for accomplishing an intrinsic strength to the success. The manufacturing sectors with global influence and covered by the use of advanced technologies with resources to support the research and development (R&D) cell are expected to move forward. Many more sectors are expected to fade away as the market needs continually advanced explanations.

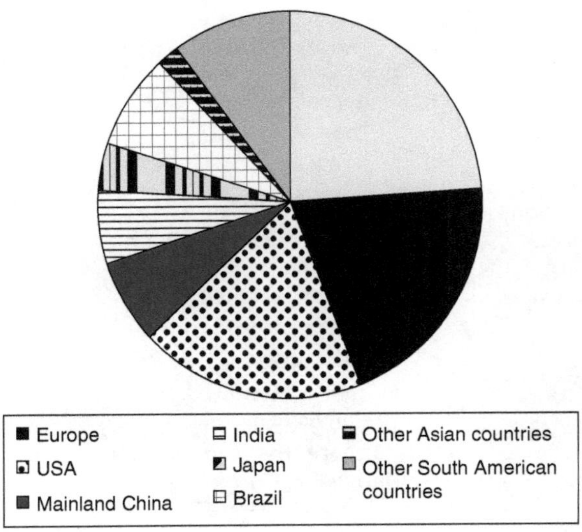

FIGURE 8.1 World consumption of organic color and pigments – year of 2022 [8].

Globally, China, Taiwan, India, Japan, Korea, and Pakistan are the major dyestuff-producing countries in the industry. In terms of market share, Europe is the leading producer due to its allegiance toward specialty products and the countries in Europe have remained the largest players owing to specialty products.

8.3 THREE ASPECTS OF DYE PRODUCTION AND DYEING PROCESS

Sustainability is an important key factor given three aspects: economic, environmental, and social (Figure 8.2). These aspects are affected by the selection of dyes and dyeing process along with possible dye removal methodology. Another fact, a fundamental knowledge of dyeing manufacturing and techniques may reduce energy and time to enhance the overall efficacy of dye industrialism.

8.3.1 Environmental Aspects

Today, the textile industry is considered one of the foremost environment-polluting segments, with an estimated ~20% of all water pollution caused by textile treatments, such as dye manufacturing and various dyeing processes. A large number of different types of chemicals, most notably, sulfuric acid, chromium, copper, and other metallic elements are being used for dye manufacturing and are harmful to humans, agriculture, and animals. The variation in chemical use is closely tied to the high demand for variable patterns and unique colors for clothing and other textiles. About ~140 k tons of synthetic dyes are released into the environment openly every year from

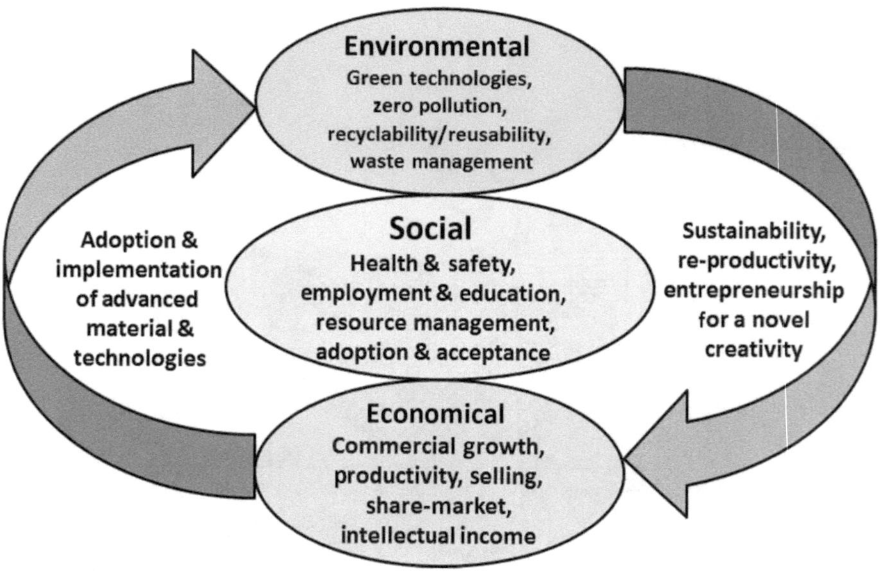

FIGURE 8.2 Three aspects of dye manufacturing and dyeing process [13].

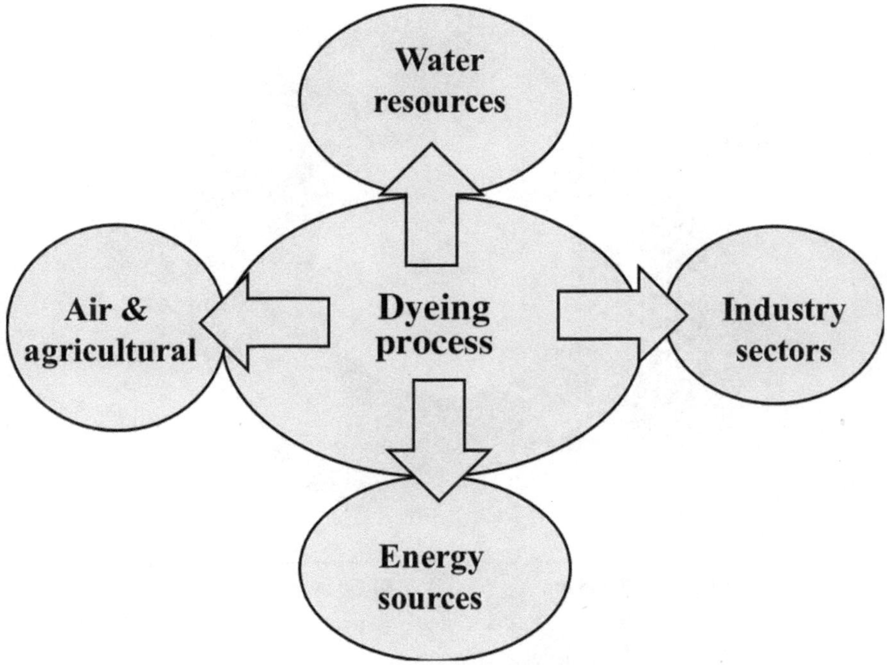

FIGURE 8.3 Dyeing process and affected resources [13].

the different dyeing methods; it results in almost ~20% of all water pollution in the world, primarily caused by textile dyeing waste [19–23].

The textile industry is one of the leading sectors globally and produces a bewildering ~60 billion kilograms of fabric annually, using up to ~9 trillion gallons of water [24–26]. This gigantic amount of water being used is a vital component of pollution.

Therefore, it seems, the dye industry is contributing a major participant in creating environmental pollution and potentially putting many millions of lives at risk (Figure 8.3). The majority of problematic dye industry sites are well established in Asian countries as global centers of textile production and also spread over many different countries. Though the organized dye industry does dominate the market, many unorganized small-scale plants disproportionately add to the problem of pollution (Figure 8.4).

Textile dyeing uses large quantities of water, of which ~93% water from the chemical dyeing process cannot be reused. Natural dyeing is an eco-friendly dyeing process that uses plants as the main source of dye. Unlike chemical dyeing, 97% of the water from natural dyeing can be reused. In conventional textile dyeing, 1 tonne of fabric could result in the pollution of up to 200 tonnes of water. The wastewater produced in textile processes is highly colored and contains complex concentrations of chemicals, such as salt, dye, detergents, peroxides, and heavy metals [4, 27–29].

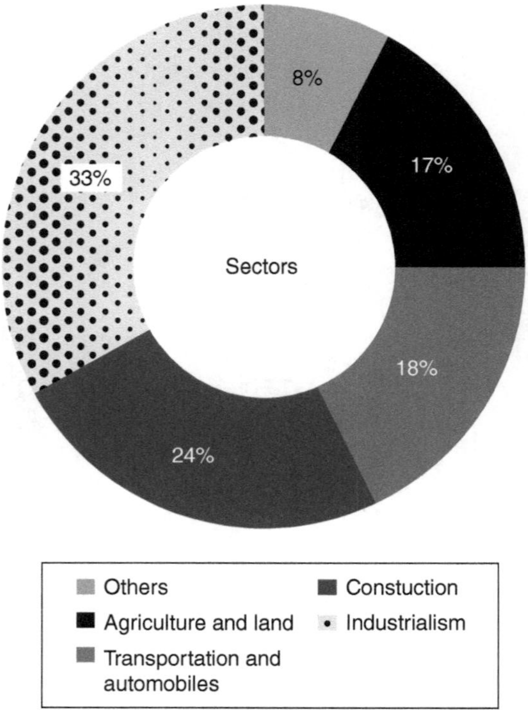

FIGURE 8.4 Global gas emission from the various growing sectors [27].

Reports of a new potential huge source of hazardous contaminants in textile wastewater will come as a shock to many apparel brands and retailers (Figure 8.5).

In the dyeing treatment, if effluents are not properly treated or exposed before being released into the environment, they can go into the food chain and be shifted to living bodies via bioaccumulation [30]. It has been reported that in industrialized countries treated wastewater is around 50–95%, while in emerging countries 80% of effluents are released into water resources without proper treatment. Trends in dye industry effluent treatment and recovery of value-added products [4, 31].

The used textile effluents contained hazardous chemicals (phthalates, chlorobenzene, toluene, and other restricted chemicals) and they become more polluting and dangerous when come to mix with other polluting sources [32, 33]. It causes acute or chronic effects that are warning bells for human health and environmental resources as well. In addition, some of them are corrosive, can cause severe burns, and can react riskily with other reagents. A more treacherous problem is uncontrollable fire threats, which can get up from the use of easily flammable liquids.

Thus, statutory requirements and inclusive environmental restrictions demand alterations in the processes and in the chemicals used in textile processing. The implementation of cleaner technologies for the treatment of effluents is essential to the recovery and improvement of water resources. Conventional wastewater treatment technologies involve physical, chemical, and biological methods that have certain

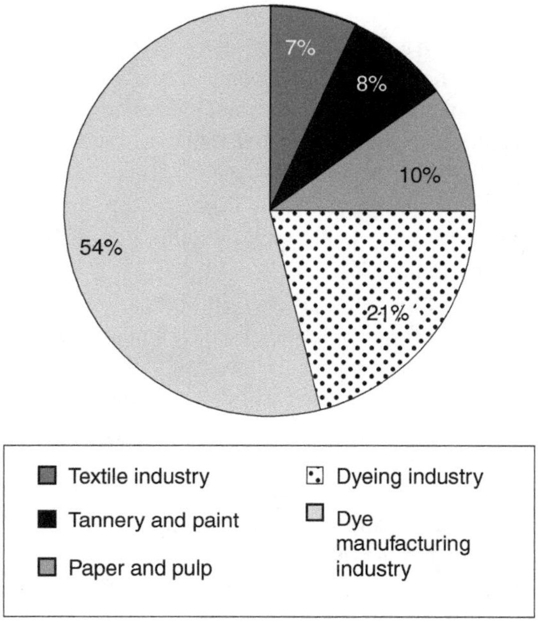

FIGURE 8.5 Comparison of dye effluent discharge from various industries [27–29].

disadvantages, such as high capital investment and maintenance costs [35]. However, nowadays many of the existing conservative treatment methods and materials are not much efficient for the removal of pollutants [36]. Furthermore, a high consumption of energy resources is seen to be another problem associated with the dyeing process through operational conditions. The United Nations' Intergovernmental Panel on Climate Change stated that 10% of global greenhouse gas (GHG) emissions are caused by the textile industry. Polluting gases producing textile manufacturing process are identified as the second biggest pollution problem for the textile industry [37].

Therefore, to minimize energy utility with the concern of environmental health affected from the unusual textile dyeing process, variables that directly affect the process including some experimental parameters and instruments must be sensibly assessed.

8.3.2 Economic Aspects

The future of dye and dyestuff, a part of the chemical industry, has good prospects in the coming years owing to its high demand. The growth of the dye sector in the future will continue to depend on the performance of end-user industries like paints, textiles, printing inks, paper, plastics, and foodstuffs [9].

To achieve global standards the industry needs to put efforts in critical areas so as to adopt aggressive growth and focus on exports, R&D, co-marketing alliances, up-gradation of manufacturing facilities, contract manufacturing with companies having established markets, identification of areas of core competence, consolidation, collaboration by cluster development, outsourcing, environmental consciousness, cost reduction, etc. The industry is likely to see many new dyeing technologies coming into the market with the help of good technical expertise and R&D achievements. Globally the high usage of cotton, polyester, and the banned vat and azo dyes in some of the countries has paved the way for reactive and dispersed dyes. It is now expected that in the future these two dye sectors will lead the global market. The industry feels that unless the labor laws, power supply, and infrastructure are improved, it would be very difficult to compete globally with rapidly declining duty differentials and appreciation in the value of currency [38].

India exports mainly to the United States, Europe, and the Far East. Exports from India make up for 4–5% of global trade in dyes and pigments. The comparative advantages of cheap labor, intelligent manpower, a well-qualified pool of scientists, and a grasp of technology are expected to open up new vistas for the industry on the export front. World demand for dyes and organic pigments is forecast to grow at around 6.5% (Figure 8.6) [39].

The production volume of dyes and pigments across India was around 398,000 metric tons. Some of the commonly manufactured products under this category were disperse dyes, optical whitening agents, and reactive dyes. The Indian chemical industry is highly diversified, producing over 80,000 products [39].

A review of economic aspects shows economic performance, market share, and hidden impacts of dyes. Traded on the open market by dealers, and often repackaged under different trade names, these bulk commodity chemicals are often bought based

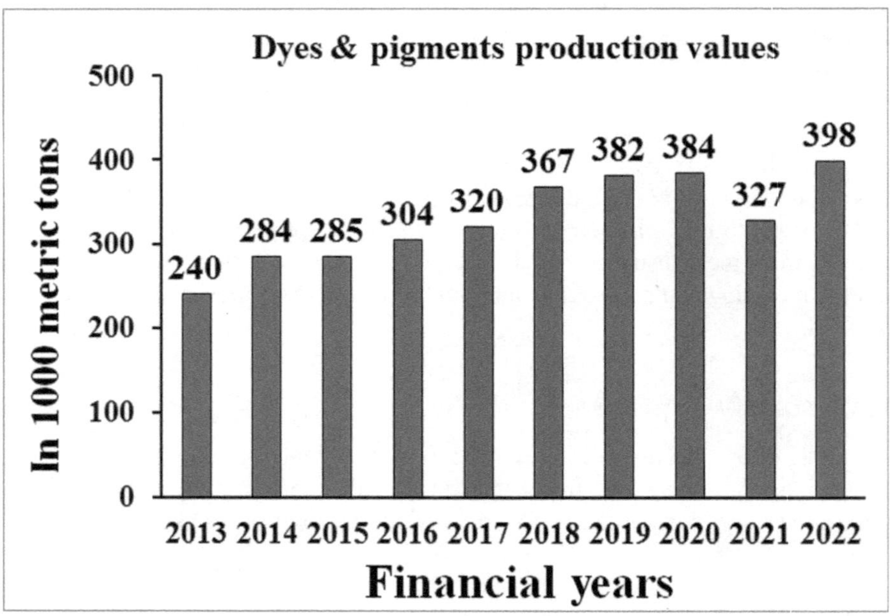

FIGURE 8.6 Production volume of dyes and pigments in India from financial year 2013 to 2022 [39].

on price only and therefore with price being directly related to the purity of the product.

8.3.3 A Positive Recovery from the Dyeing Process

As reported, wastewater contains many types of polluting agents, but it also contains valuable components like useful chemicals, precious metals, nutrients, important salts, fuels, etc. This contaminant can be regained from wastewater [30, 40–42]. Apart from these components, many more contents like algae, microbes like some bacteria *Rhodopseudomonas palustris*, *Rhodopseudomonas gelatinosa*, *Rhodopseudomonas faecalis*, *Moorella thermoautotrophica*, etc. have also been studied as obtained of value-added products [30].

8.3.4 Social Aspects

Social aspects of the sustainability of dye manufacturing and dyeing process related to acceptable employed conditions, identical learning and earning openings, consistency with collective benefits, public association, policy of health and safety for consumers, and social rights [7, 42–44]. The working atmosphere is the most demanded sub-division that reveals the significance of industrialism in terms of sustainability. The direct and/or indirect risks and fears associated with the dye manufacturing and dyeing process through mechanical, physical, chemical, ergonomic, and biological are creative issues with overtime, wages, and working conditions. However, the dye and textile sectors are now becoming integral parts of the Indian economy as it could be predictable that one in six families depends on the earnings from these industries. Other non-titled issues such as low and delayed payment overtime, high workload, verbal exploitation, job uncertainty, premises restrictions and regulations, and employment unions, also exist.

In the case of the textile industry in Bangladesh, the workers regularly work for 76 hours per week which is seen to exceed the limits. However, it is said that the norms for workers are that they should be paid within seven working days of completing work, but a large proportion of industries do not fulfill this. In addition, the remunerations committee is considering some concerns to prepare an equal level of minimum pay/benefit such as regular living standards, cost to survive/living, cost of goods produced, inflation rates, types of occupational and aptitude, and most importantly socioeconomic status. However, it seems that the scheme of the minimum remuneration frequently does not reproduce the reality in many of the dyes industry. It should be followed through the Bangladesh Labour Act of 2006 [43].

8.4 ECONOMICAL TECHNOLOGIES AS ALTERNATES FOR DYEING PROCESS AND DYE REMOVAL

Many more materials and technologies have been emerging for treating and controlling dye-contaminated water resources, apart from the existing methods such as biological treatments, reverse osmosis methods, chemical and electrochemical processes, membrane technologies, ion exchange approach, electrodialysis and electrolysis, and adsorption techniques. Among these, adsorption approaches have extensively been working for dye removal due to their comparatively simple design, safe conditional practice, good handling efficiency, cost-effectiveness, and sludge-free cleaning exercise [13, 47–50].

In the view of efficient adsorbents, alumina-zeolites, silica, clays, activated carbon, nano-composites, biomasses, and carbon-based polymeric adsorbents have been studied for the removal of dyes from aqueous pollutants [51, 52].

8.5 CASE STUDIES

The organization entitled "Makers Loft, India" [53] has trained students working on the thought of upgrading the natural dyeing process and tried to introduce it as the mainstream dyeing technique. In this process, the raw material is crushed, vaporized, and then condensed to form dye. A color sensor has been used to give feedback on whether the dye was of the customized shade or not otherwise it could be reformed. The present upgraded version of natural dyeing is found to be more efficient as it reduces the reformation process and increases the chance of getting the correct shade by detecting it using a color sensor. Here, the use of water can be minimized as much as possible and also reduce processing hours following through principle of sustainability.

Two European companies, namely, Archroma and Colorifix Ltd., are working on technical innovations for sustainable textile coloration. Both innovations have exposed numerous possibilities for forward-thinking dye-houses that could potentially figure out natural dyeing into their existing operations in terms of health and safety of environment and living [54].

8.6 CONCLUSIONS

As it is discussed about the rapidly growing industrialism through global development, rapid propagation of information and trends, the possibilities of modern technologies and society's requirements for dyes, textiles, and dyestuff products affect the environment and economy as well as due to which use and accumulation of a large amount of harmful products and wastes are accumulated throughout the living atmosphere today. In a similar way of living, as a society, we are openly eye witnessing the disproportionate productivity and utility of the dyes and their raw materials as part of the needs of clients (as we) whose behaviors are determined by different impacts, but at the same time, the society is showing an interest toward the alertness for the hazards and risk on living health from the unreasonable dye manufacturing process and their uses.

Here, the thoughts of a sustainable system in terms of economy, environment, and social values should be implemented through the community for each industrialism. It may contain sustainable technologies that create zero or fewer hazards and risks, and also sustainable materials with optimized efficiency. Thus, nowadays,

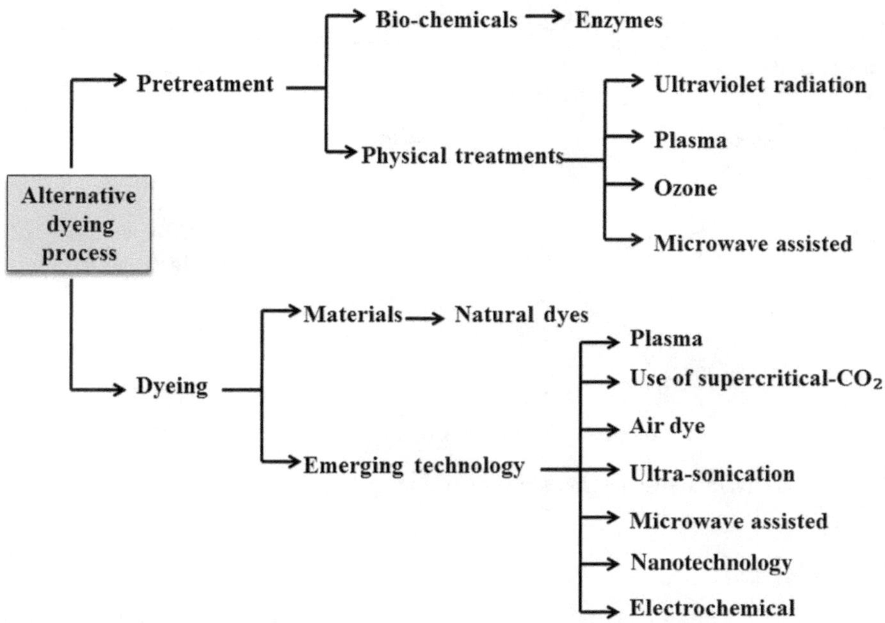

FIGURE 8.7 Existing dyeing process as alternative for conventional processes.

sustainable/environmentally friendly concepts should be taken into consideration in industrial education and practice as well.

We believe that today's lifestyle and our civilization are now totally dependent on technology; however, it should be regarded as a predictable constituent of the environment where living ones are present. One more point we cannot ignore is that technology affects and interacts with the economic dimension that permits new professional clarifications that benefit the natural resources of society (Figures 8.7 and 8.8). Particularly, in the practical use of dyeing and printing, natural dyes are more fairly good compared to synthetic ones. The use of new dyeing products and use of advanced dyeing processes create supplementary challenges for the industrial sectors because of the structure of an organization and their qualitative experimental tests, as synthetic dyes are improbable to be completely substituted.

Today, numerous efforts are now being applied to more improvement for the existing tasks related to the process of dyeing and removal, as many of the chapters of this book have discussed in detail. The change to a circular economy needs an essential universal change not only industrial innovation to have enhanced efficiency and diminish an environmental issue, but also subterranean sociological change and development in way of ideal work-ship models.

Thus, a more sustainable attitude to industrial manufacturing protocol needs to be merged with suitable policies such as rules and regulations, recognized by local Governments and Constitution bodies. More preciously, social awareness and responsibility can play a crucial role in the present theme.

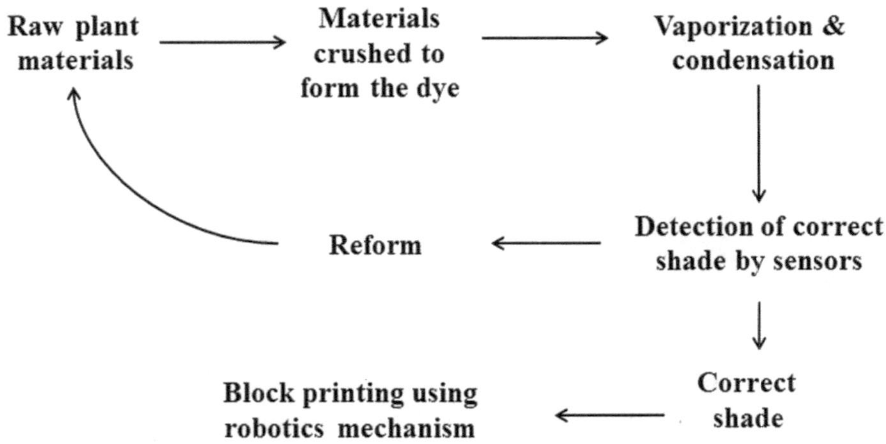

FIGURE 8.8 Natural dyeing process using robotics mechanism [53].

REFERENCES

1. Dye Manufacturing. *Pollution Prevent and Abatement Handbook*. World Bank Group (1998).
2. Siva, R. Status of natural dyes and dye-yielding plants in India. *Current Science*, 92(7), 7 (2007).
3. Phan, K., Raes, K., Speybroeck, V., Roosen, M., Clerck, K. D., and De Meester, S. Non-food applications of natural dyes extracted from agro-food residues: a critical review. *Journal of Cleaner Production*, 301, 126920 (2021). DOI: 10.1016/j.jclepro.2021.126920.
4. Kant, R., Textile dyeing industry an environmental hazard. *Natural Science*, 4(1), 22–26 (2012). DOI: 10.4236/ns.2012.41004.
5. Senthilkumar, R., Vaneshwari, V., Sathiyavimal, S., Amsaveni, R., Kalaiselvi, M., and Malayaman, V. Natural colors from dying plants for textile. *International Journal of Biosciences and Nanosciences*, 2(7), 160–174 (2015).
6. Chen, H. L., and Burns, L. D. Environmental analysis of textile products. *Clothing and Textiles Research Journal*, 24(3), 248–261 (2015), DOI: 10.1177/0887302X06293065.
7. Tkalec, M., Sutlovic, A., and Glogar, M. I. Ecological, economic and social aspects of textile dyes. In *Economic and Social Development*, 81st International Scientific Conference on Economic and Social Development – Green Economy & Sustainable Development (2022).
8. *S&P Global's Chemical Economics Handbook – Organic Color Pigments*. URL: www.spglobal.com/commodityinsights/en/ci/products/organic-color-chemical-economics-handbook.html.
9. Geissler, S., Thomas, B., and Mussak, R. Economic aspects of natural dyes. Thomas, B., Mussak, R. (Eds.), *Handbook of Natural Colorants*. Wiley. Ch. 21 (2009).
10. Matleena, K. Industrial development and economic growth: Implications for poverty reduction and income inequality. In *Industrial Development for the 21st Century: Sustainable Development Perspectives*. . United Nations, Department of Social and Economic Affairs, NY, USA. pp. 295–332 (2007).

11. Kumar, N. *East Asia's Paths to Industrialization and Prosperity: Lessons for India and Other Late Comers in South Asia*. South and South-West Asia Office. Economic and Social Commission for Asia and the Pacific (2020).
12. Yong, L. *Industrialization as the Driver of Sustained Prosperity*. United Nations Industrial Development Organization (2020).
13. Lara, L., Cabral, I, and Cunha, J. Ecological approaches to textile dyeing: a review. *Sustainability*, 14, 8353 (2022). DOI: 10.3390/su14148353.
14. Dyestuff, dyes, pigments and dye intermediates projects. URL: www.niir.org/profile-project-reports/profiles/dyestuff-dyes-pigments-dye-intermediates-projects/z,,8,0,a/index.html.
15. Organic pigments market source (synthetic and natural), type (azo, phthalocyamine, HPPs), application (printing inks, paints & coatings, plastics), and region (North America, Europe, APAC, MEA, and South America) – Global Forecast to 2026. URL: www.marketsandmarkets.com/Market-Reports/organic-pigments-market-1076.html.
16. Organic pigments market by type (azo pigments, phthalocyanine pigments, high performance pigments (HPPs), alizarin, arylide, others), by end use industry (paints and coatings, automotive, plastics, printing inks, packaging, textile, others): global opportunity analysis and industry forecast, 2021–2031. URL: www.alliedmarketresearch.com/organic-pigments-market-A12122.
17. India brand equity foundation: 2010–2023. URL: www.ibef.org/industry/chemicals-presentation.
18. Exports of Indian chemicals register growth of 106% in 2021–22 over 2013–14 (2023). URL: www.pib.gov.in/PressReleasePage.aspx?PRID=1820478.
19. Jayaswal, K., Sahu, V., and Gurjar, B.R. Water pollution, human health and remediation. In: S. Bhattacharya, A. Gupta, and A. Pandey (Eds.), *Water Remediation, Energy, Environment, and Sustainability*. Springer, Singapore, pp. 11–27 (2018). DOI: 10.1007/978-981-10-7551-3_2.
20. Tara, N., Arslan, M., Hussain, Z., Iqbal M., Khan, Q., and Afzal, M., On-site performance of floating treatment wetland macrocosms augmented with dye-degrading bacteria for the remediation of textile industry wastewater. *Journal of Cleaning Production*, 217, 541–548 (2019). DOI: 10.1016/j.jclepro.2019.01.258.
21. Ranade, V. V., and Bhandari,V. M. Industrial wastewater treatment, recycling, and reuse – past, present and future. In: *Industrial Wastewater Treatment, Recycling and Reuse*. Elsevier, Butterworth-Heinemann, pp. 521–535 (2014).
22. Biswal, T., and Priyadarsini, M. *Dyeing Processing Technology: Waste Effluent Generated From Dyeing and Textile Industries and Its Impact on Sustainable Environment*. IGI Global Publishing, Beijing, China (2020). DOI: 10.4018/978-1-7998-0311-9.ch006.
23. Routoula, E., and Patwardhan, S. V. Degradation of anthraquinone dyes from effluents: a review focusing on enzymatic dye degradation with industrial potential. *Environmental Science & Technology* (2020). DOI: 10.1021/acs.est.9b03737.
24. Dhanabhakyam, M., Indian textile industry – an overview. URL: www.fibre2fashion.com/industry-article/2363/indian-textile-industry-an-overview.
25. Balakumar, R. S. An overview of Indian textile industry, 2021. URL: https://textilelearner.net/an-overview-of-indian-textile-industry/.
26. Desore, A., Narula, S. A., and Shanti, A. An overview on corporate response towards sustainability issues in textile industry. *Environment Development and Sustainability*, 20(2) (2018). DOI: 10.1007/s10668-017-9949-1.
27. Dye. *Ecotextile News*. URL: www.ecotextile.com/2018102223813/dyes.

28. Velusamy, S., Roy, A., Sundaram, S., and Mallick, T. K. A review on heavy metal ions and containing dyes removal through graphene oxide-based adsorption strategies for textile wastewater treatment. *Chemical Record*, 21(7) (2021). DOI: 10.1002/tcr.202000153.
29. Agtaş, M., Dilaver, M., and Ismail, K. Ceramic membrane overview and applications in textile industry: a review. *Water Science & Technology*, 84 (2021). DOI: 10.2166/wst.2021.290.
30. Varjani, S., Rakholiya, P., Shindhal, T., Shah, A. V., and Ngo, H. *Journal of Water Process Engineering*, 39, 101734 (2021). DOI: 10.1016/j.jwpe.2020.101734.
31. Samsami, S., Mohamadizaniani, M., Sarrafzadeh, M. H., Rene, E. R., and Firoozbahr, M. Recent advances in the treatment of dye-containing wastewater from textile industries: overview and perspectives. *Process Safety & Environment Protection*, 143, 138–163 (2020).
32. Elsahida, K., Fauzi, M. A., Sailah, I., and Siregar, I. Z. Sustainability of the use of natural dyes in the textile industry. *IOP Conference Series: Earth Environment Science*, 399, 012065 (2019).
33. Lellis, B., Zani, C., Favaro-Polonio, C. Z., Pamphile, J. A. and Polonio, J. C. Effects of textile dyes on health and the environment and bioremediation potential of living organisms. *Biotechnology Research and Innovation*, 3, 275–290 (2019). DOI: 10.1016/j.biori.2019.09.001.
34. Roy, M., and Saha, R. Dyes and their removal technologies from wastewater: A critical review. In*: Intelligent Environmental Data Monitoring for Pollution Management*, pp. 127–160 (2021). DOI: 10.1016/B978-0-12-819671-7.00006-3.
35. Shukla, S., Khan, R., and Daverey, A. Synthesis and characterization of magnetic nanoparticles, and their applications in wastewater treatment: a review. *Environmental Technology & Innovation*, 24, 101924 (2021). DOI: 10.1016/j.eti.2021.101924.
36. Yahya, N., Aziz, F., Jamaludin, N., Mutalib, M. A., Ismail, A., Salleh, W. Jaafar, J., Yusof, N., and Ludin, N. A. A review of integrated photocatalyst adsorbents for wastewater treatment. *Journal of Environmental Chemical Engineering*, 6, 7411–7425 (2018). DOI: 10.1016/j.jece.2018.06.051.
37. UN Environment Programme. Sustainability and circularity in the textile value chain global stocktaking. (2020). URL: www.unep.org/resources/publication/sustainability-and-circularity-textile-value-chain-global-roadmap.
38. Project reports: business plan. *npcs*. URL: www.niir.org/profile-project-reports/profiles/dyestuff-dyes-pigments-dye-intermediates-projects/z,,8,0,a/index.html.
39. Production volume of dyes and pigments in India from financial year 2013 to 2024. *Statista*. URL: www.statista.com/statistics/726947/india-dyes-and-pigments-production-volume.
40. Wilberforce T., Sayed, E. T., Abdelkareem, M. A., Elsaid, K., and Olab, A. G. Value added products from wastewater using bioelectrochemical systems: current trends and perspectives. *Journal of Water Process Engineering*, 39, 101737 (2021). DOI: 10.1016/j.jwpe.2020.101737.
41. Yadav, A., Rene, E. R., Sharma, M., Jatain I., Mandal M. K., and Dubey, K. Valorization of wastewater to recover value-added products: a comprehensive insight and perspective on different technologies. *Environmental Research*, 214(20), 113957 (2022). DOI: 10.1016/j.envres.2022.113957.
42. Arora, K., Kumar, P., Singh, A., Patel, S. K. S., Li, X., Yang Y.-H., Bhatiam, S. K., and Kulshrestha, S. Valorization of wastewater resources into biofuel and value-added products using microalgal system. *Frontier in Energy Research*, 9 (2021). DOI: 10.3389/fenrg.2021.646571.

43. Haradhan, M. The first industrial revolution: creation of a new global human era. MPRA Paper No. 96644 (2019). URL: https://mpra.ub.uni-muenchen.de/96644/.
44. Kniivila, M. Industrial development and economic growth: Implications for poverty reduction and income inequality. In: *Industrial Development for the 21st Century: Sustainable Development Perspectives*. United Nations, Department of Social and Economic Affairs: New York, USA, Ch. 3.1, pp. 295–332 (2007).
45. Kandisa, R. V., and Narayana, S. K.V. Dye removal by adsorption: a review. *Journal of Bioremediation & Biodegradation*, 07(06) (2016). DOI: 10.4172/2155-6199.1000371.
46. Alene, A. N. Bioadsorption of basic blue dye from aqueous solution onto raw and modified waste ash as economical alternative bioadsorbent. *Journal of Chemistry*, 8746035 (2020). DOI: 10.1155/2020/8746035.
47. Dutta, S., Gupta, B., Srivastava, S. K., and Gupta, A. K. Recent advances on the removal of dyes from wastewater using various adsorbents: a critical review. *Material Advance*, 2, 4497–4531 (2021). DOI: 10.1039/D1MA00354B.
48. Aragaw, T. A., and Bogale, F. M. Biomass-based adsorbents for removal of dyes from wastewater: a review. *Frontier in Environment Science*, 9, 1–24 (2021). DOI: 10.3389/fenvs.2021.764958.
49. Jawad, S. F., Saddam, N. S., Adaami, Q. J., Kareem, M. M, Abdulredha, M., Mubarak, H. A., Kot P., Gkantou, M., and AlKhayyat, A. Dye removal from textile wastewater using solar-powered electrocoagulation reactor. *IOP Conference Series: Material Science Engineering*, 1058, 012016 (2020). DOI: 10.1088/1757-899X/1058/1/012016.
50. Karthik, V., Saravanan, K., Bharathi, P., Dharanya, V., and Meiaraj, C. An overview of treatments for the removal of textile dyes. *Journal of Chemical and Pharmaceutical Sciences*, 7(4), 301–307 (2014).
51. Sharma, S., and Kaur, A. Various methods for removal of dyes from industrial effluents – a review. *Indian Journal of Science and Technology*, 11(12) (2018). DOI: 10.17485/ijst/2018/v11i12/120847.
52. Mahmoodi, N. M., Gholami, M., Jafari, A. J., and Dalvand, A. Dye removal, energy consumption and operating cost of electrocoagulation of textile wastewater as a clean process. *CLEAN – Soil Air Water*, 39(7), 665–672 (2011). DOI: 10.1002/clen.201000233.
53. MakersLoft Pvt Ltd. Industrialization of natural dyeing and printing of textiles. www.makersloft.in/industrialization-of-natural-dyeing-and-printing-of-textiles
54. Filarowski, A. Innovation for sustainable dyeing. URL: www.textileworld.com/textile-world/features/2022/08/innovation-for-sustainable-dyeing/.

Index

H

I

L

M

N

O

P

Q

R

S

T

U

V

W

Y

Z

FSC
www.fsc.org
MIX
Papier | Fördert
gute Waldnutzung
FSC® C083411

Kolibri 360 GmbH
Ferdinand-Jühlke-Straße 7
99095 Erfurt, Deutschland
produktsicherheit@kolibri360.de